Workbook to Accompany

Body Structures and Functions

12th Edition

Ann Senisi Scott

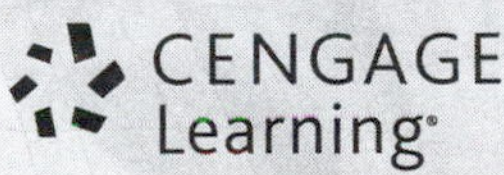

Australia • Canada • Mexico • Singapore • Spain • United Kingdom • United States

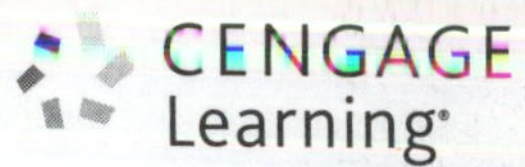

Workbook to Accompany Body Structures and Functions, 12th Edition
Ann Senisi Scott

Vice President, Careers & Computing: Dave Garza
Executive Editor: Matthew Seeley
Director, Development-Career and Computing: Marah Bellegarde
Product Development Manager, Careers: Juliet Steiner
Senior Product Manager: Debra Myette-Flis
Editorial Assistant: Melanie Chapman
Brand Manager: Wendy Mapstone
Market Development Manager: Nancy Bradshaw
Production Manager: Andrew Crouth
Senior Content Project Manager: Kenneth McGrath
Senior Art Director: Jack Pendleton
Cover image(s): Paul Cooklin/Getty Images, www.Shutterstock.com

Library of Congress Control Number: 2012948229

Workbook ISBN 13: 978-1-1336-9166-2

Cengage Learning
200 First Stamford Place, 4th Floor
Stamford, CT 06902
USA

Cengage Learning is a leading provider of customized learning solutions with office locations around the globe, including Singapore, the United Kingdom, Australia, Mexico, Brazil, and Japan. Locate your local office at: **www.cengage.com/global**

Cengage Learning products are represented in Canada by Nelson Education, Ltd.

To learn more about Cengage Learning, visit **www.cengage.com**

Purchase any of our products at your local college store or at our preferred online store **www.cengagebrain.com**

Printed in the United States of America
2 3 4 5 6 7 16 15 14 13

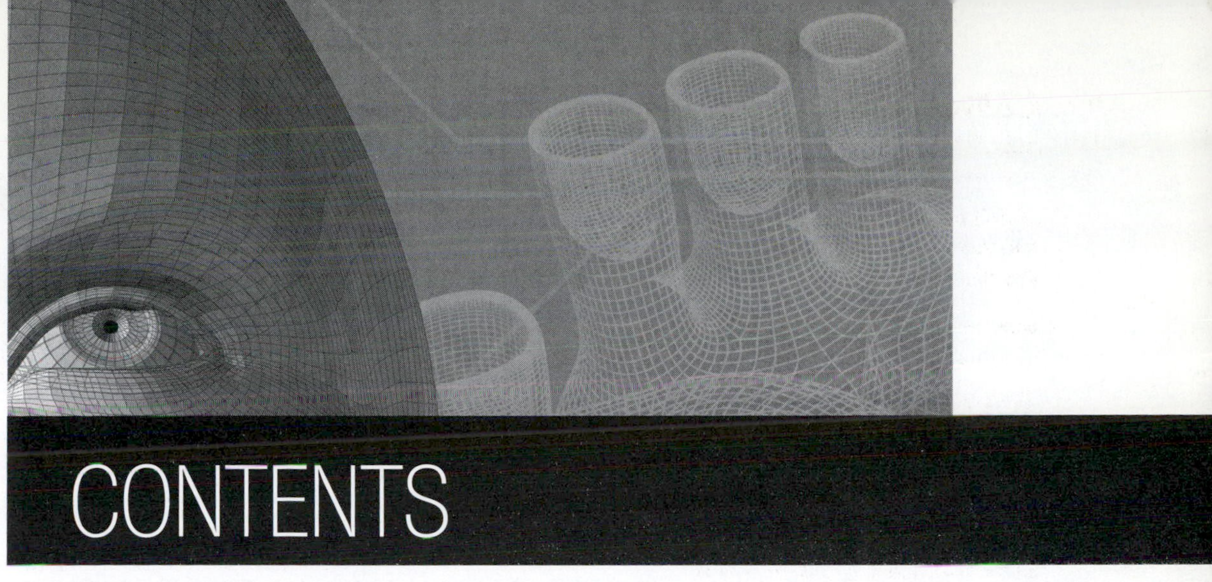

CONTENTS

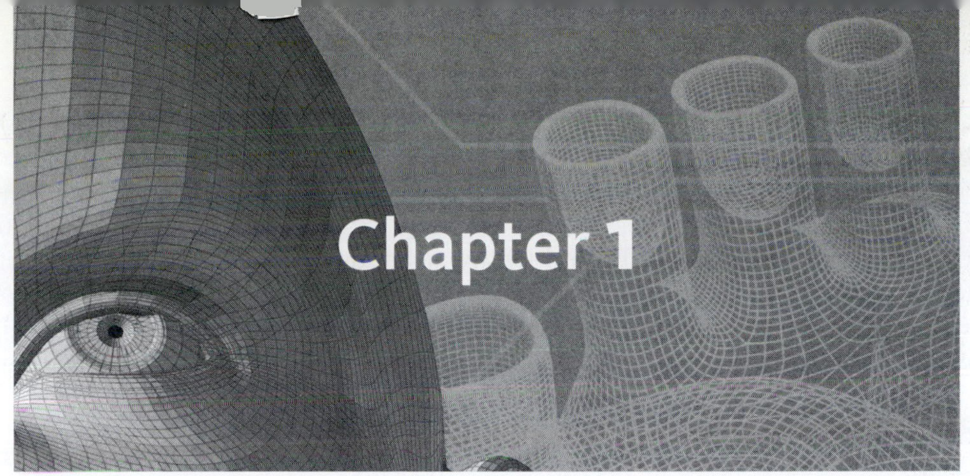

Introduction to the Structural Units

OVERVIEW

This chapter is an introduction to the study of the *structure* (anatomy) and *function* (physiology) of the body.

Anatomic Terminology

Anatomy and physiology have their own terminology to describe the parts of the body and their location, position and function.

In the anatomical position, the body is erect, the person is facing forward with arms at his or her sides, the palms are outward, and the feet are parallel.

Branches of anatomy subdivide the field depending on the information needed:

Gross anatomy can be seen by the naked eye.

Microscopic anatomy is seen with the use of a microscope.

Developmental anatomy is the study of the body from its beginning and through its lifetime.

Comparative anatomy compares human anatomy with animal anatomy.

Systematic anatomy is the study of the body organs that make up a system.

Terms that refer to the location and direction of the body usually are described in pairs:

Anterior (ventral): front/*posterior* (dorsal): back

Cranial: toward the head or top/*caudal*: toward the tail or bottom

Superior: above another part/*inferior*: below another part

Medial: toward the middle/*lateral*: toward the side

Proximal: close to the point of attachment/*distal*: away from the point of attachment

Superficial (external): at the surface of the body/*deep* (internal): deeper in the body

Body planes are imaginary dividing lines to help separate the body: *sagittal* (right and left sections), *coronal* and *ventral* (anterior and posterior portions), and *transverse* (upper and lower parts).

The organs of the body are located in cavities. The terms used to describe the body cavities are:

Dorsal: posterior, includes cranial and spinal cavities

Ventral: anterior, includes thoracic and abdominopelvic cavities

Another way of describing where the abdominopelvic organs are located is by one of the following nine regions: epigastric, right and left hypochondriac, umbilical, right and left lumbar, hypogastric, and right and left iliac (inguinal) areas.

Abdominal quadrants: the abdominal area is divided into quadrants by a median sagittal plane and one transverse plane that passes through the umbilicus; the quadrants are RUQ, LUQ, RLQ, and LLQ.

Life Functions

Life functions are the necessary activities that allow living organisms to grow and function. These activities include movement, ingestion, digestion, transport, respiration, synthesis, assimilation, growth, secretion, excretion, regulation, and reproduction.

Body Processes

Homeostasis is the ability of the body to regulate its internal environment. An imbalance results in disease.

Body processes include metabolism. **Metabolism** consists of two processes, *anabolism* and *catabolism*. Cell functioning requires a stable cellular environment; maintaining this process is known as *homeostasis*.

Metric System

The **metric system** is used in the scientific community to measure lengths in centimeters (cm); weight in kilograms (kg), grams (gm), or milligrams (mg); and volume in liters (l) or milliliters (ml).

ACTIVITIES

A. Use the words in the following list to complete the statements. Terms are used only once.

anatomy	gross anatomy
biology	histology
cytology	microscopic anatomy
dermatology	neurology
embryology	physiology
endocrinology	systematic anatomy

1. The study of all life forms is ____________________.
2. Through the study of ____________________ ____________________, we can study the minute details of body parts.
3. A study of blood tissue is called ____________________.
4. The study of the nervous system is called ____________________.
5. ____________________ ____________________ is the study of the organs that make up parts of the organ system.
6. ____________________ is the study of how our organs function.
7. The study of the cells is called ____________________.

8. The study of human cells from fertilization to birth is called ____________________.

9. The study of the size and shape of an organ is called ____________________.

10. ____________________ is the study of the hormonal system.

B. Anatomy is subdivided into many branches based on the type of knowledge sought. Identify the branch of anatomy that is described in the following statements.

1. The study of the structure and function of various organs or parts making up a particular organ system is ____________________.

2. The study of the growth and development of an organism during its lifetime is ____________________.

3. The study of anatomy at the microscopic level that is further divided into cytology and histology is ____________________.

4. The study of the different body parts and organs of humans with regard to similarities and differences of other animals in the animal kingdom is ____________________.

5. The study of the large and easily observable structures on an organism is ____________________.

C. Select the letter of the choice that best completes the statement.

1. The body in the anatomical position is
   a. standing erect, face forward, arms at the sides, palms forward, feet parallel.
   b. standing erect, face forward, arms at the back, palms forward, feet parallel.
   c. standing erect, face forward, arms at the front, palms forward, feet parallel.
   d. standing erect, face forward, arms at the sides, palms backward, feet parallel.

2. The vertical plane that divides the body into anterior and posterior sections is called the
   a. horizontal plane.
   b. sagittal plane.
   c. transverse plane.
   d. coronal plane.

3. The horizontal plane dividing the body into upper and lower sections is called the
   a. frontal plane.
   b. transverse plane.
   c. sagittal plane.
   d. coronal plane.

4. An imaginary dividing line useful in separating the areas of the body is a
   a. section.
   b. cavity.
   c. quadrant.
   d. plane.

5. The lacrimal ducts are located in the
   a. oral cavity.
   b. buccal cavity.
   c. orbital cavity.
   d. otic cavity.
6. Secretion of a substance from a cell or structure is a function of the
   a. respiratory system.
   b. endocrine system.
   c. skeletal system.
   d. nervous system.
7. The oxidation of food molecules in a cell to release energy, water, and carbon dioxide is accomplished by the
   a. respiratory system.
   b. endocrine system.
   c. skeletal system.
   d. nervous system.
8. The synthesis of simple food molecules into more complex units to help an organism build new tissue is a function of the
   a. endocrine system.
   b. respiratory system.
   c. digestive system.
   d. muscular system.
9. The building up and breaking down of cell material is called
   a. catabolism.
   b. anabolism.
   c. metabolism.
   d. homeostasis.
10. Maintenance of optimum cell functioning requires a balanced cell environment called
    a. regulation.
    b. homeostasis.
    c. metabolism.
    d. catabolism.

D. Label the diagram on this page.

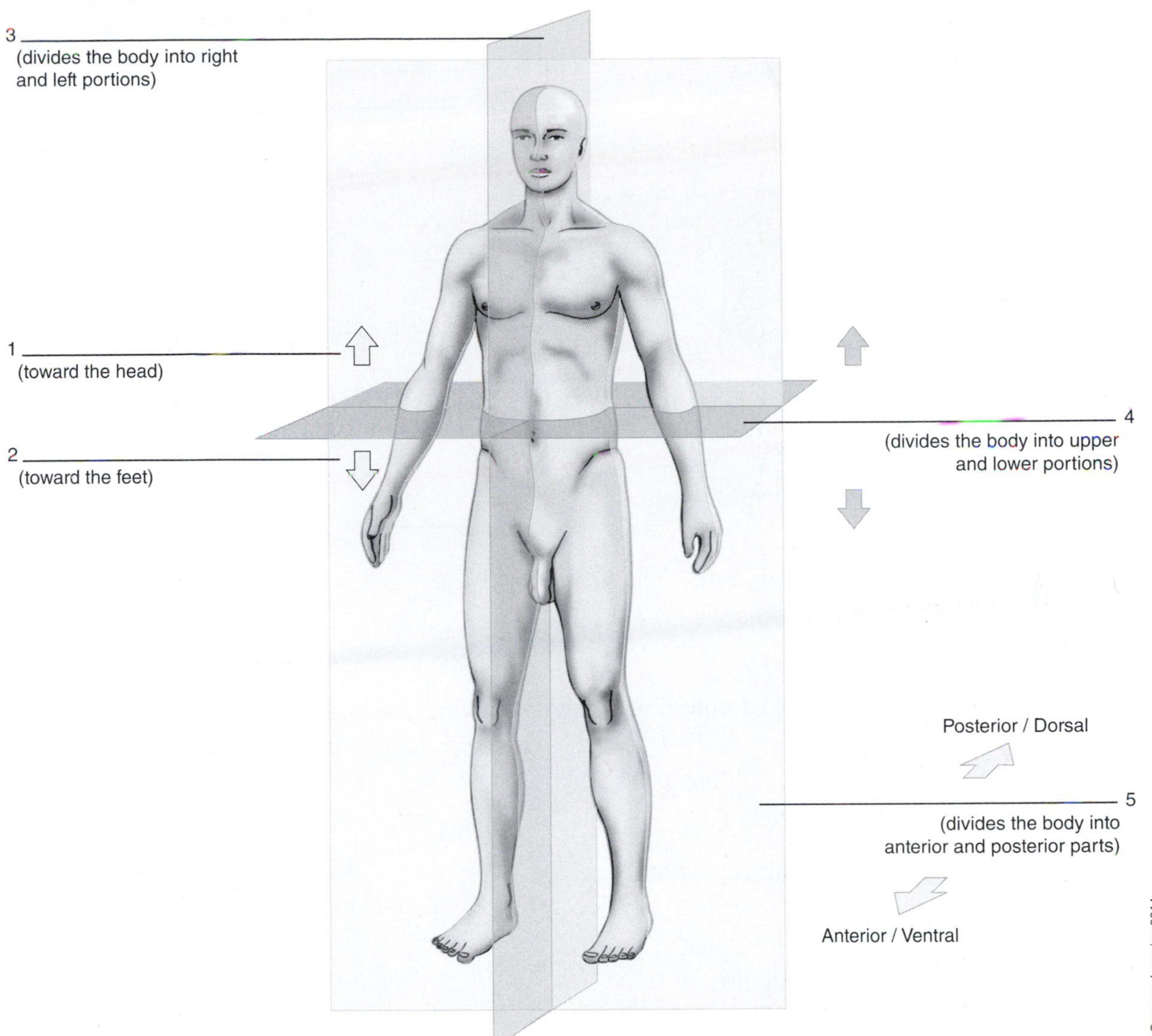

E. Match the letters in Column B with the most appropriate term in Column A.

Column A		Column B
________	1. brain	a. spinal cavity
________	2. bronchi	b. abdominal cavity
________	3. hypogastric region	c. region just below the sternum
________	4. urinary bladder	d. orbital cavity
________	5. stomach	e. pelvic cavity
________	6. mediastinum	f. pubic areas
________	7. epigastric region	g. midpoint of thoracic cavity
________	8. heart	h. pericardial cavity
________	9. vertebrae	i. thoracic cavity
________	10. eyes	j. cranial cavity

F. Label and color the cavities of the body. Color the posterior brown, the anterior yellow, the thoracic green, and the abdominopelvic blue.

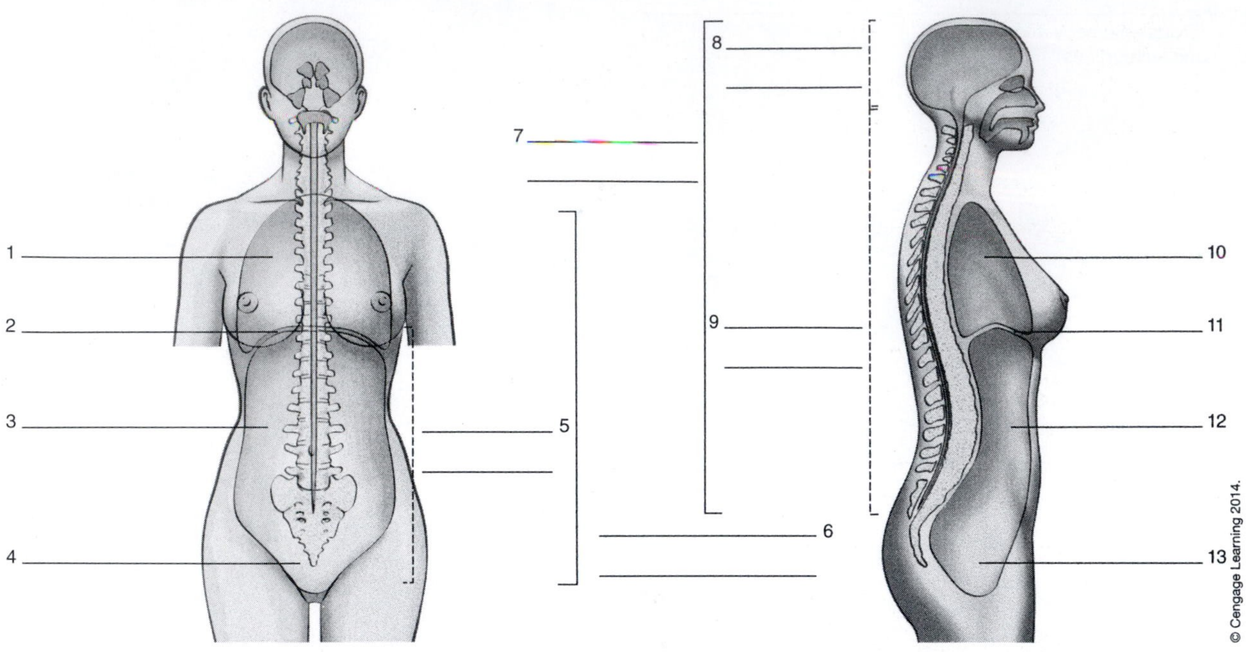

G. Match the number on the abdominal region with the correct description.

a. ________ hypogastric

b. ________ left inguinal region

c. ________ right hypochondriac region

d. ________ umbilical region

e. ________ right inguinal region

f. ________ right lumbar region

g. ________ epigastric region

h. ________ left hypochondriac region

i. ________ left lumbar region

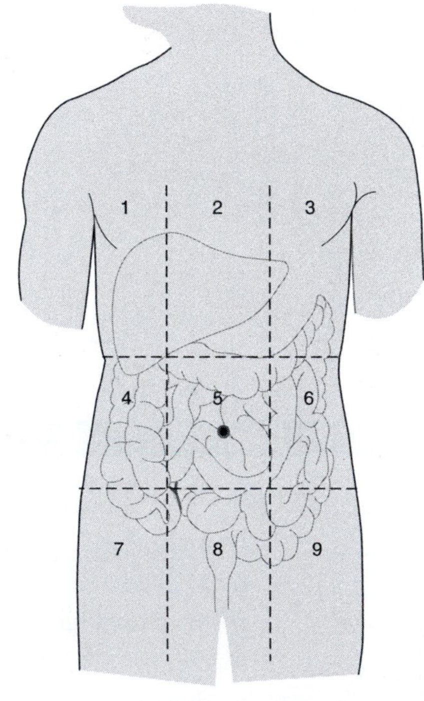

H. Unscramble the letters to define the life functions in each statement.

1. Transformation of digested food molecules into living tissue	NAATISMIOLSI	☐☐☐☐☐☐☐☐☐☐☐☐
2. The breakdown of complex food molecules into simpler food molecules	IEIDGSTNO	☐☐☐☐☐☐☐☐☐
3. The removal of metabolic waste products from an organism	ROXCNETIE	☐☐☐☐☐☐☐☐☐
4. The enlargement of an organism due to synthesis and assimilation	HGWTOR	☐☐☐☐☐☐
5. The process by which an organism takes in food	TGNOINESI	☐☐☐☐☐☐☐☐☐
6. The ability of an organism to move	VETMEMON	☐☐☐☐☐☐☐☐
7. The ability of an organism to produce offspring with similar characteristics	EORNRODUIPCT	☐☐☐☐☐☐☐☐☐☐☐☐
8. The burning or oxidation of food molecules in a cell to increase energy, water, and carbon dioxide	SITRPONIREA	☐☐☐☐☐☐☐☐☐☐☐
9. The formation and release of hormones from a cell or structure	ENTCEOSRI	☐☐☐☐☐☐☐☐☐
10. The ability of an organism to respond to its environment to maintain homeostasis (regulation)	SISNEIYTIVT	☐☐☐☐☐☐☐☐☐☐☐
11. The combination of simple molecules into more complex molecules to help an organism build more tissue	YSESISTNH	☐☐☐☐☐☐☐☐☐
12. The movement of necessary substances to, into, and around cells and wastes out of and away from cells	TOPRTARSN	☐☐☐☐☐☐☐☐☐

I. Fill in the blanks to complete the statements on body processes.

The functional activities that result in growth and repair of body tissue are called ____________________. This function consists of two processes that have opposite effects, namely ____________________ and ____________________. The taking in of food and oxygen occurs in the ____________________ state, which builds up ____________________ materials from simpler ones. The release of energy and carbon dioxide occurs in the

____________________ state, which is the breaking down of ____________________ substances into simpler ones. These functions require a stable, ____________________ environment; maintaining this internal environment is known as ____________________.

J. Mark the statements true or false. Correct any false statements.

1. In homeostasis, the negative feedback response <u>reverses</u> disturbances to our body systems.
2. The anatomical position serves as a <u>reference</u> point for body directions.
3. The <u>hypogastric region</u> is located just below the sternum
4. <u>Regions</u> divide the abdominal area into four parts.
5. Special cells that are grouped together to function are known as <u>tissue</u>.

K. Fill in the blanks relating to body planes from the following word list:

anterior	posterior
distal	proximal
inferior	superior

In the study of body parts and planes,
you need to describe the place or part by name.

If you look at the trunk it is ________________.
If the buttocks are in view it is ________________.

If the location is ________________ it is above a certain part,
whereas the navel is ________________ to the heart.

The wrist is ________________ to the shoulder joint,
whereas the elbow is ________________ to the shoulder attachment point.

Is it superficial or internal? You must know!
Or is medial or lateral the way to go?

When all is said and done,
anatomical directions can be fun.

L. Answer the following questions regarding the metric system in the clinical setting.

1. Mrs. Jones is admitted to the hospital with Type II diabetes. She is 5′4″ and weighs 220 pounds. Using the metric system, how tall is Mrs. Jones in centimeters and how much does she weigh in kilograms? ________________.
2. Riley, age 7, has a bad cough. His doctor prescribes 5 ml of children's cough medicine four times a day. How many teaspoons of cough medicine will Riley take in 24 hours? ________________.
3. In treating Mrs. Chin's pneumonia, her doctor prescribed 0.5 gm of an antibiotic three times a day. How many milligrams will Mrs. Chin take in 48 hours? ________________.
4. In the nursing home 10 residents are given 8 oz. of a nutritional supplement twice a day. How many liters of fluid will be used in one day? ________________.
5. How many tablespoons are there in 600 ml? ________________.

APPLYING THEORY TO PRACTICE

1. You are directed to an anatomical model to place the organs in the correct body cavity. Name the cavity in which you would place the following:

esophagus	____________	nose	____________
pancreas	____________	eyes	____________
appendix	____________	small intestine	____________
heart	____________	mouth	____________
spinal cord	____________	reproductive organs	____________
ribs	____________	lungs	____________
urinary bladder	____________	liver	____________
brain	____________	trachea	____________

2. Think about the following activities occurring within your body at this moment. These activities include movement, digestion, respiration, secretion, and transport. What is their function to your well-being?

   Movement: ____

   ____

   Digestion: ____

   ____

   Respiration: ____

   ____

   Secretion: ____

   ____

   Transport: ____

   ____

3. As a medical assistant in a doctor's office, you must know medical terminology. Use the correct term for the region or location to describe the following situations.
   a. Mr. David is a construction worker who comes to the office with severe pain in his back. The pain is located in the __________________.
   b. Mrs. Andrews, age 55, is scheduled to have gallbladder surgery. She wants to know where she may have a scar. __________________
   c. Kenneth is complaining of severe pains in his stomach. Where is the pain located?
      ____
   d. Leslie comes to the office complaining of having severe menstrual cramps over the last 4 months. The pain is located in the __________________.
   e. Aliya, age 10, fell while playing and has an abrasion on the lower part of his right arm. The area of the abrasion is located __________________ to the elbow.

KRISS KROSS PUZZLE

The words are listed in alphabetical order according to length. Fit them into their proper places in the Kriss Kross. The words refer to anatomical terminology.

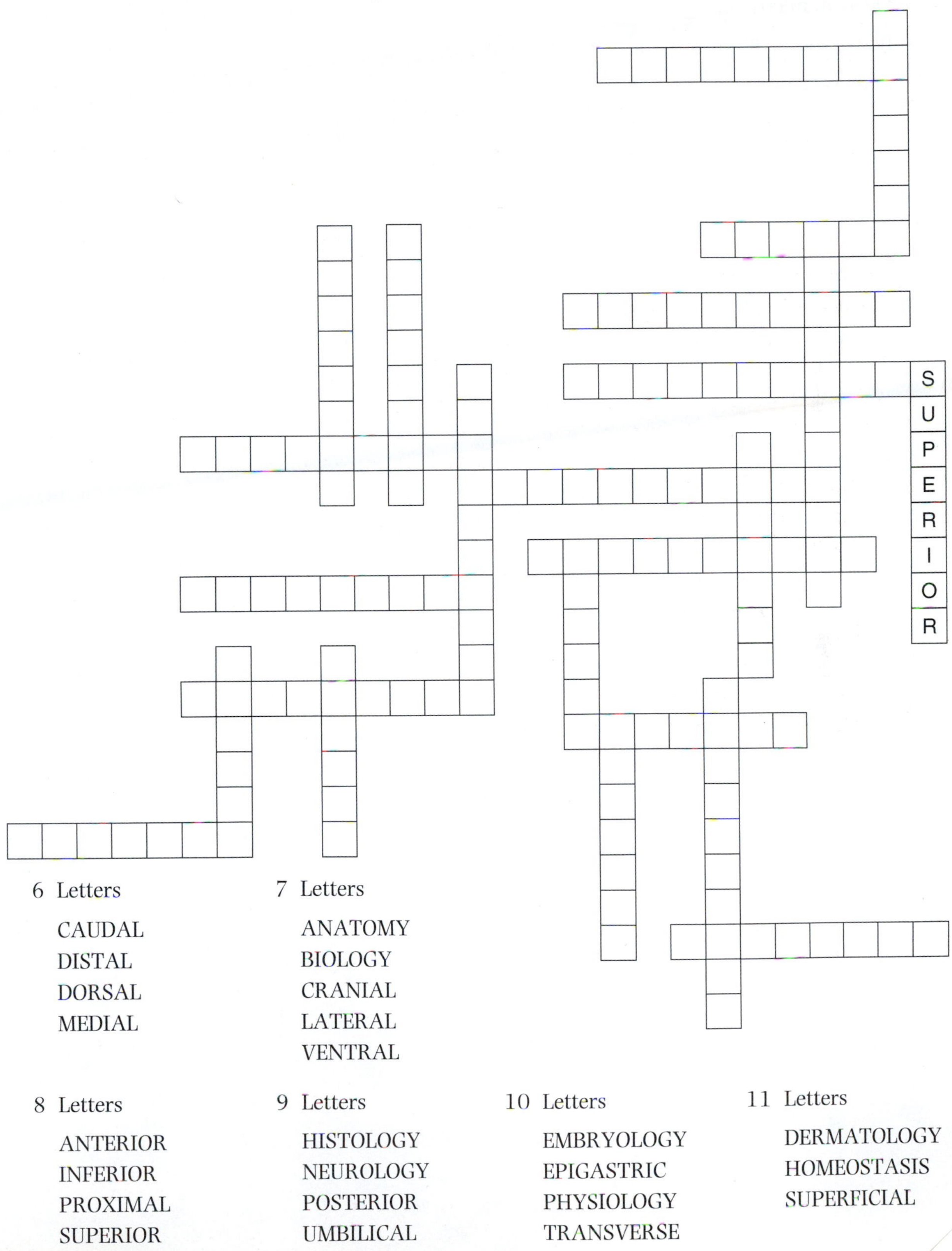

6 Letters

CAUDAL
DISTAL
DORSAL
MEDIAL

7 Letters

ANATOMY
BIOLOGY
CRANIAL
LATERAL
VENTRAL

8 Letters

ANTERIOR
INFERIOR
PROXIMAL
SUPERIOR

9 Letters

HISTOLOGY
NEUROLOGY
POSTERIOR
UMBILICAL

10 Letters

EMBRYOLOGY
EPIGASTRIC
PHYSIOLOGY
TRANSVERSE

11 Letters

DERMATOLOGY
HOMEOSTASIS
SUPERFICIAL

SURF THE NET

For additional information and interactive exercises on the Internet, use key words such as the following:

- Electron microscope
- Body planes, directions, and cavities
- Body systems
- Homeostasis
- Metabolism
- Nanotechnology

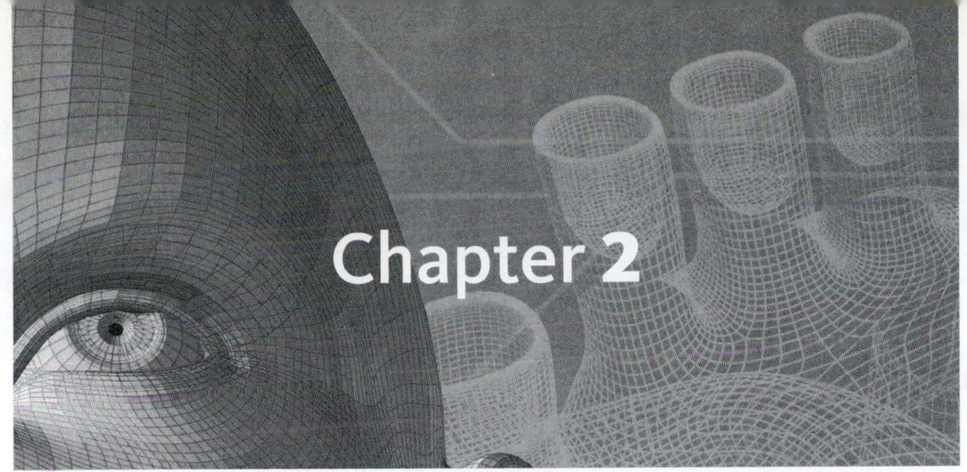

Chemistry of Living Things

OVERVIEW

Chemistry is the study of the structure of matter. **Matter** is anything that has weight and occupies space. **Energy** is the ability to do work; it can be potential or kinetic energy.

An **atom** is the smallest piece of an element. It is made of subatomic particles, namely, *protons, neutrons,* and *electrons.* The number of protons and neutrons is equal in the nucleus of the atom. **Isotopes** are atoms of a specific element that have the same number of protons but a different number of neutrons in their nuclei.

Elements are formed from atoms that are alike. **Compounds** are elements that combine in a definite proportion by weight. The smallest unit of a compound is a **molecule.**

Chemical bonds are formed when atoms share or combine their electrons with atoms of other elements. There are three types: an ionic bond is formed when one atom gives up an electron to another atom, a covalent bond is formed when atoms share their electrons to fill their outermost shell, and a hydrogen bond helps hold water molecules together by forming a bridge between the negative atom of oxygen of one water molecule and the positive hydrogen atom of another water molecule.

Ions are the smallest particles of a molecule and have a positive or negative charge. When compounds are in solution and act as if they have broken into individual pieces (ions), the elements of the compound are **electrolytes.**

Nuclear medicine is a branch of medicine that uses radioactive isotopes to prevent, diagnose, and treat disease.

Compounds

Types of compounds are *inorganic* and *organic.* Inorganic compounds do not usually contain carbon; water is the most important inorganic compound. Organic compounds always contain the element carbon. The four main groups of organic compounds are *carbohydrates, lipids, proteins,* and *nucleic acids.*

Carbohydrates consist of carbon, hydrogen, and oxygen. They are subdivided into monosaccharides, disaccharides, and polysaccharides.

Lipids are made of carbon, hydrogen, and oxygen; they differ from carbohydrates, because there is less oxygen in relation to hydrogen.

Proteins contain carbon, hydrogen, oxygen, and nitrogen, and usually some phosphorous and sulfur. *Enzymes* are specialized proteins that help control the various chemical reactions occurring in the cell; they act as catalysts.

Nucleic acids are organic compounds containing carbon, hydrogen, oxygen, nitrogen, and phosphorous; the two most important are deoxyribonucleic acid (DNA) and ribonucleic acid (RNA).

Acids, Bases, and Salts

Acids, bases, and **salts** are organic and inorganic compounds found in living organisms. An acid is a substance that, when dissolved in water, will ionize into positively charged hydrogen ions. A base or alkali is a substance that, when dissolved in water, ionizes into negatively charged hydroxide ions. When an acid and base combine they form a *salt* and *water*. This reaction is called *neutralization.*

pH Scale

To measure the acidity or alkalinity of a solution, a **pH scale** is used. pH means the potential of hydrogen. A pH of 7 is neutral; it has an equal number of hydrogen and hydroxide ions. A pH between 0 and 6.9 indicates an acidic solution; a pH between 7.1 and 14 indicates an alkaline or basic solution. Water is neutral and has a pH of 7, whereas blood is slightly alkaline, with a pH of 7.35 to 7.45. For living cells to function, their biochemical reactions must maintain homeostasis in their acid–base and electrolyte balance.

Medical Imaging

Nuclear medicine uses radionuclides to scan the body. Types include computerized axial tomography (CAT), positron emission tomography (PET), sonography, and magnetic resonance imaging (MRI). These noninvasive techniques are used for diagnostic purposes.

ACTIVITIES

A. These statements relate to matter and energy. Use the words in the following list to complete the statements. A word may be used more than once.

bone	kinetic energy
created	energy
blood	destroyed
oxygen	physical change
chemical change	potential energy

1. An example of solid matter in the body is ________________.
2. Matter can neither be ________________ nor ________________; it can change form through physical or chemical means.
3. Chewing a piece of toast is an example of a ________________ ________________ in matter.
4. An example of liquid matter in the body is ________________; an example of gaseous matter in the body is ________________.
5. Sitting in a chair is an example of ________________ ________________.
6. If ________________ is the ability to do work, a type of ________________ that results in movement or motion is ________________ ________________.

B. Select the letter of the choice that best completes the statement.

1. The ability to do work is called
   a. matter.
   b. energy.
   c. physical change.
   d. chemical change.
2. The subatomic particles with a positive (+) charge are called
   a. neutrons.
   b. electrons.
   c. protons.
   d. atoms.
3. The four main groups of organic compounds are
   a. carbohydrates, lipids, proteins, and DNA.
   b. carbohydrates, lipids, proteins, and nucleic acids.
   c. carbohydrates, lipids, proteins, and monosaccharides.
   d. carbohydrates, lipids, proteins, and RNA.
4. Lipids or fats may also be known as all of the following, *except*
   a. fatty acids.
   b. cholesterol.
   c. glycogen.
   d. triglycerides.
5. The reaction that occurs when an acid and base are combined is
   a. neutralization.
   b. dehydration.
   c. synthesis.
   d. compound.
6. Dehydration synthesis involves the synthesis of a large molecule from small ones by the
   a. addition of a molecule of H_2O.
   b. addition of a molecule of CHO.
   c. loss of a molecule of H_2O.
   d. loss of a molecule of CHO.
7. Which of the following is the correct pairing of the nitrogenous bases of the rungs of the DNA ladder?
   a. Thymine with adenine
   b. Thymine with cytosine
   c. Thymine with guanine
   d. Adenine with cytosine
8. Which of the following diagnostic tests is used to determine the effects of a stroke?
   a. Magnetic resonance imaging (MRI)
   b. Doppler scan
   c. Ultrasound
   d. Positron emission tomography (PET)

9. Specialized protein molecules that help control cell activity are
   a. triglycerides.
   b. amino acids.
   c. enzymes.
   d. nucleic acids.
10. pH measures the acidity or alkalinity of a solution. A solution with a pH of 8 is
   a. neutral.
   b. acidic.
   c. alkaline.
   d. strongly acidic.

C. Label the following diagram and color the neutrons, protons, and electrons, using a different color for each.

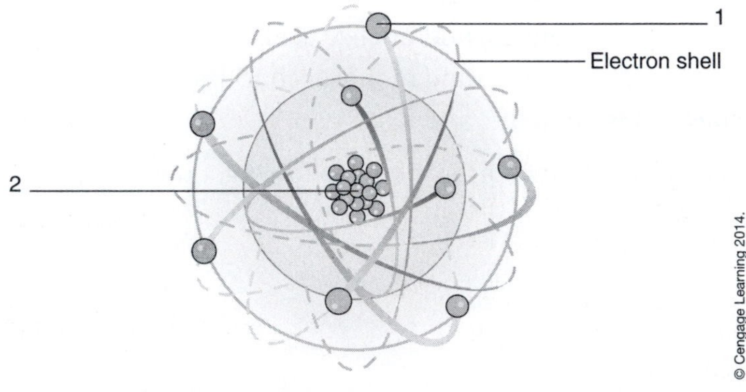

Structure of an atom

D. Answer the following questions.

1. In the previous diagram, how many protons, neutrons, and electrons are illustrated?

____

2. When an atom has six protons, six neutrons, and six electrons, is it positive, negative, or neutral?

____

3. When atom A gives up an electron to atom B, it now has more protons than electrons. What does this mean?

____

4. The atom B that took up the extra electron now has more electrons than protons. What does this mean?

____

____

5. These charged atoms are now called ____________________.

6. If an atom has an equal number of protons but a different number of neutrons it is called a(n) ______________________.

7. When a(n) ______________________ comes apart, it gives off energy in what form? How is this used for medical purposes?

____

____

____

E. Circle the correctly spelled word in each of the following statements.

1. Nuclear medicine is used to (diagnose, diagnos) and treat (disease, disese).
2. Without water our bodies would become (dehydrated, dehidrated), which is a life-threatening situation.
3. Persons with (prothetic, prosthetic) devices cannot have an MRI examination done.
4. (Separately, separatly), hydrogen and oxygen are gases, and when they unite to form the compound water, the substance now has (deferent, different) characteristics.
5. Most living organisms will take the 20 (essential, esential) elements and change them into the compounds needed by the body.
6. The smallest unit of a compound that still has the properties of the compound is called a (molecul, molecule).
7. When compounds are in a (solution, solutin) and act as if they have broken into individual pieces, the elements of the compound are called (electrolytes, electrolights).
8. The ability to record electrical charges is useful for (diegnostic, diagnostic) purposes.

F. Write the common symbol for the following elements.

1. sodium	______________	6. iron	______________
2. calcium	______________	7. magnesium	______________
3. chlorine	______________	8. phosphorous	______________
4. hydrogen	______________	9. potassium	______________
5. oxygen	______________	10. carbon	______________

G. Answer the following questions.

1. Water is the most important ________________________ compound in the body.
2. List at least five reasons why water is essential to life.

____

____

____

____

____

3. List the four main groups of organic compounds.

____

____

____

____

4. The element always found in organic compounds is ________________________.
5. Explain the differences between a monosaccharide, disaccharide, and polysaccharide.

____

____

6. An RNA nucleotide differs from a DNA nucleotide because it has the nitrogenous base of ________________________ instead of thymine.
7. The fluid between the tissues is called ________________________.
8. The sugar found in DNA is ________________________, and the sugar found in RNA is ________________________.
9. A double sugar is formed from two simple sugars that lose a molecule of H_2O; this process is known as ________________________.
10. When a large molecule is broken down into smaller molecules by the addition of H_2O, it is called ________________________.

H. Identify the compounds illustrated by the following symbols.

1. H_2SO_4 ________________________
2. NaCl ________________________
3. CO ________________________
4. HCL ________________________
5. $C_{12}H_{22}O_{11}$ ________________________
6. CO_2 ________________________

7. $CaCO_3$ ____

8. H_2O ____

9. $C_6H_{12}O_6$ ____

10. $NaHCO_3$ ____

I. Select the letter of the choice that best completes the statement.

1. A chemical bond occurs when two atoms share their
   a. electrons.
   b. protons.
   c. neutrons.
   d. elements.

2. When one atom gives up an electron to another atom, it forms a(n)
   a. hydrogen bond.
   b. compound.
   c. ionic bond.
   d. covalent bond.

3. When one atom shares an electron with another atom to fill the outermost shell, it forms a(n)
   a. hydrogen bond.
   b. compound.
   c. ionic bond.
   d. covalent bond.

4. Which of the following is a type of nonessential amino acid?
   a. Lysine
   b. Phenylalanin
   c. Proline
   d. Valine

5. __________ is the process by which amino acids are arranged through the involvement of messenger RNA, transfer RNA, and ribosomes.
   a. Neutralization
   b. Buffer formation
   c. Covalent bonding
   d. Protein synthesis

J. Compare the likenesses and differences between the following pairs.

1. Matter and energy

____

____

2. Acid and base

____

____

3. Element and compound

____

____

4. Ion and electrolyte

____

____

5. Protein and carbohydrate

____

____

6. Glucose and starch

____

____

7. CAT scan and MRI

____

____

8. DNA and RNA

____

____

K. Carbohydrates are divided into three main groups: monosaccharides, disaccharides, and polysaccharides. Identify the group for each of the following sugars.

1. ribose	________________	6. sucrose	________________
2. cellulose	________________	7. glycogen	________________
3. maltose	________________	8. lactose	________________
4. fructose	________________	9. glucose	________________
5. starch	________________		

L. Match the words in Column A with the most correct statement in Column B.

	Column A	Column B
________	1. fats	a. consists of the elements C, H, O, and N
________	2. DNA	b. contains ribose sugar
________	3. phospholipid	c. triglycerides
________	4. protein	d. found in brain and nervous tissue
________	5. steroid	e. consists of the elements of C, H, O, N, and P
________	6. amino acid	f. genes for heredity
________	7. lysine	g. contains the elements C, H, and O
________	8. nucleic acid	h. essential amino acid
		i. the smallest molecule of protein
		j. contains cholesterol

M. Mark the following statements about acids, bases, and salts either true or false. Correct any false statements.

________ 1. An acid dissolved in water ionizes into positively charged hydronium ions or hydrogen ions and negatively charged ions of some other element.

________ 2. Blue litmus paper does not change color in the presence of an acid.

________ 3. A base is also called an alkali.

________ 4. When dissolved in water, a base ionizes into negatively charged hydroxide ions and positively charged ions of a metal.

________ 5. A base turns blue litmus paper red.

________ 6. An acid and a base combine to form a salt and water; this reaction is called a neutralization or exchange reaction.

________ 7. In a neutralization reaction, hydrogen ions from the acid and hydroxide ions from the base join to form water.

________ 8. In a neutralization reaction, the positive ions of the acid combine with the negative ions of the base to form a salt.

N. Complete the following chemical reactions and state whether each is an acid, base, or neutralization reaction.

1. $HCl + H_2O \rightarrow$ __________ $+ Cl^-$

   Reaction: ____

2. $NaOH \rightarrow Na^+ +$ __________

   Reaction: ____

3. Hydrochloric acid + __________ __________ → salt + water

   __________ + NaOH → __________ + __________

   Reaction: ____

O. The pH scale measures whether a solution is an acid or alkaline. Circle the correct answer for each of the following.

1. Which pH is the most acidic?
   a. 5
   b. 7
   c. 9
2. Which pH is the most alkaline?
   a. 5
   b. 7
   c. 10
3. Distilled water has a pH of
   a. 7.
   b. 7.3.
   c. 6.9.
4. Blood has a pH of
   a. 7.0–7.1.
   b. 7.35–7.45.
   c. 6.9–7.0.
5. A pH of 7 is considered
   a. neutral.
   b. acidic.
   c. basic.

P. Next to the following substances, state whether each is an acid or a base.

1. Milk ____________________
2. Baking soda ____________________
3. Gastric juice ____________________
4. Bleach ____________________
5. Egg white ____________________
6. Black coffee ____________________
7. Vinegar ____________________
8. Household ammonia ____________________
9. Tomatoes ____________________
10. Milk of magnesia ____________________

Q. Circle the key words related to the chemistry of living things.

o r g a n i c c a t a l y s t d a n

r b a s e c o m p o u n d r b i c e

g d y r t s i m e h c o i b e s e u

a m i n o a c i d f h g j k t a l t

n g m n o e l u c e l o m e a c e r

i e m y z n e l p y q u d s r c d a

c d n u c l e i c a c i d t d h i l

c i s p l u v e n e r g y w y a r i

o x t r x t r y m a t t e r h r a z

m o e o z i i a h b e z i n o i h a

p r r p d c d c f r e f f u b d c t

o d o e i m c o e n z y m e r e c i

u y i r o a j k m l i p i d a l a o

n h d t s n a b s a l t e f c a s n

d n a y u n i c e l l u l a r c o a

c d l e r f g h a l k a l i t s n c

l o r e t s e l o h c n i a j h o i

p h o s p h o l i p i d f k r p m d

Key Words

acid
alkali
amino acid
atom
base
biochemistry
buffer
carbohydrate
cholesterol
coenzyme
compound
disaccharide
DNA
energy
enzyme
fat
hydroxide
ionize
lipid
matter
molecule
monosaccharide
multicellular
neutralization
nucleic acid
organic catalyst
organic compound
pH scale
phospholipid
polysaccharide
property
RNA
salt
triglyceride
unicellular

APPLYING THEORY TO PRACTICE

1. When we say an ion has a positive charge, what does this mean? The expression "opposites attract" occurs in chemistry. What does the expression mean when it applies to ions?

____

____

____

2. As a society we worry about cholesterol, because we know it may clog the arteries and cause other health problems. Cholesterol has many functions in our bodies. Name at least four functions of cholesterol. Explain why it is also considered a health risk.

____

____

____

____

3. You are employed in a group practice center. What nuclear medicine test would you expect to be ordered for the following conditions?
   a. stroke ______________________________
   b. cerebral palsy ______________________________
   c. heart disease ______________________________
   d. inflammation of the liver ______________________________
   e. brain tumor ______________________________

4. Explain the following tests.

Name of Test	Explanation	Special Instructions for the Patient
a. Sonography		
b. Positron emission tomography (PET)		
c. Computerized axial tomography (CAT)		
d. Magnetic resonance imaging (MRI)		

5. In which of the tests noted in Question 4 is an injection of a radionuclide given?

____

6. Margaret is pregnant. At her obstetrics appointment, she reports a history of irregular menstrual cycles. To help determine her delivery date, the obstetrician will order what type of test?

____

7. Diane is a young mother who brings her 7-year-old son to the pediatrician. She reports that he stares at the computer monitor and occasionally shakes. Diane reports that her son is addicted to video games. What type of diagnostic test will the doctor order for the child?

____

8. John is a 70-year-old patient who has been complaining of abdominal pain. He has been in good health except for knee replacement surgery about a year ago. What must the doctor know about the knee replacement surgery before a nuclear imaging diagnostic test can be ordered?

____

9. Steve has been complaining of pain and cramping in his legs. After examining Steve, the doctor makes a diagnosis of peripheral artery disease. What type of test did the doctor perform on Steve?

____

____

Was this an invasive or noninvasive procedure?

____

10. Ann has been trying to lose weight. Her problem is that she is addicted to sweets. What can she substitute for candy in a weight-reducing diet, to help satisfy her craving for sweets?

____

SURF THE NET

For additional information and interactive exercises, use the following key words:

- how atoms work
- chemical bonds
- carbohydrates, fats, and proteins
- the structure of DNA and RNA
- acids, bases, neutralization
- medical imaging

LAB HOME ACTIVITIES

1. Conduct a taste test at home for foods that contain acids or seem to be neutral. Invite another family member or friend to join you in this experiment. Taste a piece of grapefruit, lemon, orange, strawberry, and banana.
   a. Which fruits seem to have an acid taste?
   b. Which fruits seem to be neutral?
   c. What tastes are you experiencing?
   d. Is your family member having the same reactions?

Effects of an Acid on a Base

In this activity, you will use vinegar to remove an egg's shell without cracking it. Vinegar contains an acid, and the main material of the eggshell is calcium carbonate, a base.

Items needed

Small self-sealing plastic bag
1 uncooked egg
16 fluid ounces of vinegar
1 glass

Steps in the experiment

1. Place the egg in the bag and add enough vinegar to completely cover the egg.
2. Hold the bag and look closely at the egg's shell; the bubbles you can see are carbon dioxide gas. This gas is given off as the vinegar reacts with the shell.
3. Turn the bag so that the egg is in one corner, and slip this part of the bag into the glass.
4. Let the egg sit overnight.
5. The following day, lift the egg carefully out of the bag and it will feel soft.
6. Let the egg sit in the vinegar for 2 more days, and the egg will be completely soft.
7. What caused the shell of the egg to disappear?

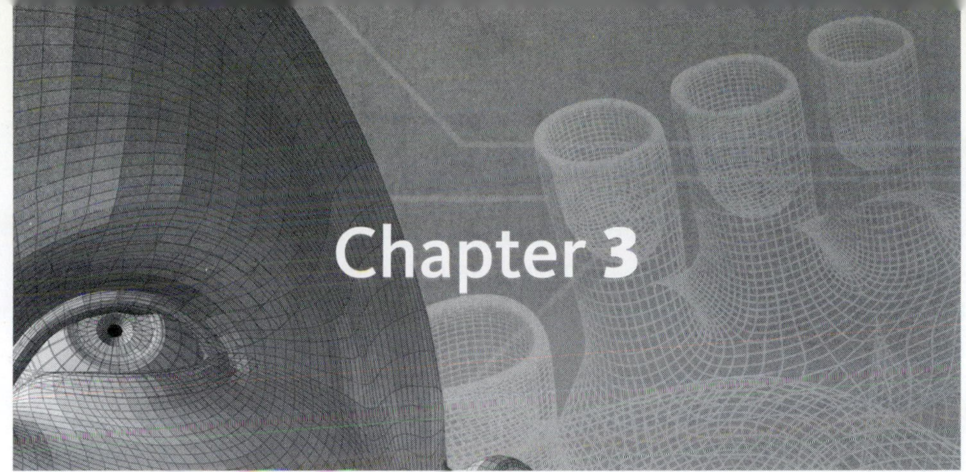

Cells

OVERVIEW

To study anatomy it is essential to understand the basic structure and function of the cell, the main parts of the cell, and the organelles. It is important to understand how the cell obtains nutrients and reproduces through the process of mitosis.

Protoplasm

The basic unit of structure and function of all living things is the cell. All cells are composed of **protoplasm**. The cell has three major parts: cell/plasma membrane, nucleus, and cytoplasm.

Cell/Plasma Membrane

The **cell membrane**, or *plasma membrane,* is selective and semipermeable.

Nucleus

The **nucleus** is the control center of the cell; it has a nuclear membrane around it and contains the nucleoli and DNA.

Cytoplasm

Cytoplasm is a semifluid material between the cell membrane and the nucleus. Embedded in the cytoplasm are *organelles* that help a cell to function. The organelles include the *centrosomes, ribosomes, cilia and flagella, Golgi apparatus, endoplasmic reticulum, mitochondria, lysosomes, cytoskeleton,* and *peroxisomes.*

The organelles have the following functions:

Centrosomes are active during mitosis.

Endoplasmic reticulum is a channel for transport of material in and out of the nucleus and cytoplasm.

Mitochondria supply energy for the cell in the form of ATP.

The *Golgi apparatus* stores secretions for the cell.

Lysosomes digest protein molecules.

Ribosomes are the sites for protein synthesis.

Peroxisomes digest fats and detoxify harmful substances.

The *cytoskeleton* of microtubules and microfilaments is the internal framework.

Cilia and *flagella* are hair-like projections that beat and vibrate.

Cell Division

There are two types of cell division. **Mitosis** is an orderly series of steps by which the DNA is precisely distributed to two new daughter cells, each with 46 chromosomes.

Meiosis is a special type of cell division of the germ cells, the ova and sperm. Each cell reduces to 23 chromosomes; when the ova and sperm unite there are 46 chromosomes.

Movement of Materials Across Cell Membranes

Movement of cell material through the semipermeable membrane occurs through passive and active processes. Passive processes that do not require energy are as follows:

Diffusion: molecules move from an area of greater concentration to lesser concentration.

Osmosis: diffusion of water occurs across a semipermeable membrane from an area of higher concentration of a solution to an area of lower concentration of a solution.

Filtration: solutes and water move across a semipermeable membrane as a result of a mechanical force.

Active processes that require an energy source are the following:

Active transport: requires the energy of ATP to move molecules from an area of lower concentration to an area of higher concentration.

Phagocytosis: the cell engulfs particles; also known as *cell eating.*

Pinocytosis: the cell engulfs particles in solution; also known as *cell drinking.*

Disorders of Cell Structure

Tumors are abnormal cell growths. They may be benign, confined to a local area, or malignant (cancer), when the cells move rapidly from one place to another.

Cancer staging is a method used to describe the extent of the cancer. The most common types of staging used are TNM (tumor, nodes, metastasis) and Roman numerals.

The Effects of Aging on Cell Structure

There are 30% fewer cells in the elderly.

ACTIVITIES

A. Answer the questions or complete the statements regarding parts of the cell.

1. Name the three major parts of the cell.

____

____

____

2. The cell plasma membrane is a double layer that regulates passage of molecules into and out of the cell; it is therefore called a ______________, ______________ ______________.

3. State the two major functions of the nucleus.

____

____

4. The nucleus contains ____________________ and protein.

5. The number of chromosomes in the nucleus is ____________________.

6. The outer layer of the nuclear membrane is continuous with the ____________________ ____________________ of the cytoplasm.

7. Name the structure in the nucleus that contains the ribosomes.

____

8. Describe the cytoplasm.

____

____

9. The structures embedded in the cytoplasm that help cells to function are the ____________.

10. Do cells of the body have identical substances in their cytoplasm? Explain.

____

B. Organelles perform specific functions within the cell. Next to the following statements, write the name of the organelle involved in that function from the list provided. A word may be used more than once.

centrosome	lysosome
cytoskeleton	mitochondria
endoplasmic reticulum	peroxisomes
Golgi apparatus	ribosomes

1. Attached to the walls of the endoplasmic reticulum ____________________
2. Detoxifies harmful substances ____________________
3. The center for cellular digestion ____________________
4. Forms internal framework ____________________
5. Manufactures CHO and packages secretions ____________________
6. Site for protein synthesis ____________________
7. Transport of substances through the cytoplasm ____________________
8. Site of cellular respiration and energy production ____________________
9. Enzymes oxidize cell substances ____________________
10. "Suicide bags" ____________________
11. Role in cholesterol synthesis and fat metabolism ____________________

12. Found in cells that need the most energy ________________

13. Abundant in gastric glands ________________

14. Plays an important role in mitosis ________________

C. Label and color the parts of the cell and the organelles. Use different colors for each part and organelle.

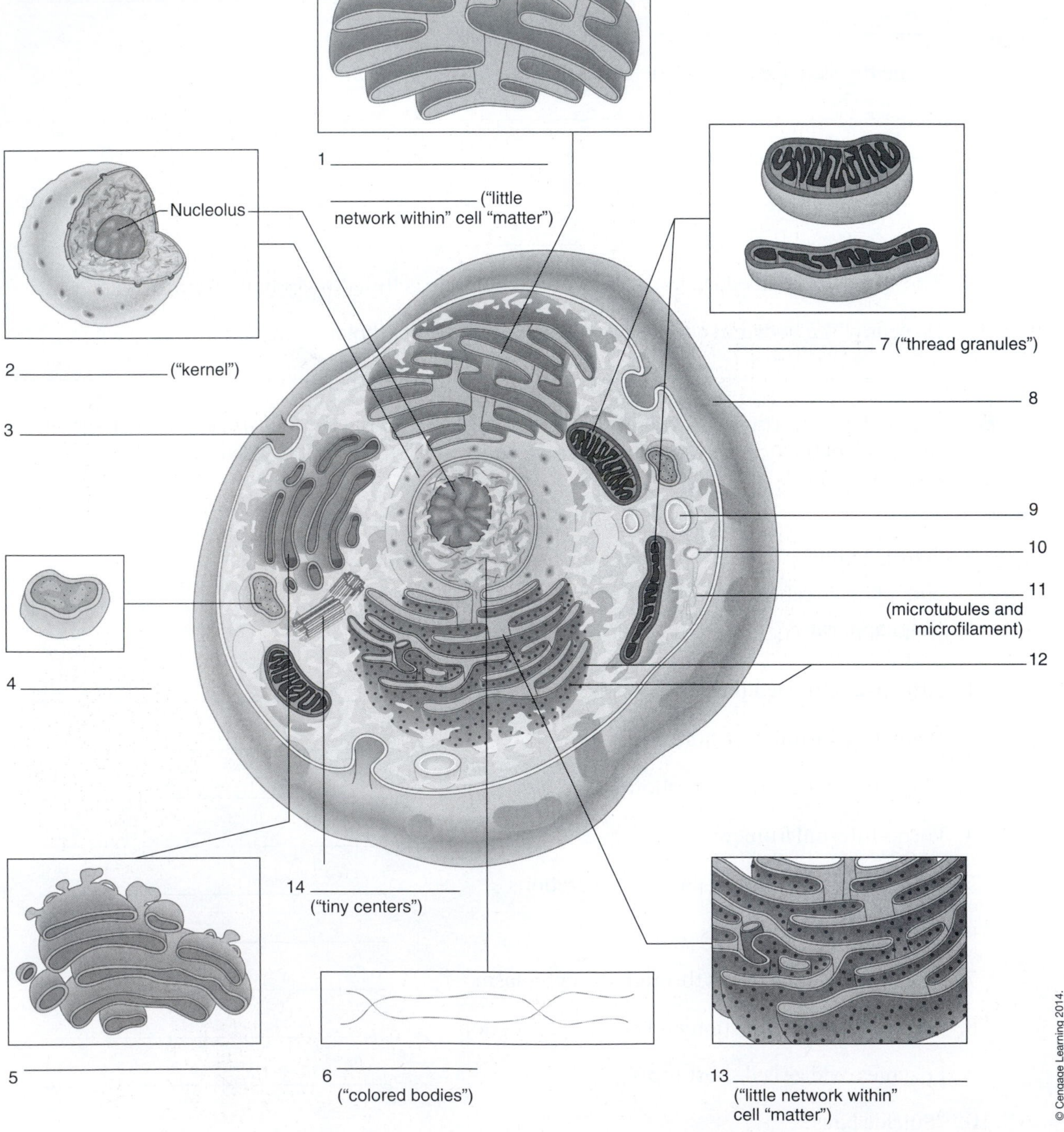

D. Label and describe the structure of the cell/plasma membrane.

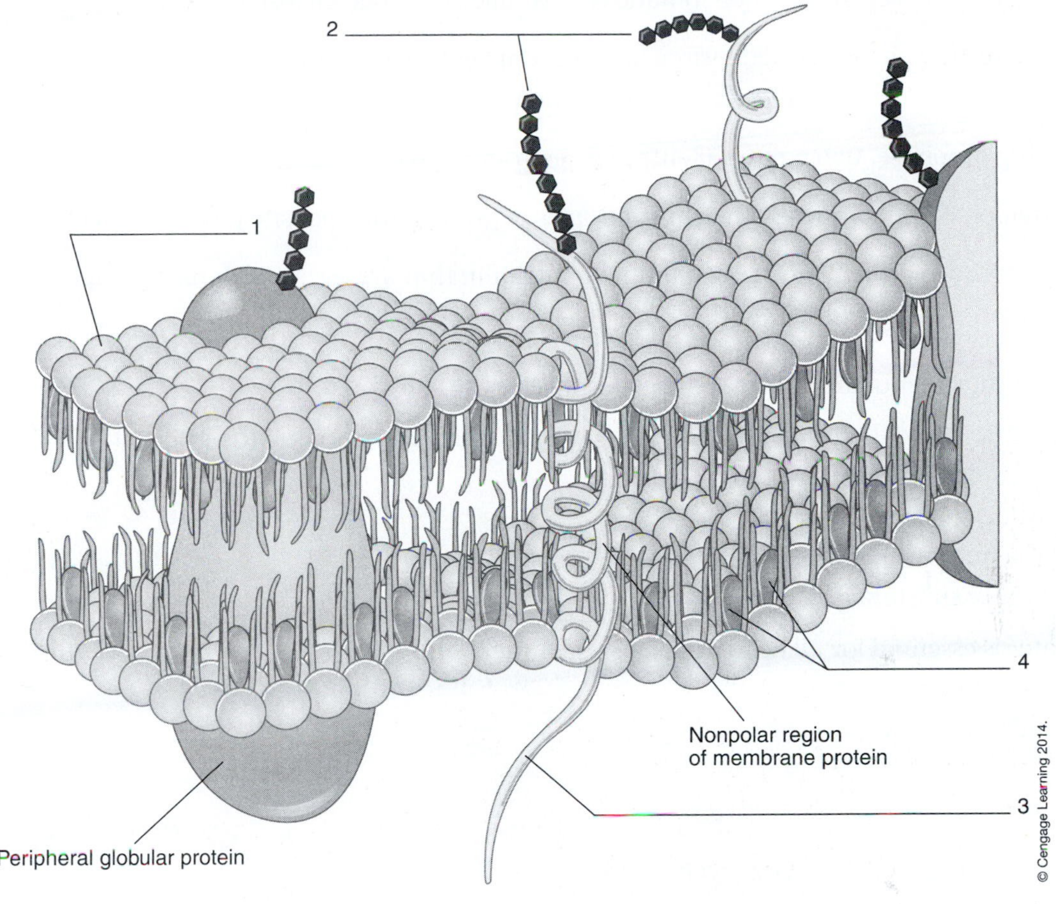

E. Label the stage of mitosis and describe what is occurring in each stage.

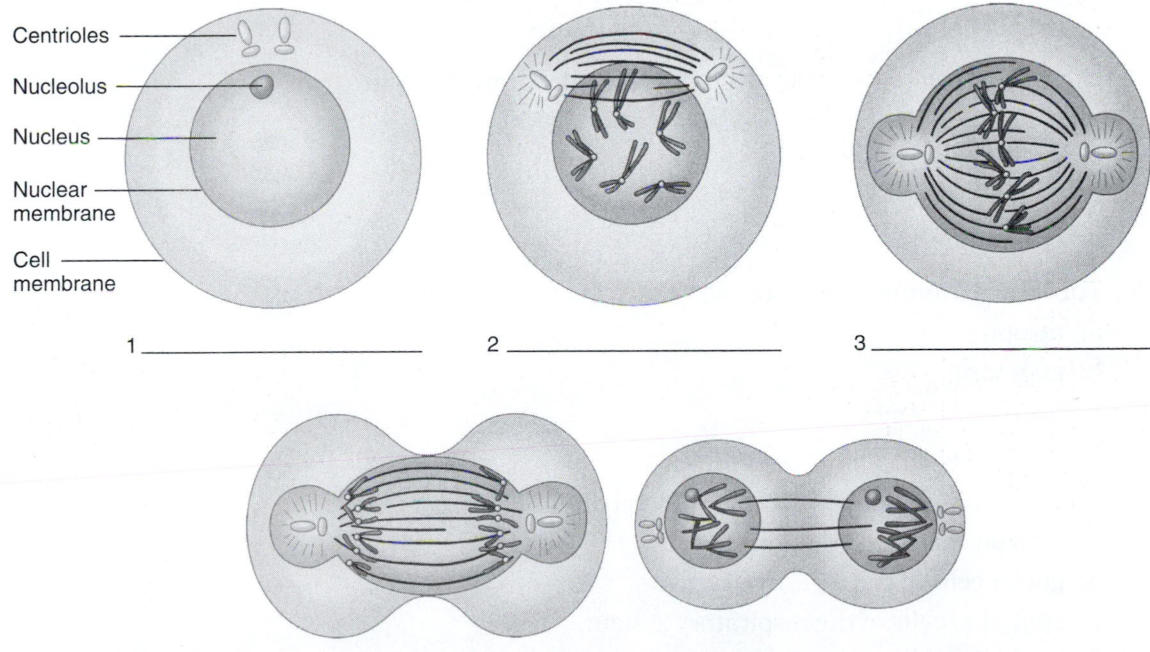

F. Circle the correct word in each of the following statements.

1. The process of cell division for somatic cells is called (mitosis, meiosis).
2. In the resting phase of cell division, an exact duplicate of each nuclear chromosome is made; this activity is called (replication, reproduction).
3. During prophase, two pairs of (centrioles, sentrioles) go to opposite ends of the cell.
4. In (telophase, metaphase), the chromosomes migrate to the opposite poles of the cell.
5. Cells produce proteins, such as albumin or globulin that are essential to life through a process called protein (synthesis, synthisis).

G. Select the letter of the choice that best completes the statement.

1. The clear liquid fluid that fills the spaces around the chromatin and the nucleoli is
   a. cytoplasm.
   b. nucleoplasm.
   c. the nuclear membrane.
   d. a fatty substance.
2. Water is essential for all cellular life, as water makes up ____________________ of cytoplasm.
   a. 50% to 70%
   b. 60% to 70%
   c. 70% to 80%
   d. 70% to 90%
3. The orderly process by which cells die is
   a. atrophy.
   b. apoptosis.
   c. necrosis.
   d. dysplasia.
4. Hair-like projections of the cell that beat and vibrate are called
   a. lysosomes.
   b. ribosomes.
   c. cilia.
   d. mitochondria.
5. The unprogrammed death of cells and living tissue is called
   a. atrophy.
   b. apoptosis.
   c. necrosis.
   d. dysplasia.
6. All of the following types of cells undergo mitosis, *except*
   a. neurons of the nervous system.
   b. goblet cells of the digestive system.
   c. epithelial cells of the respiratory system.
   d. epithelial cells of the reproductive system.

7. The diffusion rate of molecules for a gas is
   a. slower than that for liquids.
   b. quicker than that for liquids.
   c. slower than that for solids.
   d. quicker than that for liquids and solids.

8. Most intravenous fluids ordered by physicians are __________ solutions.
   a. hypertonic
   b. isotonic
   c. hypotonic
   d. glucose and water

9. The type of fluid ordered by the physician for a person with dehydration would be a(n) _______ solution.
   a. hypertonic
   b. isotonic
   c. hypotonic
   d. glucose and water

10. Cancer that occurs in the bone marrow is known as
    a. sarcoma.
    b. lymphoma.
    c. carcinoma.
    d. leukemia.

H. Indicate whether the underlined word or phrase makes the statement true or false. If the statement is false, correct it.

_________ 1. Active transport that moves material across a cell membrane <u>does not require energy</u>.

_________ 2. An example of <u>diffusion</u> that moves molecules from an area of higher concentration to an area of lower concentration occurs when oxygen goes from the lungs to the bloodstream.

_________ 3. Osmosis is the diffusion of water through the cell membrane from an area of <u>higher</u> concentration of the solution to an area of lower concentration of the solution.

_________ 4. If a solution has the same number of sodium particles as the solute, the solution is said to be <u>hypertonic</u>.

_________ 5. In the process of <u>filtration</u>, the blood pressure forces the blood through the kidneys.

_________ 6. In the process of <u>phagocytosis</u>, the substances engulfed by the cell membrane are in solution.

_________ 7. Nerve cells are specialized to <u>respond</u> to stimuli.

_________ 8. Muscle cells <u>reproduce continuously</u>.

_________ 9. A wart is a type of <u>benign</u> tumor.

_________ 10. A papilloma is a type of <u>malignant</u> tumor.

I. Match the activity with the correct word or phrase from the following list. An answer may be used more than once.

active transport	filtration	pinocytosis
biomarker	osmosis	
diffusion	phagocytosis	

1. ________________ The aroma of coffee percolating
2. ________________ Blood passing through the kidney
3. ________________ Cell drinking
4. ________________ Exchange of oxygen from the blood to extracellular fluid
5. ________________ Cell eating
6. ________________ Putting sugar into a cup of tea
7. ________________ Diffusion of water through a selective semipermeable membrane
8. ________________ Process that requires the energy of ATP
9. ________________ Process by which white blood cells destroy bacteria
10. ________________ Normal substance found in blood or tissue in small amounts

J. Answer the following questions.

1. Describe what occurs in a hypertonic solution.

____

____

2. Describe what occurs in a hypotonic solution.

____

____

3. Describe what occurs in an isotonic solution.

____

____

K. Fill in the blanks with the appropriate word.

Active transport is a way in which cells may obtain nutrients and excrete their waste products. In this process, molecules move across the cell membrane from an area of ________________ concentration to an area of ________________ concentration, which requires ________________ in the form of the compound ________________.

Think of the cell membrane as a bridge. A molecule from ________________ the cell wants to cross over the bridge and get ________________ the cell. To do this, the molecule needs an escort called a ________________ molecule. Arm in arm they go across the cell membrane;

once inside the cell, the escort ____________________ the molecule at the ____________________ surface of the membrane. The escort then returns to the other side of the bridge to wait for the next molecule that wants to cross the bridge or cell membrane.

L. Complete the story on the cell using the following list of words.

cell	lysosomes
cell membrane	mitochondria
centriole	nucleus
cytoplasm	organelles
cytoskeleton	peroxisomes
DNA	phagocytosis
endoplasmic reticulum	ribosomes
Golgi apparatus	RNA

THE C.E.L.L.

The employment agency sent Ms. Glucose to a new plant that was hiring temporary help for the season. When Ms. Glucose arrived at the C.E.L.L. Plant Company, she noticed that the entryway had a most peculiar door. It appeared to have little holes throughout and a sign posted that read: "Do not push anything through this ____________________."

As a huge gap appeared on the side of the entryway and engulfed her, she heard a voice say, "Do not worry about that; it is only ____________________ up to his old tricks." Ms. Glucose was finally inside this strange company; the air was very humid and all the surfaces felt slippery. A receptionist, Mr. RNA, appeared and said the atmosphere was especially suited for the kind of work done at the C.E.L.L. Company; this slippery substance is called ____________________ .

The receptionist said, "Stick with me; I am called Mr. ____________________, and I will take you on a tour of the plant." They hopped aboard a tramlike car labeled E.R.T., which meant ____________________ . Along the way, Ms. Glucose was introduced to the various departments.

Mr. RNA said, "We are like chipmakers; we manufacture peppy little proteins that are then changed into many other products." The first stop was a place where they synthesized the protein; it was called the ____________________ department. As they traveled, Ms. Glucose noticed scaffolding throughout. She was told it was ____________________, which forms the internal framework of the plant.

In one area the air was hot and full of energy. The head of the department was dressed like a superhero, in keeping with the ____________________ or powerhouse division of the plant. In quick order they went to the packing plant, or ____________________ division, which uses carbohydrate packing material to send packages from the factory.

Before a product is shipped, it passes through two quality-control rooms. One is the ______________________ room, which bathes the product in oxidase material; this helps to remove harmful impurities. The other is the ______________________ room, which checks to see whether additional cellular digestion is required for the final product.

The final destination was a special walled room in the center, called the president's office. It was guarded by two identical-looking secretaries called Ms. and Mr. ______________________. The president's office is also known as the ______________________ of the plant. The president of the company is known as ______________________, because he dictates what happens in that factory. Ms. Glucose thanked Mr. RNA for the tour, but she really did not think she was ready for a job at C.E.L.L., the home of the ______________________.

M. Match the terms in Column B with the statements in Column A.

	Column A	Column B
________	1. necrosis	a. ability to change into another type of cell
________	2. hydrophobic	b. change in size/shape of cell as a result of a stimulus
________	3. biomarker	c. cancer of internal of external lining of body
________	4. atrophy	d. an unprogrammed death of cells
________	5. dysplasia	e. decrease in amount of oxygen to cell
________	6. neoplasia	f. cancer that occurs in plasma cells of bone marrow
________	7. hypoxia	g. normal substance found in blood in small amounts
________	8. metaplasia	h. repels water
________	9. myeloma	i. uncontrolled growth pattern of cell
________	10. carcinoma	j. decrease in size of cell

APPLYING THEORY TO PRACTICE

1. In the classroom Rebecca dropped her purse and her bottle of nail polish fell out and broke. The smell of nail polish soon permeated throughout the classroom. This is an example of the process of ______________________.
2. When preparing coffee, the coffee is placed into a lined basket in a holder, very hot water is poured over the coffee, and the liquid and some of the solids pass through to the serving container. This is an example of the process of ______________________.
3. Courtney has an infection in her right ear. Her white blood cells will help control the infection by eating up the harmful bacteria. This process is known as ______________________.
4. Ben, age 20, has been lifting weights at the gym. He notices his arm muscles getting bigger. What name is given to this change of the size of his muscles? What is the name given to the opposite of this condition?

____

5. Anthony had a biopsy done on a mole removed from his left shoulder. The doctor reported that the mole was the size of a quarter, was localized, there was no lymph node involvement, and it had not metastasized. The doctor was using the classification system known as ____________________.

6. Lucille has been diagnosed with leukemia. The doctors will use her stem cells as therapy to treat her particular type of leukemia. The type of stem cells found in adults is ____________________ stem cells.

7. Our body cells do not all reproduce at the same rate. How frequently do our intestinal, skin, muscle, and nerve cells reproduce?

____

____

____

8. The doctor has just told your aunt that she has a lump in her breast and that it must be biopsied. If the biopsy is positive, the doctor has told her that she may need surgery and other treatment.

   a. Define *tumor*.

   ____

   ____

   ____

   b. Describe the types of tumors.

   ____

   ____

   ____

   c. What is the implication of a positive biopsy?

   ____

   ____

   ____

   d. List some early signs of cancer.

   ____

   ____

   ____

   e. Explain cancer staging and its purpose.

   ____

   ____

   ____

f. Discuss some of the treatment modalities for cancer.

g. List some of the major problems involved with cancer treatment.

9. After the birth of their son Riley, his parents were asked if they wanted to bank his cord blood. Describe to the parents how the procedure could help Riley.

10. There is much controversy over stem cell research.
   a. What is the function of stem cells?

   b. How do adult stem cells differ from embryonic stem cells?

   c. Why do parents hesitate to donate their child's cord blood for research?

SURF THE NET

For additional information and interactive exercises, use the following key words:

- cell, organelle
- cell division
- passive and active transport of cell material
- stem cell research
- cancer, classification of, treatments
- proteomics

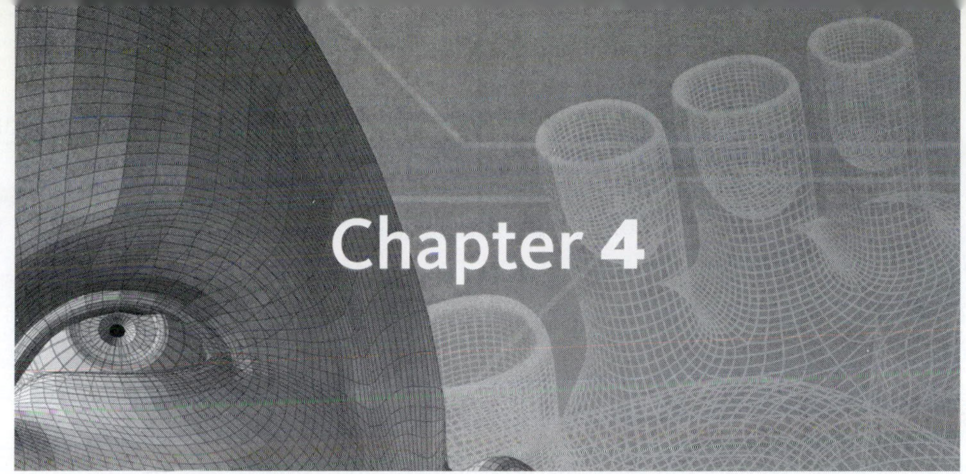

Tissues and Membranes

OVERVIEW

Tissues are groups of cells similar in shape, size, structure, intercellular material, and function. Two layers of tissue form membranes. A group of organs acts together to form an organ system.

Tissues are groups of cells that are similar in shape, size, structure, intercellular material, and function. Four main types of tissue are as follows:

Epithelial tissue protects the body by covering internal and external surfaces. Covering and lining types include *squamous, cuboidal,* and *columnar*; glandular or secretory types include *exocrine* and *endocrine* glands.

Connective tissue includes cells whose intercellular material (matrix) supports and connects organs. Types include adipose areolar, dense fibrous, supportive (bone and cartilage), and vascular (blood and lymph).

Muscular tissue provides movement and produces body heat.

Nervous tissue reacts to stimuli and conducts messages.

Membranes are formed by two layers of tissues. Types of membranes are *epithelial,* which produces either mucous or serous secretions, *cutaneous,* and *connective.*

Mucous membranes are also called mucosa, and include the respiratory mucosa, gastric mucosa, and intestinal mucosa.

Serous membranes are the pleural (lining thoracic cavity), pericardial (lining heart cavity), and peritoneal (lining abdominal cavity).

Cutaneous membranes are related to the skin.

Connective membranes are made of two layers of connective tissue. Synovial membrane is one type; it lines the joint cavities.

Organs and Systems

The formation of the human organism progresses from different layers of complexity: from atom to molecule to organelle to cell to tissue to organ to organ system to human organism. Organs are several tissues grouped together to perform a single function.

Organ systems are groups of organs that act together to perform specific related functions. The following are types of organ systems:

Skeletal: serves as the framework; forms blood components and stores minerals.
Muscular: provides for movement and produces body heat.
Digestive: prepares food for absorption by the body through mechanical and chemical means.
Respiratory: takes in oxygen and gives up carbon dioxide.
Circulatory: carries oxygen and nutrients to the cells and carries waste away from the cells.
Reproductive: reproduces organisms.
Excretory: eliminates the waste products of metabolism.
Endocrine: manufactures hormones to regulate body activity.
Nervous: communicates, coordinates, and controls body activities through response to stimuli.
Integumentary: protects the body and is a sensory organ.

Degree of Tissue Repair

The degree of tissue repair depends on the damage or injury and where it is located. Types of repair include the following:

Primary repair takes place in a clean wound; a scab will form if a larger area of tissue is involved. Damage to deeper tissues requires the edges of the wound to be brought together with sutures.

Secondary repair is required in deeper and larger wounds; healing takes place by the process of granulation.

Vitamins necessary for tissue repair include A, B, C, D, E, and K.

ACTIVITIES

A. Answer the following questions regarding tissues.

1. Cells, when grouped according to their structure, intercellular material, and function, are called ____________________.

2. Name the four major types of tissue and their primary functions.

____

____

____

____

3. Circle the mismatched pairs.

Squamous/outer layer of skin
Cuboidal/lining of digestive tract
Columnar/part of the respiratory tract
Glandular/secrete hormones
Exocrine/thyroid gland
Endocrine/adrenal gland

B. Each diagram illustrates the structure of epithelial tissue. Label the diagram with the name of epithelial tissue and its function in the body.

1. Cube-shaped cells

   Name of tissue: ______________________________

   Function: ______________________________

   ____

   ____

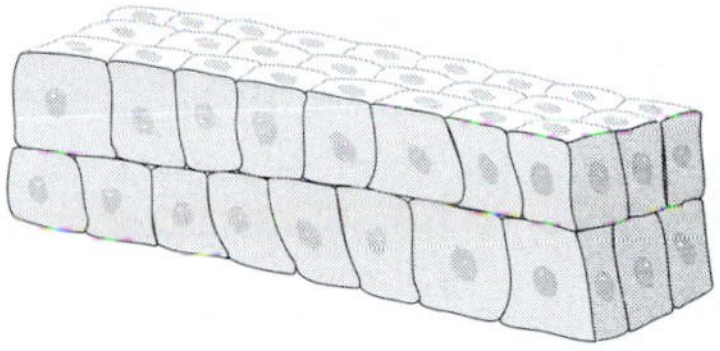

© Cengage Learning 2014.

2. Elongated cells, with the nucleus generally near the bottom; often ciliated

   Name of tissue: ______________________________

   Function: ______________________________

   ____

   ____

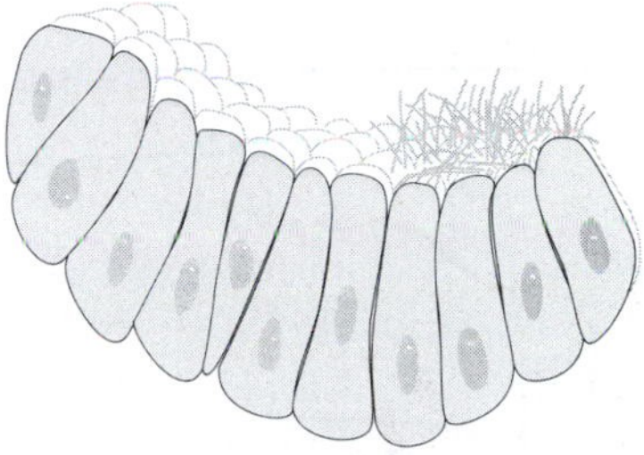

© Cengage Learning 2014.

3. Flat, irregularly shaped cells

   Name of tissue: ______________________________

   Function: ______________________________

   ____

   ____

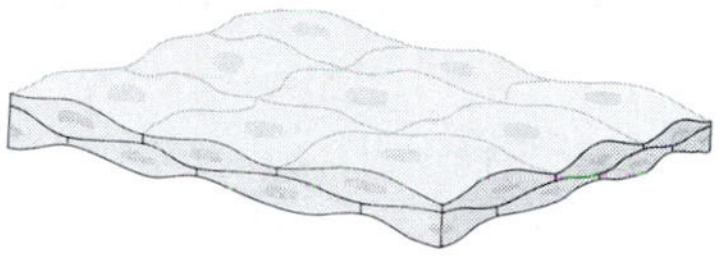

© Cengage Learning 2014.

4. Glandular tissue specialized to secrete hormones

   Name of tissue: ______________________________

   Function: ______________________________

   ____

   ____

Duct (where secretions leave)

Secretory cells

Exocrine (duct) gland cell e.g., sweat and mammary glands

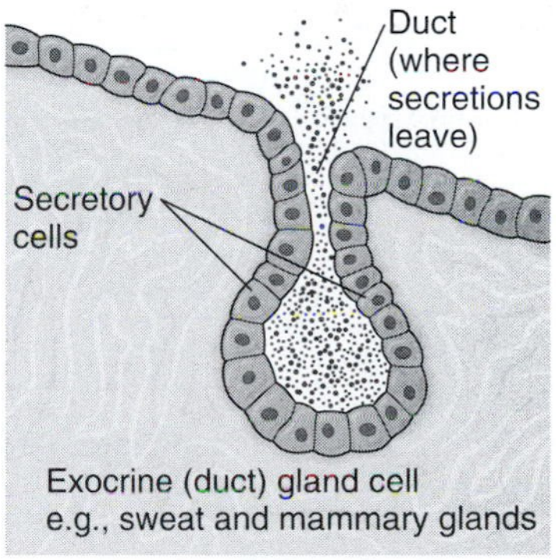

© Cengage Learning 2014.

C. In the glandular type of epithelial tissue there are two types of glands that secrete: exocrine and endocrine. In the following list, write EX next to exocrine glands and EN next to endocrine glands.

________ mammary gland

________ thyroid gland

________ sweat gland

________ salivary gland

________ adrenal gland

D. Connective tissue ranges from the loose, ordinary type to that which can bear weight. Write one or two sentences describing each type of connective tissue and where it is located in the body.

1. Adipose tissue

   Description: ______________________________

   Location: ______________________________

2. Areolar (loose connective) tissue

   Description: ______________________________

   Location: ______________________________

3. Dense fibrous tissue

   Description: ______________________________

   Location: ______________________________

4. Supportive—bone tissue

   Description: ______________________________

   Location: ______________________________

5. Supportive—cartilage tissue
   a. Hyaline

   Description: ______________________________
   ____
   ____
   ____

   Location: ______________________________
   ____
   ____

   b. Fibrocartilage

   Description: ______________________________
   ____
   ____
   ____

   Location: ______________________________
   ____
   ____

   c. Elastic cartilage

   Description: ______________________________
   ____
   ____
   ____

   Location: ______________________________
   ____
   ____

6. Vascular tissue
   a. Blood

   Description: ______________________________
   ____
   ____
   ____

   Location: ______________________________
   ____
   ____

b. Lymph

Description: ____

____

____

____

Location: ____

____

____

E. Match the description in Column A with the type of tissue in Column B.

	Column A	Column B
______	1. blood	a. adipose tissue
______	2. fibroblast	b. fasciae
______	3. elastic, single fibers	c. ligaments
______	4. tissue sheet that wraps around muscle bundles	d. bone tissue
		e. collagen
______	5. flexible, white fibrous protein	f. simple squamous tissue
______	6. holds bones together at joints	g. vascular tissue
______	7. connects muscle to bone	h. areolar tissue
______	8. calcified by mineral salts	i. tendon
______	9. fat	j. elastin
______	10. lymphocytes and granulocytes	k. columnar epithelial tissue
		l. lymph tissue

F. Complete the following statements in reference to muscle tissue.

1. Cardiac muscle tissue is ____________________ and involuntary; it makes up the ____________________ of the heart.
2. Smooth muscle tissue is nonstriated and ____________________.
3. Skeletal muscle tissue is ____________________ and ____________________.

G. Nervous tissue has two unique characteristics. Describe them.

____

____

____

H. Circle the correctly spelled word in each of the following statements about membranes.

1. (Epithelial, Epethelial) membranes are classified as mucous or serous depending on their secretion.
2. The mucous membranes line (surfuses, surfaces) and spaces that lead to the outside of the body.
3. The type of secretion of the mucous membrane is mucus, which (lubicates, lubricates) and protects the lining, especially of the (respiratory, risporatory) tract.
4. The portion of serous membrane that covers the organs is called (viseral, visceral) lining, and the portion that lines the cavity is called (parietal, parital).
5. Lining the thoracic cavity is the (plural, pleural) membrane.
6. The (precardial, pericardial) lining is in the heart cavity.
7. The lining of the abdominal cavity is the (peritoneal, peratoneal) membrane.
8. The connective membrane lining the joint cavity is (sinovial, synovial).

I. Label and color the following diagram. Color the serous membranes blue and the mucous membranes red.

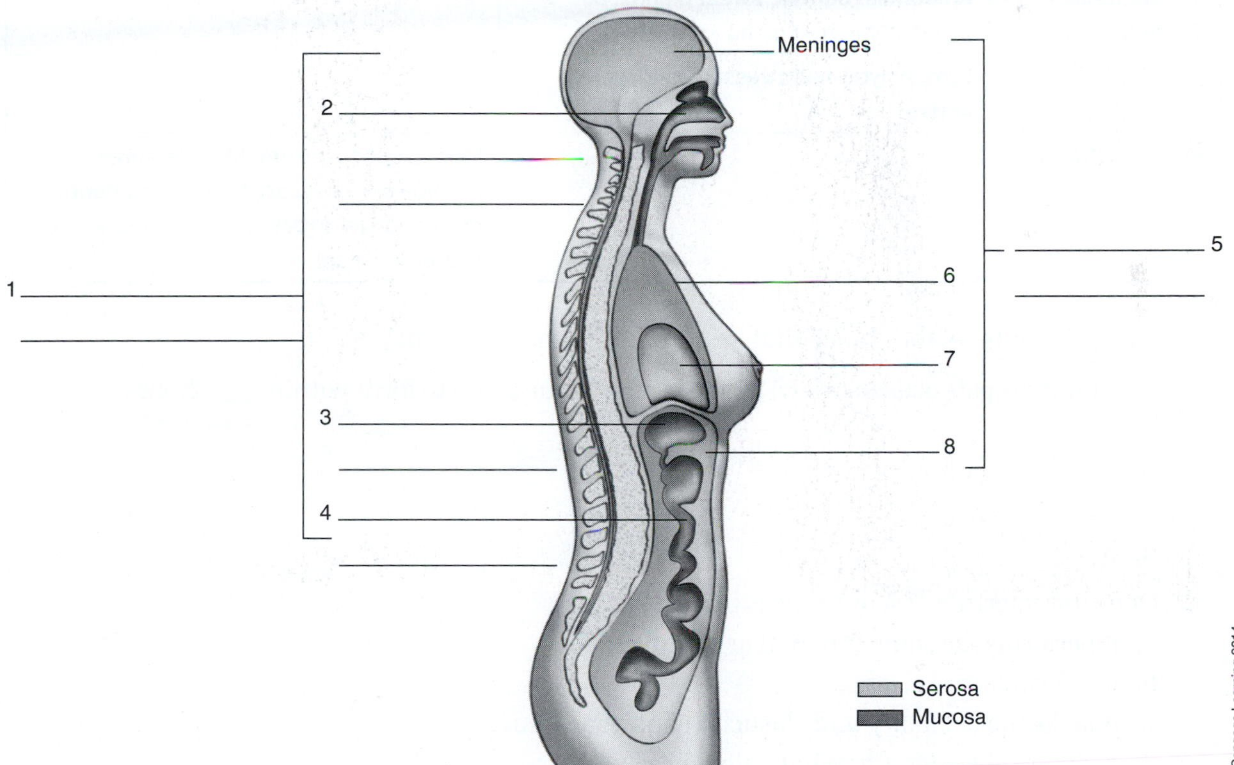

J. Refer to figure 4-2 in the textbook to describe the formation of the human organism from simple to complex.

K. Complete the following table on the body systems.

BODY SYSTEM	MAJOR STRUCTURES	MAJOR FUNCTIONS
Skeletal	Bones, joints and cartilage	
		Makes movement possible. Moves body fluids and generates heat.
Digestive system	Mouth, salivary glands, teeth, pharynx, esophagus, stomach, intestines, liver, gallbladder, and pancreas	
Respiratory		
Circulatory	Heart, arteries, veins, capillaries, and blood	
		Filters blood to eliminate waste products of metabolism.
Nervous	Nerves, brain, and spinal cord	
Special Senses		
		Manufactures hormones to regulate body activities.
Integumentary System	Epidermis, dermis, sweat glands, oil glands, hair, and nails.	
	Lymph, lymphatic vessels, and lymph nodes	
Reproductive		Reproduces new life. Manufactures hormones necessary for development of reproductive organs and secondary sex characteristics.

L. Select the letter of the choice that best completes the statement.

1. In primary repair of deep tissue, new vascular tissue starts to form within ____ hours.
   a. 12
   b. 24
   c. 48
   d. 72
2. One characteristic of scar tissue is that
   a. it performs the same function as normal tissue.
   b. it is flexible and elastic.
   c. it lacks the flexibility and elasticity of normal tissue.
   d. collagen fibers lengthen in healing process.
3. In primary repair of deeper tissues, fibroblast cells help make new collagen fibers within ____ hours.
   a. 24–48
   b. 48–72
   c. 72–96
   d. 96–120

4. In secondary repair, an open wound with large tissue loss heals by the
   a. granulation process.
   b. division of stratified squamous epithelial cells.
   c. drying of capillary fluid, which seals the wound.
   d. edges of the wound being sewn together.

5. A bactericidal action helps to reduce the risk of infection by
   a. reducing the number of bacteria.
   b. destroying bacteria.
   c. keeping the area clean.
   d. increasing the blood supply to the area.

M. Specify which vitamins (A, B, C, D, E, or K) help in each healing process.

________ 1. This vitamin is necessary for healing bones because it enhances calcium absorption from food.

________ 2. This vitamin is important for the normal production of collagen and repair of connective tissue.

________ 3. This vitamin is helpful in the replacement of epithelial tissues, for example, in the lining of the respiratory tract.

________ 4. Thiamine, nicotinic acid, and riboflavin are vitamins of this group and generally promote the well-being of the individual.

________ 5. This vitamin aids in blood clotting and helps to prevent excessive blood loss.

________ 6. This vitamin promotes healing by its action as an antioxidant protector.

APPLYING THEORY TO PRACTICE

1. Name the type of tissue:
   a. on the end of your nose ________________
   b. in the lining of your mouth ________________
   c. on your skin ________________
   d. on the lobe of your ear ________________
   e. on your fingers ________________

2. You are working in an assisted living facility. Your resident, Mr. Gianco, age 80, asks you why he is getting these funny brown spots on his arms. What is your response?

   ____

   ____

3. Tamika, age 4, has a bad cold and cough. She is seen by the nurse practitioner in the outpatient clinic. The type of membrane involved with Tamika's cold is ________________.

4. Juan, age 9, has had surgery for a ruptured appendix. The doctors fear he may get an inflammation of the lining of the abdomen. The name of this lining is the ________________.

5. Corey slid into second base when playing baseball. He complains of pain in his left ankle. The team doctor says Corey has probably strained the ligaments in his ankle. What is the function of the ligaments?

   ____

6. Molly has been vomiting for 10 hours. Her father brings her to the emergency room, where she is diagnosed with gastritis. The tissue involved in the inflammation of the stomach is ________________________.

7. Mrs. Givia, age 85, resides in a skilled nursing facility. She complains of being cold even though the temperature in the room is 24°C (76°F). Mrs. Givia may have lost some of her subcutaneous fat, which is part of ________________________ tissue.

8. Victoria has been exercising and lifting weights. Her right shoulder develops pain and stiffness. The doctor states she has bursitis of the shoulder joint. The membrane lining the shoulder joint is called ________________________.

9. Mrs. Nancy, age 60, has been a heavy smoker for 30 years. She now has severe shortness of breath, which limits her activities of daily living. Treatment has not improved her condition. She is scheduled for a lung transplant. The doctor tells her she must stay near her home to await the transplant.
   a. What is the reason for this instruction?

   ____

   ____

   ____

   b. Mrs. Nancy does receive a successful lung transplant. What is the major complication of an organ transplant?

   ____

   ____

   c. Mrs. Nancy must continue medical treatment for the rest of her life. She is also cautioned to avoid large crowds.
      1. List a reason for lifelong medical treatment.

      ____

      ____

      2. Why would Mrs. Nancy be told to avoid large crowds?

      ____

      ____

10. What methods are under investigation by researchers to help the immune system to accept an organ transplant?

    ____

    ____

SURF THE NET

For additional information and interactive exercises, use the following key words:

- tissues, types of tissue
- epithelial membrane, mucous membrane, serous membrane
- how tissue heals
- transplants, types of transplant
- life after a transplant

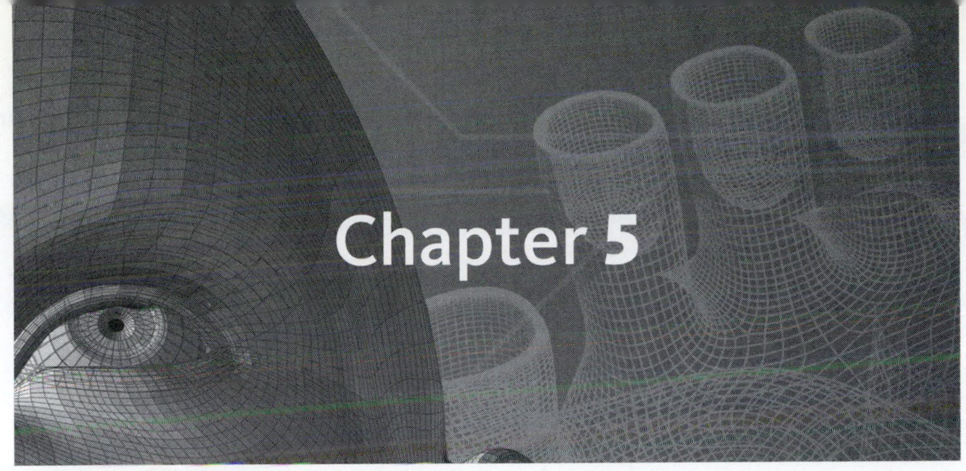

Integumentary System

OVERVIEW

The integumentary system is made up of the skin and its appendages—hair, nails, sebaceous glands, and sweat glands. The skin is our protective covering; it is tough, pliable, and multifunctional.

Functions of the Skin

Functions of the integumentary system include the following:

- Covering and protecting tissue from infection and dehydration
- Regulating body temperature
- Helping to manufacture vitamin D
- Acting as a site for nerve receptors
- Acting as a site for temporary storage of fat, glucose, water, and salts
- Screening out harmful rays of sunlight
- Absorbing certain drugs and other chemicals

Structure of the Skin

Skin consists of two basic layers: the epidermis and the dermis. The *epidermis*, or epithelial tissue, is the outermost layer of skin. It is avascular and contains keratin and melanocytes. The *dermis* is connective tissue containing collagen, elastic fibers, nerve endings, hair follicles, and oil and sweat glands. The *subcutaneous* or hypodermal layer is not a true part of integumentary, but is made of loose connective and adipose tissue.

Skin color depends on the presence of three pigments: melanin, carotene, and hemoglobin.

Appendages of the Skin

Characteristics of the skin include appendages such as hair, nails, and certain glands. *Hair* consists of the hair root, shaft, and three layers. *Nails* are keratinized plates that cover the ends of the fingers and toes. *Sweat glands*, or sudoriferous glands, help to cool skin through perspiration. *Sebaceous glands* secrete sebum, which lubricates the skin and hair.

The Integument and Its Relationship to Microorganisms

Handwashing is the number one way to prevent the spread of disease. If soap and water are not available, a hand sanitizer that has at least a 60% alcohol content may be used.

Representative Disorders of the Skin

Skin can be host to numerous disorders, including the following:

Acne vulgaris—oversecretion of the sebaceous glands; mostly seen in adolescents
Athlete's foot—contagious fungal infection, usually found between the toes
Dermatitis—inflammation of the skin
Eczema—noncontagious, inflammatory skin disease
Impetigo—acute, inflammatory, and contagious skin disease mostly seen in babies and young children
Psoriasis—chronic inflammatory disease
Ringworm—contagious fungal infection with circular patches
Urticaria or *hives*—skin reaction of itchy wheals, usually the response to an allergen
Boils—bacterial infection of a hair follicle
Rosacea—inflammatory disease characterized by chronic redness and irritation of the face.
Shingles (herpes zoster)—skin eruption due to a viral infection of the nerve endings
Herpes—viral infection seen as a fever blister or cold sore
Genital herpes—viral infection of the genital area

The Effects of Aging on the Integumentary System

As the sebaceous glands secrete less sebum, skin becomes fragile and dry. Loss of subcutaneous fat results in lines and wrinkles. The vascular network decreases in response to heat and cold.

Disorders of the Hair and Nails

Head lice—parasitic insects on the heads of people
Ingrown nails—usually the great toe
Fungal infections—make up 50% of nail disorders
Warts—human papilloma viral infections affecting the skin around or under the nail

Skin Cancer

Skin cancers are the most common combined cancer in the United States; they include the following types:

Basal cell—most common and least malignant
Squamous cell—arises from the epidermis, grows rapidly
Melanoma—malignant, occurs in the pigmented cells of the skin; may appear as a brown or black irregular patch

All are associated with overexposure to ultraviolet light.

Burns

Burns result from radiation, heat, chemicals, or electricity. First-degree burns involve the epidermis; redness, swelling, and pain are present. Second-degree burns may involve the epidermis and dermis; pain, redness, swelling, and blistering are present. Third-degree burns involve complete destruction of the skin; they are life threatening because of fluid loss and infection.

Skin Lesions

Different types of skin lesions include abrasion, fissure, laceration, bulla, macule, nodule, papule, pustule, pressure or decubitus ulcer, tumor, vesicle, and wheal.

ACTIVITIES

A. Answer the following questions regarding skin functions.

1. List the seven functions of the skin.

____

____

____

____

____

____

____

2. Which functions provide protection for the body?

____

3. How does the skin regulate body temperature?

____

____

B. Match the letter from Column B that best completes the statement in Column A.

Column A	Column B
One square centimeter of skin contains	
________ 1. nerve endings to record pain	a. 3,000
________ 2. sensory apparatuses for heat	b. 4
________ 3. sensory cells at the end of nerve fibers	c. 25
________ 4. yards of nerves	d. 200
________ 5. pressure apparatuses	e. 12

C. Complete the following statements about skin layers.

1. The stratum corneum is replaced by a nonliving substance that forms a waterproof covering. It is called ________________.

2. The stratum corneum destroys bacteria because it is slightly ________________.

3. The stratum germinativum displays ridges known as ________________. They are more pronounced on the palms of the hands and soles of the feet. This characteristic is used for ________________ in newborns.

4. Blood vessels in the dermis aid in the regulation of ________________.

5. The muscle attached to the hair follicle is known as the ___________________ ___________________ muscle.
6. Another name for the dermis layer is the ___________________.
7. Sudoriferous glands are exocrine glands that produce ___________________. Their ducts extend to form ___________________ on the skin.
8. Complete cell turnover in the stratum corneum occurs every ___________________ to ___________________ days in young adults.
9. The hypodermis layer contains fat and is also called the ___________________ layer.
10. Sebaceous glands produce ___________________, which lubricates the skin, keeping it ___________________ and ___________________.

D. Label the following diagram of the skin.

1. ______________________	9. ______________________
2. ______________________	10. ______________________
3. ______________________	11. ______________________
4. ______________________	12. ______________________
5. ______________________	13. ______________________
6. ______________________	14. ______________________
7. ______________________	15. ______________________
8. ______________________	16. ______________________

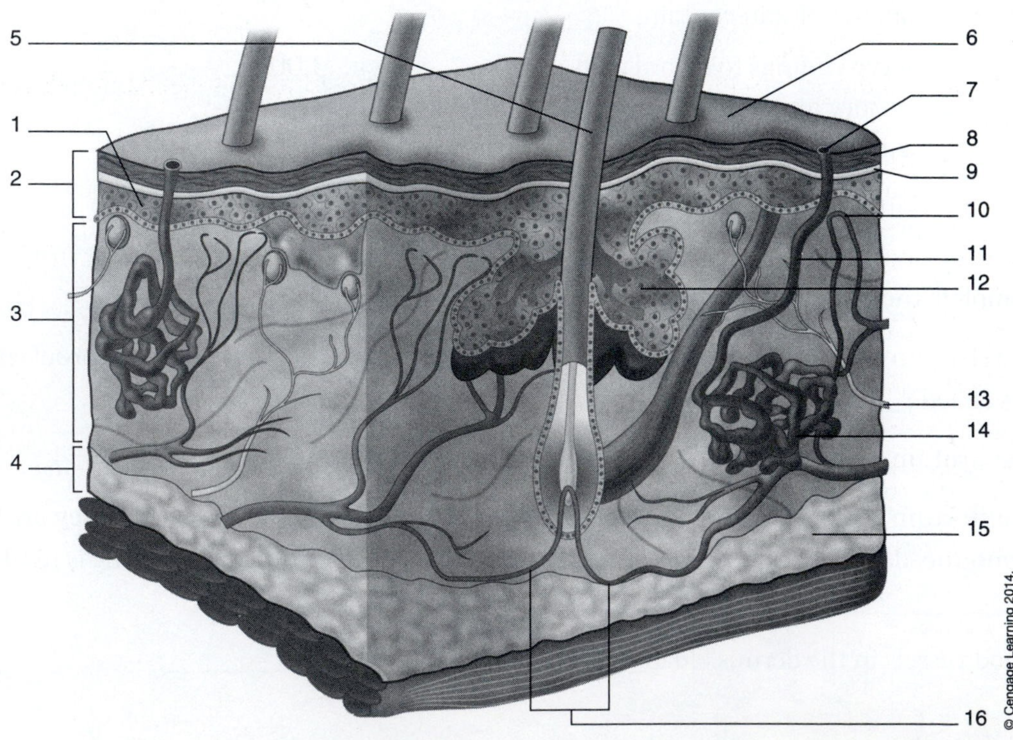

E. Next to each structure, state whether it is part of the hair or nails.

1. Cuticle layer or cortex ______________________
2. Hard, keratinized plate ______________________
3. Shaft in dermis ______________________
4. Medulla or inner layer ______________________
5. Elongated epidermal cell ______________________

F. Select the letter of the choice that best completes the statement.

1. The body's first line of defense is formed by the
   a. stratum germinativum.
   b. stratum corneum.
   c. stratum spinosum.
2. Light-skinned people generally have a greater proportion of
   a. keratin in the skin.
   b. pheomelanin in the skin.
   c. eumelanin in the skin.
3. The hair is composed of three layers, the
   a. cuticle, cortex, and medulla.
   b. keratin, cuticle, and cortex.
   c. cuticle, cortex, and dermis.
4. The name given to glands found in the ear canal is
   a. sebaceous.
   b. mammary.
   c. ceruminous.
5. The epidermal layer containing melanocytes, keratinocytes, and Langerhans cells is the
   a. stratum granulosum.
   b. stratum spinosum.
   c. stratum lucidum.
6. The best way to prevent the spread of infection is by handwashing for ____ seconds.
   a. 20
   b. 25
   c. 30
7. Underarm odor is caused by the interaction of bacteria and secretions from the
   a. sudoriferous glands.
   b. hair follicles.
   c. ceruminous glands.

8. Athlete's foot, which is characterized by itching and blisters between the toes, is caused by
   a. shoes that are too tight.
   b. a fungus.
   c. inflammation of the sweat glands.

9. A pregnant mother may infect her baby during a vaginal delivery if she has
   a. impetigo.
   b. genital herpes.
   c. eczema.

10. ________ is a painful condition that occurs around the nerve endings.
    a. Herpes simplex
    b. Shingles
    c. Psoriasis

G. Complete the table relating to skin color and condition.

SKIN COLOR	CAUSE	CONDITION
Erythema		Fever, allergic reaction, or embarrassment
Cyanosis	Decrease in oxygen in capillary network	
	Accumulation of bile in capillary network	
Pallor		Emotional stress or anemia

H. Unscramble the letters to fit the following statements.

1.	chronic disorder of the sebaceous glands	NAEC	☐☐☐☐
2.	destruction of tissue by freezing	RGSCROUYYER	☐☐☐☐☐☐☐☐☐☐☐
3.	pressure ulcer	ESUCIDUTB	☐☐☐☐☐☐☐☐☐
4.	chronic noncontagious inflammation of the skin	AMEZEC	☐☐☐☐☐☐
5.	blackened area of the skin usually as a result of burns	CERSHA	☐☐☐☐☐☐
6.	fungal infection with raised, itchy, circular patches	MORNRGWI	☐☐☐☐☐☐☐☐
7.	viral infection of nerve endings	SIGHENSL	☐☐☐☐☐☐☐☐
8.	human papilloma virus affects the nail bed	SRAWT	☐☐☐☐☐
9.	intensely itchy wheal resulting from an allergen response	RIURAITCA	☐☐☐☐☐☐☐☐☐
10.	inflammatory disease of the skin characterized by redness of the face	CAASROE	☐☐☐☐☐☐☐

I. Write the correct disorder or condition next to each description.

abrasion
acne vulgaris
boils or carbuncles
cherry angiomas
dermatitis
eczema
fissure
genital herpes
impetigo
laceration
psoriasis
ringworm

1. This nonspecific rash could be caused by chemicals such as soap, or by stress. ________________
2. This disorder of the sebaceous gland plugs the opening of the gland and occurs primarily during adolescence. ________________
3. An injury in which the superficial layers of the skin are scraped. ________________
4. As one ages, these benign red bumps may appear on the skin. ________________
5. This bacterial infection of a hair follicle or sebaceous gland becomes deeply embedded in the skin. ________________
6. The onset of this chronic inflammatory condition affects mainly the elbows and knees, and may be triggered by stress or trauma. ________________
7. This chronic noncontagious inflammation of the skin often occurs in the first year of life. ________________
8. This term refers to a torn or jagged wound. ________________
9. This term refers to a groove or crack-like break in the skin. ________________
10. This inflammatory contagious skin condition seen in babies is characterized by the appearance of vesicles that rupture and develop distinct yellow crusts. ________________

J. Mark the following statements as either true or false; correct the false statements.

________ 1. The most common type of cancer is skin cancer.

________ 2. Basal cell carcinoma usually has a recovery rate of 75%.

________ 3. Squamous cell cancer is usually found on the face.

________ 4. Malignant melanoma is a tumor that may appear as a brown or black irregular patch.

________ 5. Squamous cell cancer rarely metastasizes.

________ 6. The usual treatment for skin cancer is surgical removal and radiation.

K. Match the words in Column A with the most correct statement in Column B.

	Column A	Column B
________	1. ringworm	a. solid, abnormal mass of cells
________	2. papule	b. loss of skin surface may extend to the dermis
________	3. wheal	c. fluid-filled raised area
________	4. pustule	d. raised, itchy, circular patches with crusts
________	5. macule	e. brown or black irregular patch
________	6. vesicle	f. flat spot, flush with skin area, that is a different color
________	7. melanoma	g. elevated solid area
________	8. psoriasis	h. discrete pus-filled area
________	9. ulcer	i. reddish patches with silvery scales
________	10. tumor	j. itchy, temporarily elevated area

L. State whether the treatment or statement applies to first-, second-, or third-degree burns.

________ 1. Life-threatening situation

________ 2. Pain medication and dry, sterile dressing

________ 3. Application of cold water

________ 4. Prevention of contracture and fluid replacement

________ 5. Healing generally complete in 2 weeks

________ 6. Eschar present

________ 7. Redness, swelling, and blistering

M. Label and describe the following skin lesions.

© Cengage Learning 2014.

1. ________________________________

____

____

____

Example: Lipoma, erythema, cyst

© Cengage Learning 2014.

2. ________________________________

____

____

____

Example: Stage 2 pressure ulcer

© Cengage Learning 2014.

3. ________________________________

____

____

____

Example: Insect bite or a wheal

4. ____________________

____

____

____

Example: Freckle

5. ____________________

____

____

____

Example: Benign epidermal tumor

6. ____________________

____

____

____

Example: Herpes simplex, herpes zoster, chickenpox

7. ____________________

____

____

____

Example: Acne, impetigo, furuncles, carbuncles, folliculitis

8. ____________________

____

____

____

Example: Contact dermatitis, large second-degree burns, bulbous impetigo, pemphigus

9. ____________________

____

____

____

Example: Warts, elevated nevi

N. Use the words from the following list to complete the rhyme about functions of the skin.

bacteria	evaporation	receptors
bones	harmful	sunburn
difference	hot	vitamin D
elastic	protective	wrinkled

Think about your skin and what comes to mind?
How does your protective coat stand the test of time?

From baby's skin, smooth, ________________, and smelling so sweet
to aging skin, ________________, dry, and not feeling too neat.

It helps protect us from the ________________ rays of the sun,
but your skin thinks a ________________ is definitely not fun.

The skin helps us manufacture ________________ for free,
and that keeps our ________________ strong and healthy.

When our bodies are ________________, it cools us by perspiration,
a process completed by ________________.

The sense ________________ present let us know the
________________ between a soft touch or a hard blow.

All this time you never thought too much about your skin.
It keeps us well by preventing ________________ from getting in.

APPLYING THEORY TO PRACTICE

1. Mr. John, age 70, is fair skinned. He visits his doctor because his face gets very red at times, especially his nose. He wants to know what is wrong. The doctor's diagnosis is rosacea. As the medical assistant in the office, the doctor wants you to explain this condition and what causes it.
____
____
____
____
____

2. A friend obtains a nicotine patch to help her stop smoking. She asks you how something put on her skin can work. How do you reply?
____
____
____
____

3. Skin disorders are visible for all to see. Parents whose children have eczema worry about what others will think when they see patches on the skin. What could you do to relieve a parent's stress?
____
____
____
____

4. Alan is very distraught when he brings his son, Jack, to the emergency center with first- and second-degree burns. Jack has no third-degree burns. Describe the appearance of first-, second-, and third-degree burns and treatment. Name the major complications that result from second- and third-degree burns. When a person has third-degree burns, he or she is not in pain; explain the reason.

____

____

____

____

5. Bryan, age 15, visits the school nurse because of his cysts and pimples. What condition does Bryan have and what is the cause? Is there a treatment for this condition?

____

____

6. Jodi gets a note home from the school stating that her daughter Kayla, in fourth grade, has been exposed to head lice. The note includes what the symptoms are and the treatment for head lice.
   a. What is the cause of head lice?

   ____

   b. What are the symptoms?

   ____

   c. How is head lice treated?

   ____

   ____

7. As a health care professional, you are advised to wash your hands with soap and water for at least 20 seconds. How do you know when 20 seconds has passed?

____

8. Your neighbor tells you his prescription says something about "photosensitive." He asks you what that means.

____

____

____

____

9. Your 90-year-old grandmother had a stroke and has been in a nursing home for about 3 months. On your last visit you noticed a red, blistered area on the back of her leg. Name your grandmother's skin condition, its stage of development, and the proper treatment.

____

____

____

____

10. List at least one way in which the integumentary system interacts with the following body systems: skeletal, muscular, nervous, endocrine, circulatory, lymphatic, digestive, respiratory, urinary, and reproductive.

SURF THE NET

For additional information and interactive exercises, use the following key words:

- integumentary system, layers of the skin
- hair, nails, sudoriferous glands, sweat glands
- effects of aging on the skin
- diseases of the skin and appendages—acne vulgaris, athlete's foot, dermatitis, eczema, impetigo, psoriasis, ringworm, hives, boils, herpes, rosacea, shingles, head lice, ingrown nails, and fungal infections
- skin cancer
- effects of sunlight
- burns, types and treatment

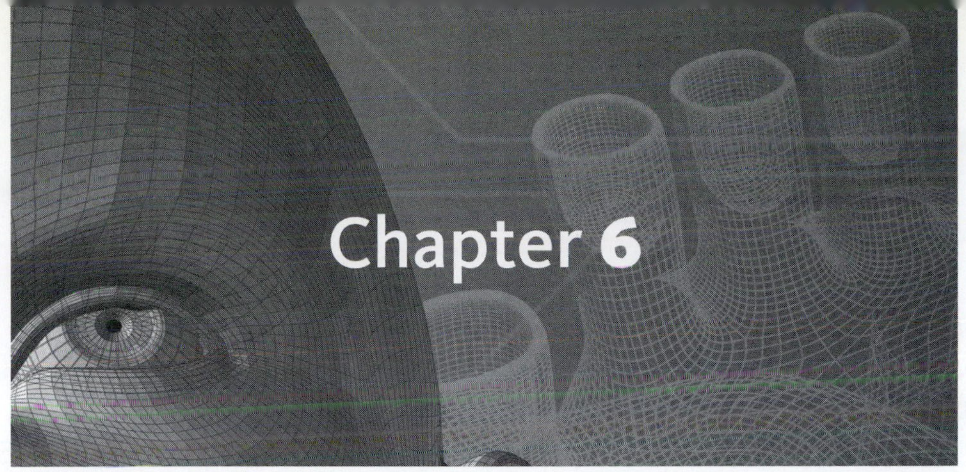

Skeletal System

OVERVIEW

The **skeletal system** is the bony framework within the body. It is composed of 206 bones.

Functions

Functions of the skeletal system are as follows:

- Supporting body structures
- Protecting internal organs
- Serving as an attachment for muscles
- Storing minerals, calcium, and phosphorous
- Acting as a hematopoietic site of blood cell formation
- Aiding movement

Structure and Formation of Bone

Bone is made of organic and inorganic material.

Structure of Long Bone

Long bone consists of the following:

- The *diaphysis* is the hollow, cylindrical shaft of a long bone.
- The *epiphysis* is at each end of the diaphysis; it contains the red marrow.
- The *medullary canal* is the center of the shaft, and has yellow marrow. The lining is called the *endosteum.*
- *Compact bone* is hard bone surrounding the medullary canal.
- *Spongy bone* is that which remains when some of the hard bone dissolves.
- *Periosteum* is fibrous tissue covering the outside of the bone.

Growth

Long bone grows from the diaphysis to the epiphysis. Bone cells include the following:

Osteoblasts are bone cells that deposit new bone.

Osteoclasts are bone cells that secrete enzymes that split the bone minerals into calcium and phosphorous.

Osteocytes are bone cells that help to maintain bone as a living tissue.

Bone Types

Long, flat, irregular, and short are types of bones.

Parts of the Skeletal System

Axial. The axial skeleton includes skull, vertebral column, sternum, ribs, and hyoid.

The *skull* is divided into cranial and facial bones.

The cranium has 8 bones in the frontal, parietal, temporal, occipital, ethmoid, and sphenoid areas.

The face has 14 bones in the nasal, maxilla, mandible, lacrimal, zygomatic, and palatine areas.

The *vertebral column* includes cervical (7), thoracic (12), lumbar (5), sacrum (1), and coccyx (1) bones.

The *sternum* includes the breastbone (1).

The *ribs* include true ribs (7), false ribs (3), and floating ribs (2).

The *hyoid* is a U-shaped bone (1) in the neck.

Appendicular. The appendicular skeleton includes the shoulder girdles, arms, wrists, hands, pelvic girdle, legs, ankles, and feet.

The *shoulder girdle* includes the clavicle (2) and scapula (2).

The *arm* includes the humerus (2), a bone in the upper arm; the radius (2), which runs up the thumb side of the forearm; and the ulna (2), a larger bone of the forearm.

The *hand* has carpals (16), 8 small bones that make up each wrist; metacarpals (10), each hand has 5, which make up the palm; and phalanges (28), each hand has 14, which make up the fingers.

The *pelvic girdle* (1) is made up of the ilium, ischium, and pubis bones.

The *upper leg* is the femur or thigh bone, the longest and strongest bone in the body.

The *lower leg* has the tibia, or shin bone, and fibula, the smaller bone of the lower leg.

The *ankle* has tarsals (14), each ankle having 7 tarsals; the *calcaneus* is the heel bone.

The *foot* has metatarsals (10), each foot having 5 bones arranged to make up the arch; and phalanges (28), each foot having 14, which make up the toes.

Ligaments connect bones and cartilage; tendons connect muscles to bones.

Joints and Related Structures

A **joint** is the point of contact or articulation between two bones. Related structures of joints are as follows:

Articular cartilage is the smooth, slippery cap of cartilage that covers the two joint surfaces.

The *articular capsule* is the fibrous connective tissue that encloses the two joint surfaces; it is lined with synovial membrane.

Types of joints include diarthroses, amphiarthroses, and synarthroses.

Diarthroses are freely movable joints. Types of diarthroses are ball and socket, which has the greatest degree of freedom (hip); hinge, which moves in one direction (elbow, knee); pivot, which has an extension rotating in a second arch-shaped bone (axis); and gliding, in which flat surfaces glide across each other (vertebrae).

Amphiarthroses are partially movable joints (symphysis pubis).

Synarthroses are immovable joints; they connect bone by fibrous connective tissue (sutures of the skull).

Types of Motion

Following are the various types of joint movement:

Flexion decreases the angle between two bones.

Extension increases the angle between two bones.

Abduction is movement away from the midline.

Adduction is movement toward the midline.

Circumduction includes flexion, extension, abduction, and adduction.

Rotation moves bones around a central axis.

Pronation is the palm downward or backward.

Supination is the palm forward or upward.

The Effects of Aging on the Skeletal System

After the age of 40, bone mass and density begin to shift, which leads to osteoporosis and a change in posture. Joints also become less mobile and flexible.

Disorders of the Bones and Joints

Fractures. A **fracture** is a break in the bone. Types of fractures include greenstick, simple, compound, and comminuted.

Bone and Joint Injuries. Bone and joint injuries include the following:

Dislocation—bone is displaced from its proper position in a joint.

Sprain—an injury to a joint caused by a sudden motion. The ligaments are either torn from or torn across their attachments to bones.

Hammer toe—refers to a toe that is flexed due to a bend in the middle joint of one or more toes.

Whiplash—trauma to the cervical vertebrae.

Diseases of the Bones

The body can be afflicted with various bone diseases, such as the following:

Arthritis is an inflammatory condition of one or more joints. Types include *rheumatoid*, a chronic autoimmune disease, and *osteoarthritis*, articular cartilage degeneration.

Gout occurs due to deposits of uric acid crystals in a joint cavity; the most commonly affected site is the great toe.

Rickets is when bones are soft due to lack of vitamin D.

Abnormal curvatures of the spine include *kyphosis*, a humped curvature in the thoracic area of the spine; *lordosis*, an exaggerated inward curvature in the lumbar region of the spine; and *scoliosis*, a lateral curvature of the spine.

Osteoporosis is loss of calcium and phosphorous in the bone, causing brittleness.

Osteomyelitis is inflammation of the bone.

Osteosarcoma is cancer of the bone.

ACTIVITIES

A. List the five functions of the skeletal system.

____

____

____

____

____

B. Mark the following statements as either true or false. Correct any false statements.

________ 1. The cranium protects the brain, the outer ear, and parts of the eye.

________ 2. Bones act as passively operated levers to move the body.

________ 3. Bone is constantly renewed through a process of remodeling that consists of resorption and formation.

________ 4. Tendons are fibrous cords that connect bone to bone.

________ 5. Red marrow, which manufactures blood cells, is found in irregular bones, the sternum, and the hip bones.

C. Select the letter that best completes each statement.

1. Bones are formed of microscopic cells called
   a. osteoblasts.
   b. osteoclasts.
   c. embryonic cells.
   d. osteocytes.
2. On average, bone growth in females continues to about ____ years of age.
   a. 18
   b. 20
   c. 16
   d. 24

3. Bone cells that develop new bone are called
   a. osteoblasts.
   b. osteoclasts.
   c. embryonic cells.
   d. osteocytes.
4. Ossification, or bone creation, is the process by which
   a. mineral matter replaces cartilage.
   b. cartilage is deposited between collagen fibers.
   c. osteoclasts begin to secrete enzyme.
   d. the articular cartilage covers the epiphysis.
5. The inorganic portion of bone is made from all the following mineral salts, *except*
   a. calcium phosphate.
   b. calcium carbonate.
   c. calcium chloride.
   d. calcium fluoride.

D. Label the long bone diagram and match the number that corresponds to the description.

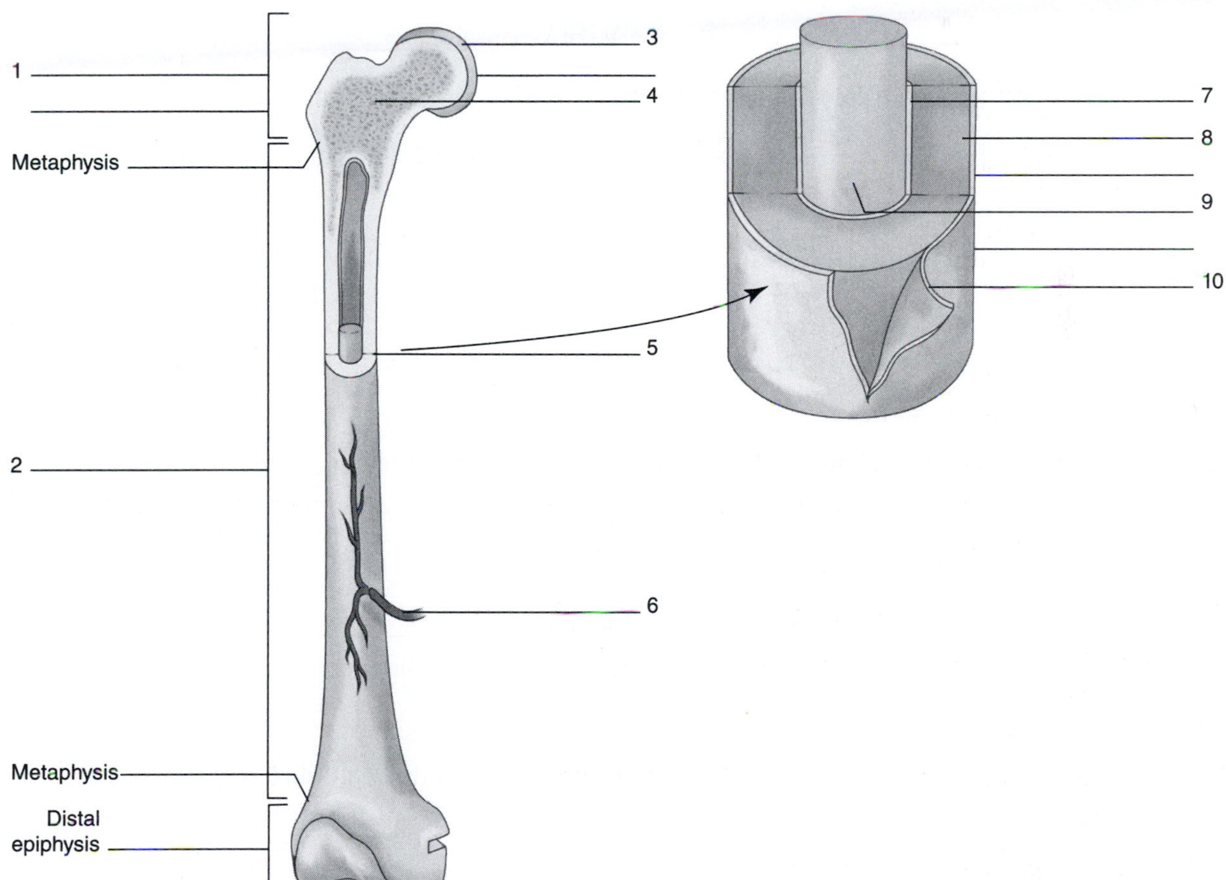

________________ a. Lining of the marrow cavity

________________ b. Located in the center of the shaft

________________ c. Shaft

________________ d. Containing red bone marrow

________________ e. Articular layer covering epiphysis

________________ f. Proximal end of long bone

________________ g. Carries blood supply to the bone

________________ h. Tough, fibrous covering of bone

________________ i. Fat storage center

________________ j. Bone surrounding the medullary canal

E. Complete the statements with the correct word or words.

1. One function of the skeletal system is to store minerals such as calcium; this helps maintain the blood ________________ ________________.
2. The process of blood cell formation in the bones is called ________________.
3. The organic substance of bone gives it a degree of ________________.
4. The ________ shape of the cranium affords a better protection than a flat surface.
5. Blood vessels that nourish the osteocytes, or bone cells, travel to the area through the ________________ ________________.
6. The wrist and ankle are cubelike in shape; they also may be classified as ________________ bones.
7. Irregular bands of connective tissue that hold the bones in place during infancy are called ________________.
8. The **cranial** bone that forms part of the nasal cavity is called the ________________.
9. On the ________________, or second cervical vertebrae, is the ________________ process, which permits us to nod our heads.
10. On the lower cartilaginous part of the breastbone or ________________ is the ________________ process, an important landmark in cardiopulmonary resuscitation (CPR).

F. Label and color the bones of the skeleton. Color the bones of the axial skeleton blue and the bones of the appendicular skeleton yellow. How many bones are in the skeleton?

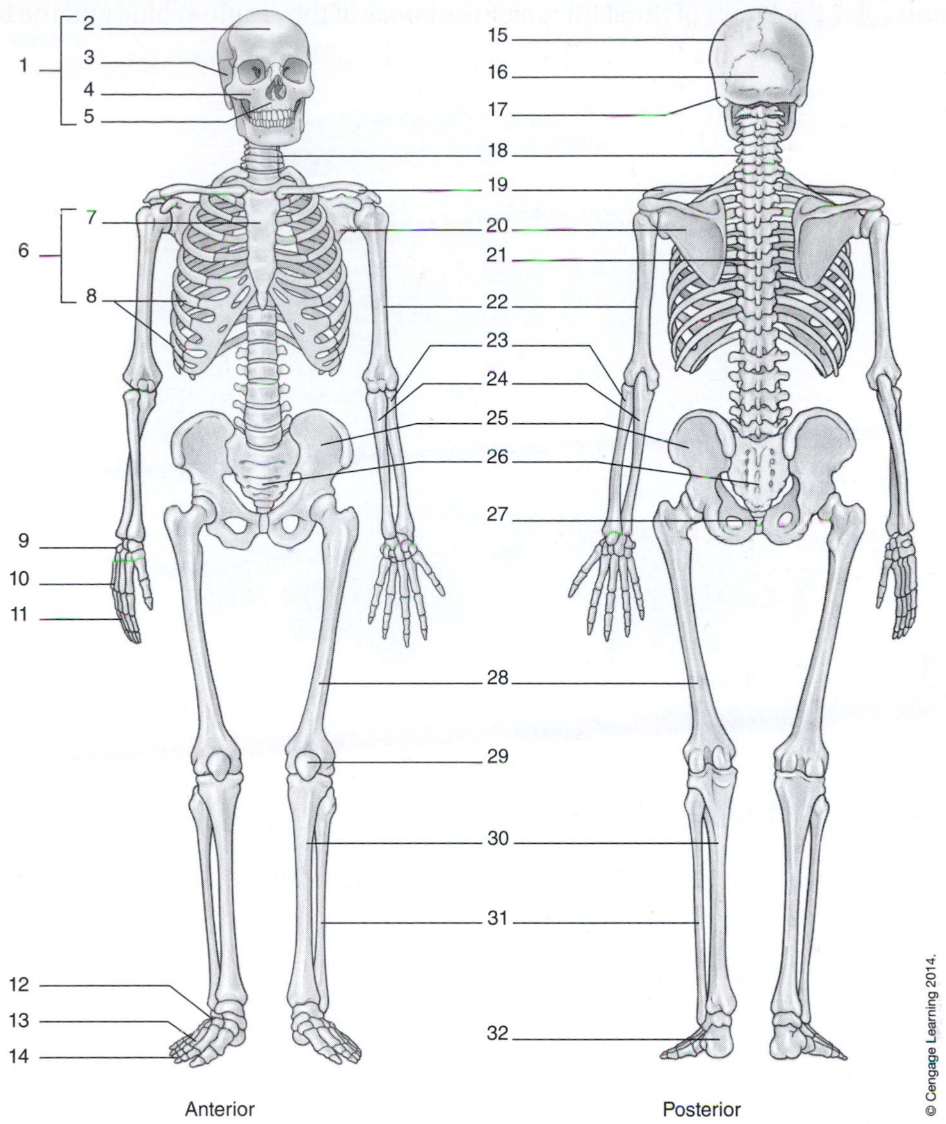

Axial

1. ____________________
2. ____________________
3. ____________________
4. ____________________
5. ____________________
6. ____________________
7. ____________________
8. ____________________
9. ____________________
10. ____________________
11. ____________________
12. ____________________
13. ____________________
14. ____________________
15. ____________________
16. ____________________

Appendicular

17. ____________________
18. ____________________
19. ____________________
20. ____________________
21. ____________________
22. ____________________
23. ____________________
24. ____________________
25. ____________________
26. ____________________
27. ____________________
28. ____________________
29. ____________________
30. ____________________
31. ____________________
32. ____________________

G. Label and color the bones of the skull. Color the bones of the cranium blue and the bones of the face yellow.

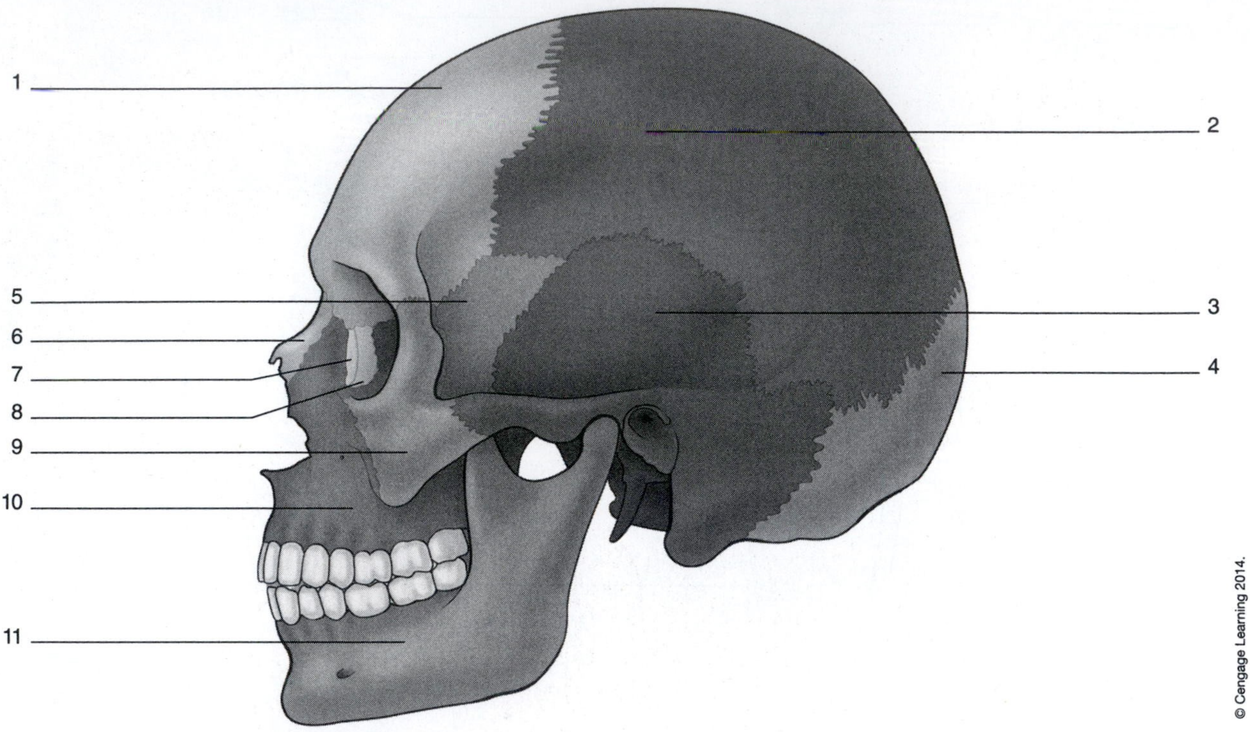

H. Using the diagram of the cranial bones, match the name of the bone with the following information. Also indicate the quantity of each structure.

A. The dome shape of all of these bones protects this. ________________

B. This bone forms part of the nasal cavity. ________________ # _____

C. Organs of hearing are protected by this bone. ________________ # _____

D. Forms the roof and sides of the cranium. ________________ # _____

E. Protector of the anterior portion of the brain, the forehead. ________________ # _____

F. Features the foramen magnum, the opening through which the spinal cord connects with the brain. ________________ # _____

G. All of the bones of the cranium connect with this. ________________ # _____

I. The face has two palatine bones, which form the roof of the mouth with the maxilla. The hyoid bone is a U-shaped bone in the posterior portion of the mouth. Write the names of the other bones of the face in the statements that follow. Include the number of bones involved.

A. The cheek bones also form the prominence of the cheek. ________________ # _____

B. These bones hold the ducts from which our tears fall. ________________ # ____________

C. The upper jaw, which also forms the hard palate. ________________ # _____

D. These bones make up the side walls of the nasal cavity. ________________ # _____

E. These bones join to form the bridge of the nose. ____________________ # ______

F. Lower jaw; the only movable bone in the face. ____________________ # ______

G. Forms part of the nasal septum. ____________________ # ______

J. Label and color the bones of the vertebrae. Color the cervical vertebrae red, the thoracic vertebrae green, the lumbar vertebrae blue, the sacrum yellow, and the coccyx orange.

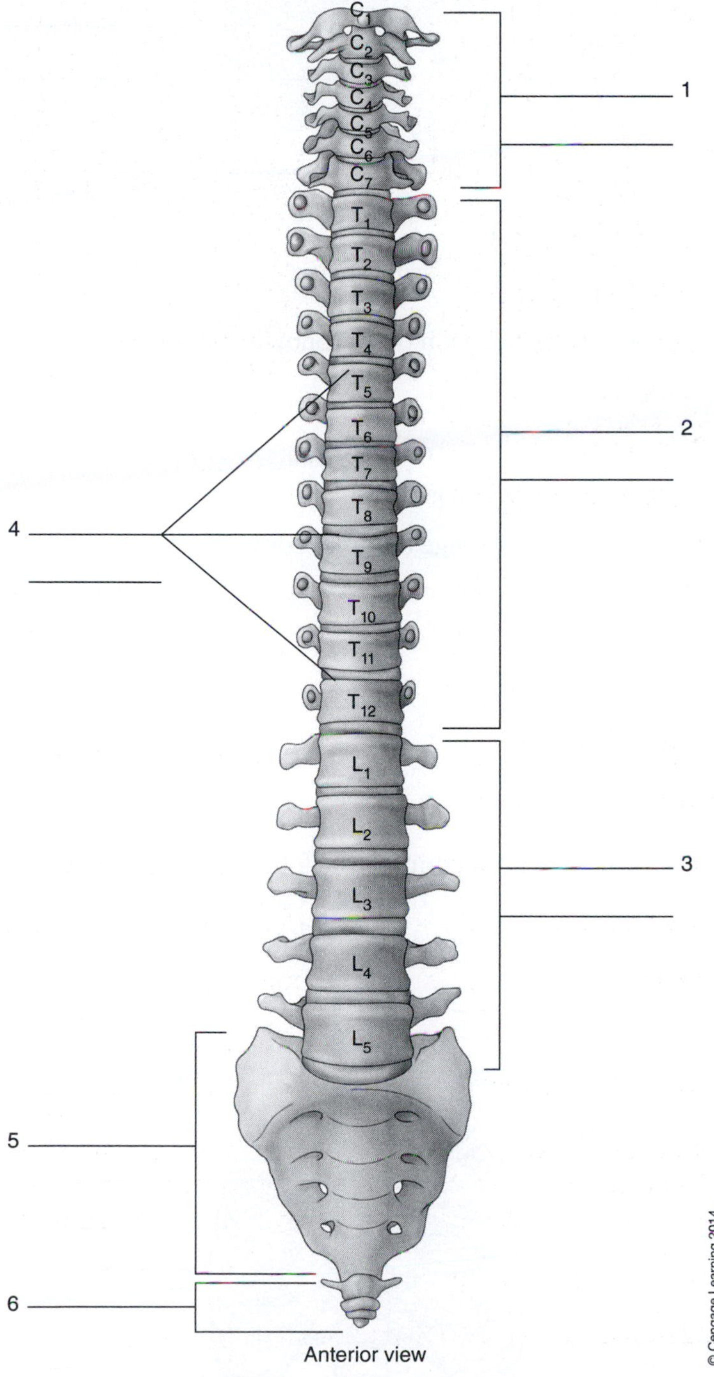

Anterior view

K. Label a typical vertebra: **body, foramen,** and **transverse process.**

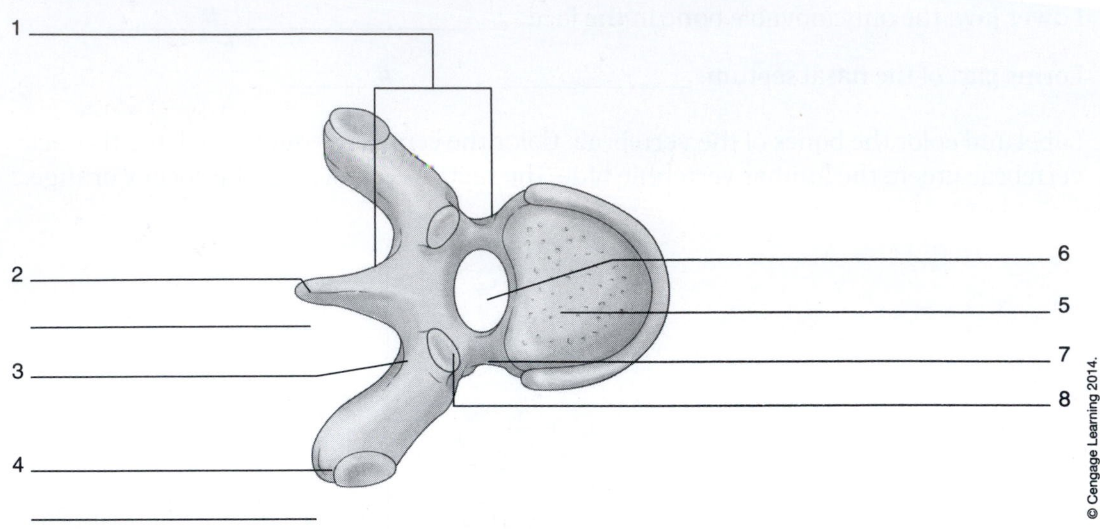

L. Fill in the term that best describes each of the following statements.

1. Large solid part of the vertebrae ________________
2. Second cervical vertebra ________________
3. Forms posterior portion of the pelvic girdle ________________
4. Opening in a vertebra to allow passage of spinal cord ________________
5. Tailbone ________________
6. Pads of cartilage between disks ________________
7. Articulate with the ribs ________________
8. Have large and heavy bodies ________________
9. First seven vertebra ________________

M. Label and color the rib cage and sternum in the following diagram. Color the true ribs blue, the sternum green, the false ribs gold, the costal cartilage gray, and the floating ribs brown. Why do the ribs have the names *true, false,* and *floating*? ____________________________

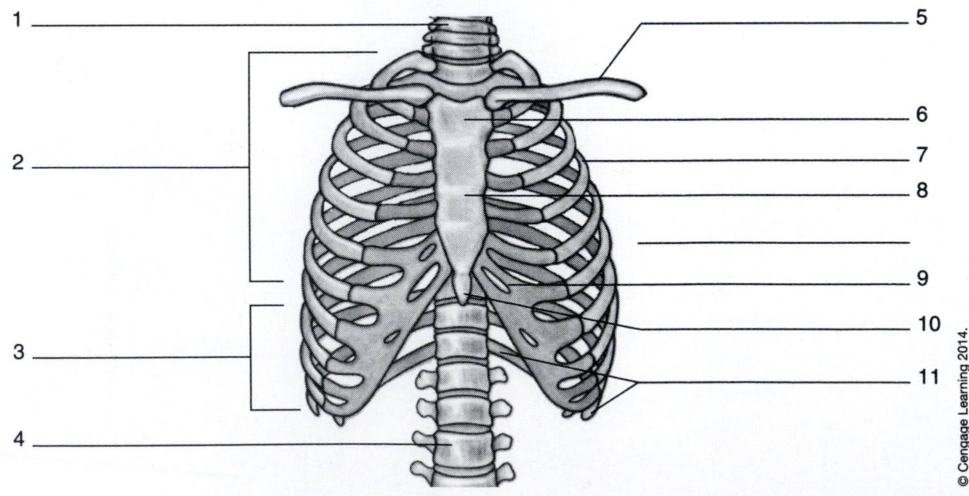

N. Answer the following questions regarding the appendicular skeleton.

1. The two bones that form the shoulder girdle are the ________________ or ________________ ________________, and the ________________, or ________________ ________________. Feel these bones on yourself. The location where they meet serves as the attachment point for the arms.

2. Label the following diagram of the lower arm.

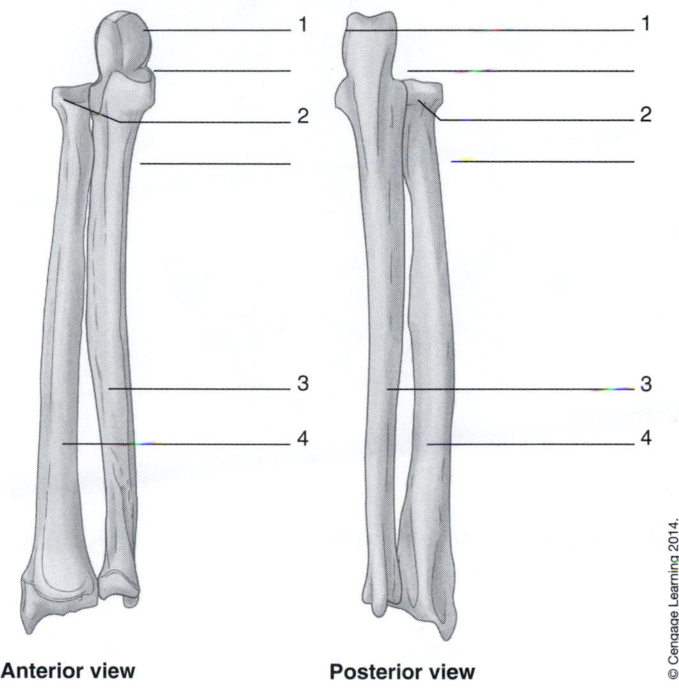

3. Label the following diagram of the left hand and state the number of bones for each.

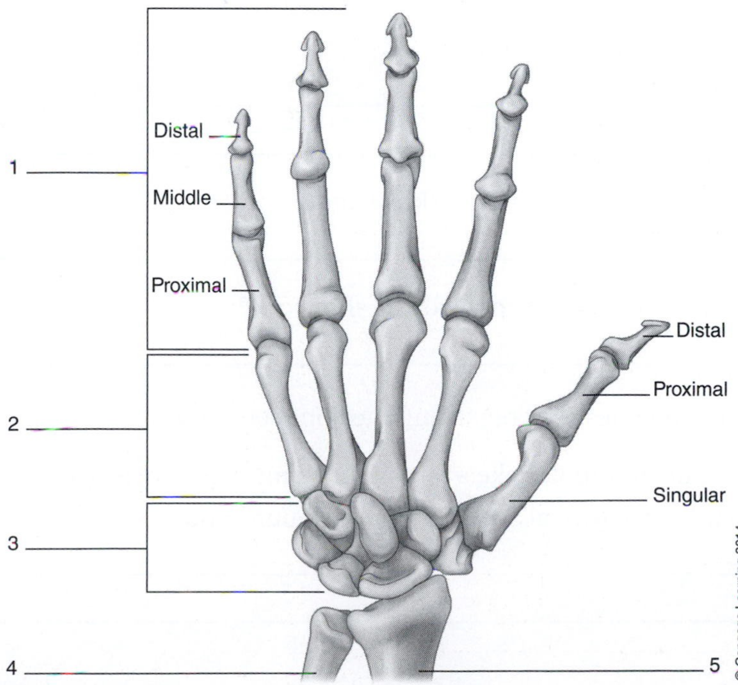

1. ____________________ #__________ 4. ____________________ #__________
2. ____________________ #__________ 5. ____________________ #__________
3. ____________________ #__________

O. Label the diagrams of the bones and structures of the pelvic girdle.

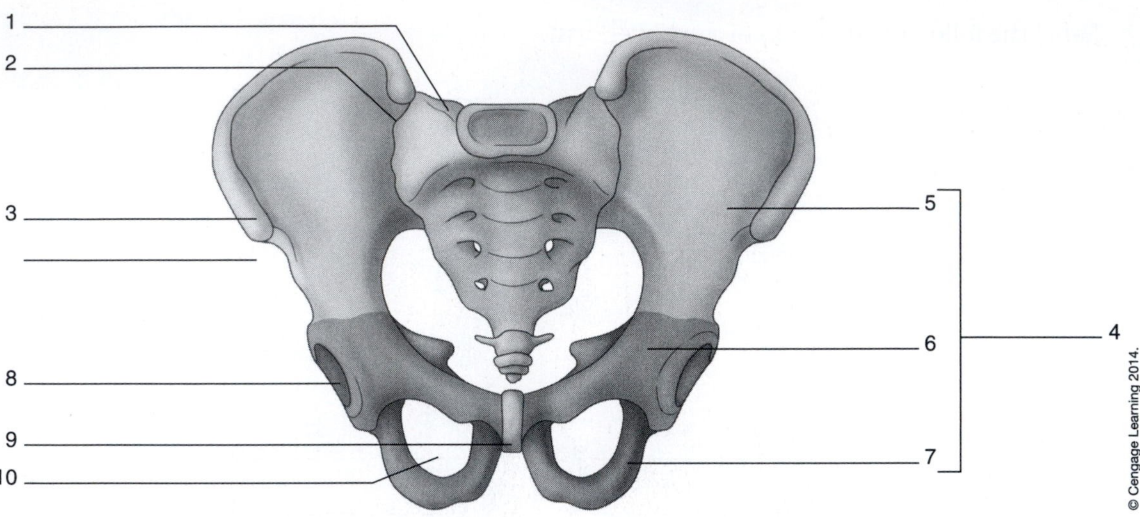

P. Answer the following questions.

1. Name the bones that fuse together to form the innominate or hip bone. ____________________

2. The hip bone fuses with what axial bone to form the pelvic girdle? ____________________

3. Name the part on the pelvic girdle where the head of the femur fits in to form a ball-and-socket joint. ____________________

4. List two characteristics of the femur.

5. Name the sesamoid bone in front of the knee joint.

6. Which bone of the lower leg is known as the shin bone?

Q. Answer the following questions regarding the bones of the feet.

1. Look at the bones of your foot. Take a few steps. What structure is responsible for giving spring to your step? Is this structure also in the palms of your hands?

2. Label and color the diagram of the foot bones. Color the tarsals red, the metatarsals yellow, and the phalanges blue. Coloring the phalanges blue indicates that what condition may be developing?

____

____

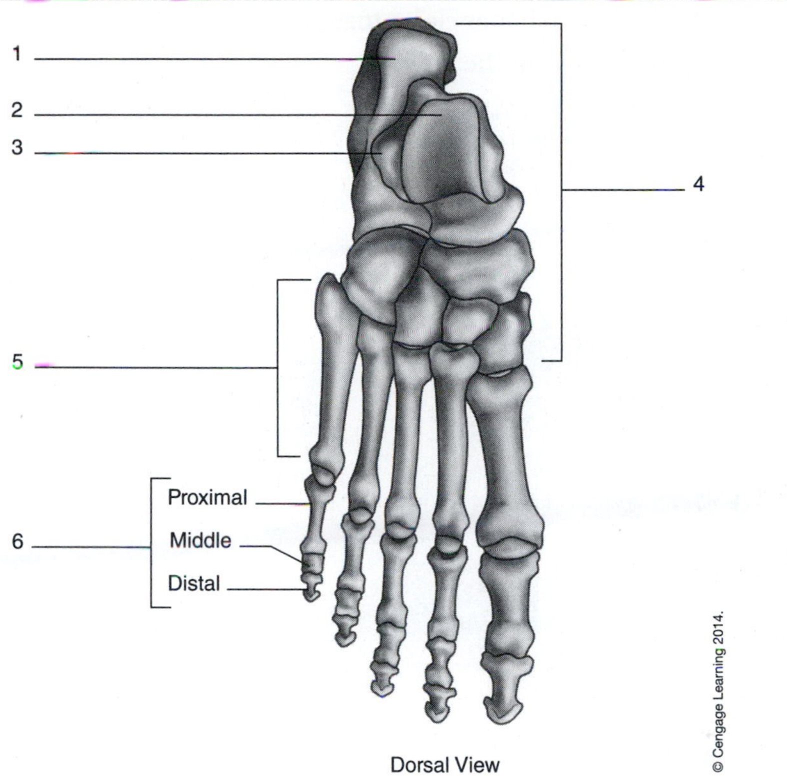

Dorsal View

R. Match the terms in Column B with the statements in Column A regarding joint structure, tendons, and ligaments.

	Column A	Column B
________	1. movable joint	a. amphiarthrosis
________	2. immovable joint	b. synovial membrane
________	3. fibrous band that binds joints	c. disk
________	4. partially movable joint	d. tendon
________	5. lining the articular cartilage	e. diarthrosis
________	6. example of pivot joint	f. suture of the skull
________	7. fibrous cord connects muscle to bone	g. ligament
________	8. elastic material between vertebrae	h. radius and ulna

S. In the following diagram, label the joint movement illustrated and match the letter to the correct statement.

_________ 1. Allows a bone to move around one central axis

_________ 2. Act of increasing the angle of two bones

_________ 3. Movement toward the midline

_________ 4. Act of bringing two bones closer together

_________ 5. Movement away from the midline

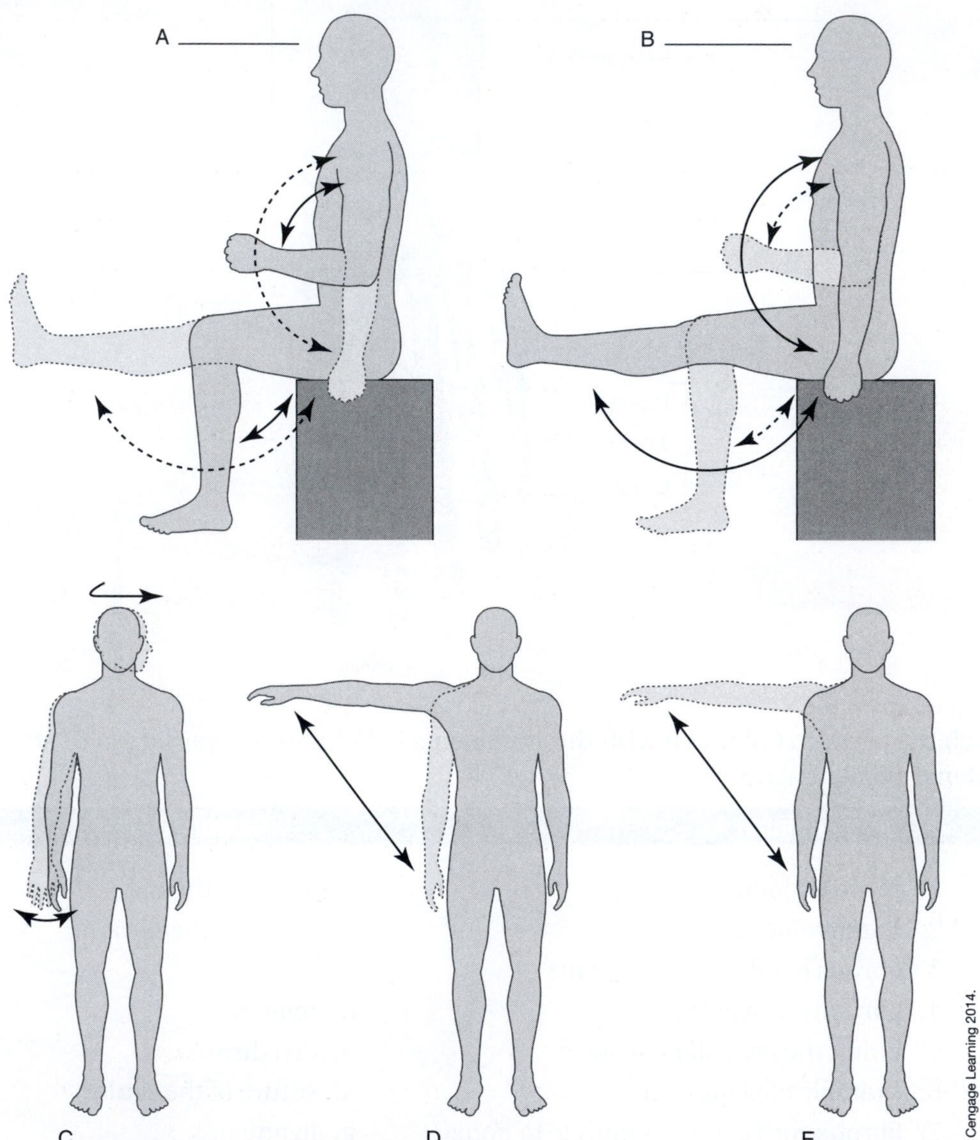

T. Compare the differences between each of the following:

1. Male pelvis and female pelvis

____

____

____

2. Ball-and-socket joint and hinge joint

____

____

____

3. Synarthrosis joint and amphiarthrosis joint

____

____

____

4. Axial skeleton and appendicular skeleton

____

____

____

5. Kyphosis and lordosis

____

____

____

U. Select the letter of the choice that best completes each statement.

1. An inflammation of the clefts in the connective tissue between muscle, tendons, and ligaments is called
   a. arthritis.
   b. bursitis.
   c. osteoarthritis.
   d. rheumatoid arthritis.
2. A fracture in which the bone is partly bent but never penetrates through the skin is called a __________ fracture.
   a. compound
   b. simple
   c. greenstick
   d. comminuted
3. The treatment for a fracture may be closed reduction, which is bringing the bony fragments into alignment by
   a. manipulation.
   b. surgical intervention.
   c. devices such as wires or screws.
   d. a pulling force.

4. A chronic autoimmune disease that affects the joints is
   a. bursitis.
   b. tendinitis.
   c. osteoarthritis.
   d. rheumatoid arthritis.
5. An exaggerated inward curvature of the spine is
   a. scoliosis.
   b. lordosis.
   c. hunchback.
   d. kyphosis.
6. In osteoporosis, the mineral density of the bone is reduced; by age 55, the average woman has lost about ______ of her bone mass.
   a. 20%
   b. 25%
   c. 30%
   d. 35%
7. Rickets, a disease in which bones become soft, is caused by lack of
   a. vitamin A.
   b. vitamin B.
   c. vitamin C.
   d. vitamin D.
8. A traumatic injury to the cervical vertebrae is
   a. whiplash.
   b. gout.
   c. kyphosis.
   d. a herniated lumbar disc.
9. ______________ is an infection of the bone.
   a. Gout
   b. Arthritis
   c. Osteosarcoma
   d. Osteomyelitis
10. An injury to the joint in which the ligaments are torn from the attachments to the bone is called a
    a. dislocation.
    b. sprain.
    c. strain.
    d. fracture.

V. Match the description in Column B with the disorder in Column A.

Column A	Column B
________ 1. hammer toe	a. infection of the bone
________ 2. scoliosis	b. degenerative joint disease
________ 3. kyphosis	c. deformity such as bowlegs
________ 4. osteoporosis	d. toe curls due to a bend in the middle joint
________ 5. gout	e. fallen arches of the feet
________ 6. rickets	f. lateral curvature of the spine
________ 7. osteomyelitis	g. the silent bone disease
________ 8. flatfeet	h. hunchback
________ 9. osteoarthritis	i. joint injury, turning the ankle
________ 10. sprain	j. acute inflammation of the big toe

W. Complete this two-part puzzle.

1. In Column B, write the correct name of the bone or bones from the descriptions in Column A.
2. Use the words from Column B for the word search. When you are finished, the remaining letters in the word search will give you a message.

M E T A C A R P A L S S
U O A M E L E H B O I N
I E I S M U L A S O V F
H T B U H B C L E T L S
C A I I P I I A H A E U
S L T D P F V N U R P E
I E N A D I A G M S A N
C U L R A R L E E A T A
S A L U P A C S R L E C
K N E L E T A L U S L L
T L O F E M U R S N L A
P U B I S S L A P R A C

Column A	Column B
wrist bones	________
fingers	________
collarbone	________
shoulder bone	________
rotates around ulna	________
kneecap	________
heel bone	________
pelvic girdle (3 bones)	________
	________
	________
palms of the hand	________
small lower leg bone	________
broad tarsal bone	________
bone with olecranon process	________
articulates with scapula	________
longest, strongest bone	________
ankle bones	________
shin bone	________
structure is different in males and females	________

APPLYING THEORY TO PRACTICE

1. Kenneth fell off a ladder trying to fix a light fixture and broke one-half of the bones in his left wrist. How many bones would be broken? ___________________

2. When you think about the skeletal system, bones come to mind. Yet there are body systems affected by the skeletal system as well. Name them and their connection to the skeletal system.

   ____

   ____

   ____

   ____

   ____

   ____

   ____

   ____

   ____

   ____

3. The patient comes to the doctor's office with a condition known as athlete's foot. If one-fourth of the toes of both feet show this condition, how many toes are involved?

   ____

4. Riley, age 7, is brought to the emergency room. He fell off his bike, and a piece of bone has broken through the skin of his lower arm. The doctor states that it is what type of fracture? Explain this type of fracture to his parents, along with the process of bone healing.

   ____

   ____

   ____

   ____

5. As people age, they are often affected by some form of arthritis. At a health fair you are asked to do a presentation on the different types of arthritis. Briefly describe the following for each type.

   Types:

   ____

   Symptoms:

   ____

   Treatment:

   ____

   A. Standard

   ____

   ____

B. Alternative

____

____

C. Arthroscopy

____

____

D. Surgical procedures

____

____

6. Employment studies indicate that there will be great career opportunities for physical therapists in the future. What are the duties of a physical therapist? Are there any obstacles to this career path?

____

____

____

____

7. Nadia, a gymnast, fell while practicing on the parallel bars. She seems to have sprained her ankle. As the school athletic trainer, you advise her to use the RICE treatment. She asks you to explain what this treatment is. How would you respond?

____

____

____

____

8. While driving home from work, Rebecca had to brake suddenly to avoid hitting the car in front of her. Rebecca's neck immediately began to hurt. What type of injury did Rebecca sustain? Explain what happens to the skeletal structures in this type of injury.

____

____

9. Michael, age 45, has difficulty in putting on his left shoe because his big toe is swollen and painful. After a visit to the doctor, Michael is diagnosed with gout. Explain to Michael the cause of and treatment for gout.

____

____

____

10. As a health care professional, you are requested to do a presentation on osteoporosis at the local senior center. The presentation should include information on the following:
    a. explanation of the disease, and why it is called the "silent bone disease"

    ____

    ____

b. the cause of osteoporosis

c. the population affected by the disease

d. the test to determine bone density

e. treatment of osteoporosis

SURF THE NET

For additional information and interactive exercises, use the following key words:

- bone formation
- skeletal system, axial and appendicular
- types of joints, joint movement
- fractures, RICE treatment
- diseases of the skeletal system—include causes, symptoms, and treatment for arthritis, osteoporosis, and recreation injuries
- benefits of massage therapy

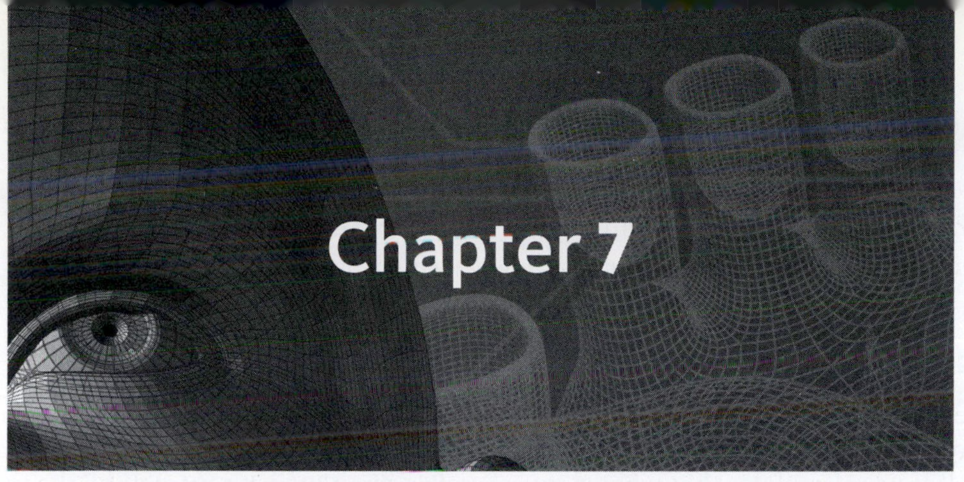

Muscular System

OVERVIEW

Muscles comprise nearly half of our body weight and are responsible for all movement.

FUNCTIONS OF THE MUSCULAR SYSTEM

Functions of the muscular system include:

Being responsible for all body movement
Giving the body form and shape
Producing most of the body's heat

Types of Muscles

Muscle is one of three types:

Skeletal is striped or striated, multinucleated, attached to the bones of the skeleton, and voluntary.
Smooth (visceral) is nonstriated, has one nucleus, and is involuntary.
Cardiac is striated and branched, found only in the heart, and is involuntary.

Characteristics of muscle are contractility, extensibility, elasticity, and irritability. Muscles only pull; they never push.

Muscle Attachments and Functions

Origin is the part of the muscle that is attached to a fixed structure, moving the least during a muscle contraction. *Insertion* means it is attached to the movable part of the bone, moving the most during a muscle contraction.

MUSCLE PAIRS

Muscles are arranged in pairs:

A prime mover creates movement in a single direction—an *antagonist* creates movement in the opposite direction (biceps and triceps).

A flexor flexes or bends a joint—an *extensor* extends or straightens a joint.

A levator raises a body part—a *depressor* lowers a body part.

Contraction of Skeletal Muscle

The sources of energy for muscle contractions are glucose, oxygen, and ATP. Movement occurs as a result of myoneural stimulation and contraction of muscle proteins.

The *all or none law* states that when a muscle cell is stimulated, it contracts all the way.

The Effects of Aging on the Musculoskeletal System

Over time, the muscle system experiences a gradual decrease in the number of muscle fibers, which results in a loss of strength and energy.

Muscle Fatigue

Muscle fatigue is caused by an accumulation of lactic acid, a waste product of muscle metabolism.

Muscle Tone

Muscles are always in a state of slight contraction and ready to pull. The following terms describe muscle tone:

Isotonic contraction—muscles shorten and contract.

Isometric contraction—tension increases; muscle does not shorten.

Atrophy—muscles shrink from disuse.

Hypertrophy—muscle fibers increase in size from overuse.

Principal Skeletal Muscles

Muscles are named by location, size, direction of fibers, number of origins, location of origin and insertion, and action.

Muscles of the Head and Neck

Examples of muscles of the head and neck include the following:

Frontalis—controls facial expressions.

Masseter—controls mastication.

Sternocleidomastoid—moves the head.

Muscles of the Upper Extremities

Examples of muscles of the upper extremities include the following:

Deltoid—moves the shoulder.

Biceps—moves the arm.

Flexor carpi—moves the wrist, hand, and fingers.

Muscles of the Trunk

Examples of muscles of the trunk include the following:

Diaphragm—helps in breathing.
Rectus abdominus—compresses the abdominal cavity.

Muscles of the Lower Extremities

Examples of muscles of the lower extremities include the following:

Gluteus maximus—moves the upper leg.
Sartorius—moves the lower leg.
Tibialis anterior—moves the ankle.
Peroneus longus—moves the ankle, foot, and toes.

See the tables in the textbook for a more complete listing of muscles.

How Exercise and Training Change Muscles

Exercise of muscles will improve the strength and efficiency of muscles and circulation.

Massage Muscles

Massage therapy may provide health benefits as well as offering a form of physiotherapy.

Electrical Stimulation

Electrical stimulation may also be used as part of physical therapy.

Intramuscular Injections

Intramuscular injections may be given in the following sites: deltoid, dorsal gluteal, and vastus lateralis.

Musculoskeletal Disorders

Rehabilitation or therapeutic exercise will help damaged or injured muscles. The following are various types of musculoskeletal disorders:

Muscle atrophy—muscles shrink in size due to insufficient usage.
Muscle strain—a tear in the muscle.
Muscle spasm—a sustained contraction of the muscle.
Myalgia—muscle pain. Fibromyalgia is a collection of symptoms, the most definite of which is chronic muscle pain lasting 3 months or more.
Dystonia—condition characterized by involuntary muscle contraction that causes repetitive movement or abnormal posture; types include tortocollis (wry neck), blepharosm (blinking), and cranio-facial dystonia.
Hernia—organ protrusion through a weak muscle wall; types are abdominal, hiatal, and inguinal.
Heel spur—a calcium deposit in the plantar fascia.
Plantar fascilitis—an inflammation of the plantar fascia causing foot or heel pain when walking or running.

Tetanus (lockjaw) —an infectious disease characterized by continuous spasms of voluntary muscles.

Muscular dystrophy—a group of diseases in which the muscle cells deteriorate.

Myasthenia gravis—progressive muscular weakness and paralysis.

Muscle injuries include the following:

Tennis elbow (lateral epicondylitis)—inflammation of the tendon that connects the arm muscle to the elbow.

Shin splints—injury to the muscle tendon in front of the tibia.

Rotator cuff disease—inflammation of the group of tendons surrounding the shoulder joint.

ACTIVITIES

A. Label the diagrams of the muscle tissue. List three structural features of each type of muscle tissue and the location in the body where each type is found.

1. Name of tissue: ______________________________

____

Features: ______________________________

____

____

____

Location: ______________________________

____

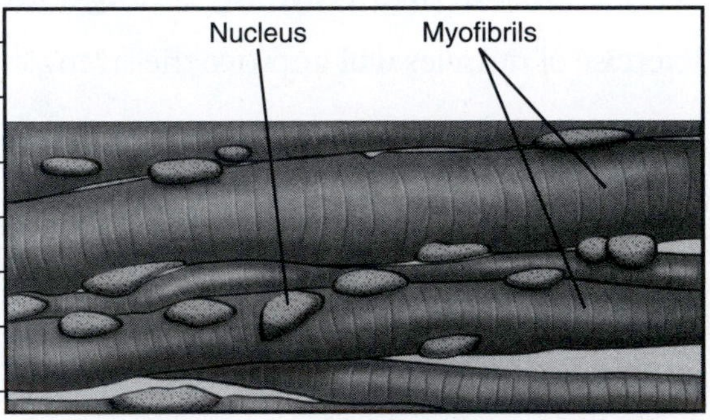

© Cengage Learning 2014.

2. Name of tissue: ______________________________

____

Features: ______________________________

____

____

____

Location: ______________________________

____

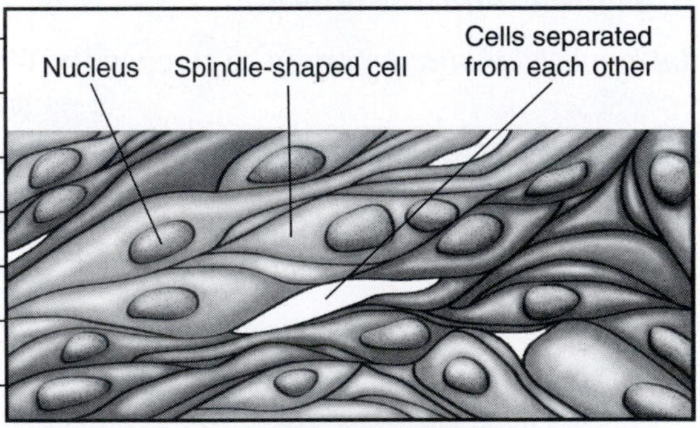

© Cengage Learning 2014.

3. Name of tissue: ______________________________

____

Features: ______________________________

____

____

____

Location: ______________________________

____

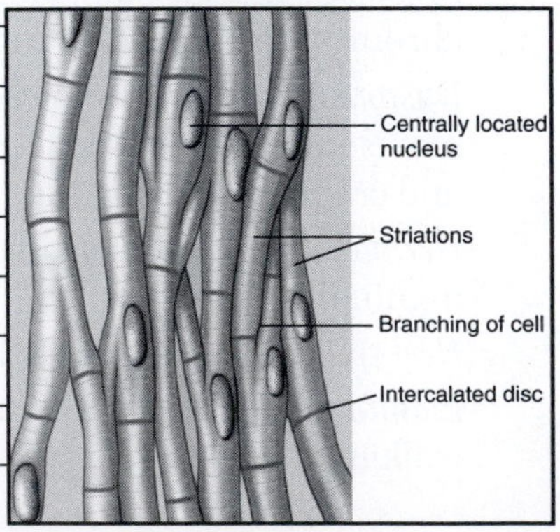

© Cengage Learning 2014.

B. Name the four common characteristics of the muscle cells.

____

____

____

C. Place the correct word or words next to the following statements; make a selection from the list provided.

antagonist	elasticity	insertion	smooth muscle
cardiac muscle	excitability	origin	synergist
contractility	extensibility	prime mover	tendons
dilator	fasciae	skeletal muscle	

1. A characteristic shared with nerve cells; the ability to respond to a stimulus. ____________
2. This structure contains membranes fused at places called intercalated disks; a communication system at the fused area will not permit the cells to act independently. ____________
3. The ability of a muscle to return to its original length after stretching. ____________
4. The ability of muscles to be stretched. ____________
5. Muscles only pull and never push; they are attached to the bones of the skeleton by nonelastic cords. ____________
6. The part of the muscle attached to a fixed point on the bones; the least movable part during a contraction. ____________
7. This muscle has the ability to cause the diameter of blood vessels to decrease on contraction. ____________
8. Muscles that open and close to control the passage of substances. ____________
9. The ability of the muscle to shorten, which reduces the distance between the parts of its contents. ____________
10. The part of the muscle attached to the movable part of the bone; it is the most movable during a contraction. ____________

D. Using the following words, complete the story about the steps in muscle contraction. Words may be used more than once.

action potential	fatigue	motor	positive
adenosine triphosphate	glucose	neurotransmitter	sarcolemma
ATP	lactic acid	original	sodium
contraction	length	pain	synaptic cleft
cramps			

For muscles to work, they need a stimulus from a ________________ nerve and a source of energy that is ________________ ________________, also known as ________________. The muscle cell also requires oxygen and ________________.

Between the nerve cell's fiber, the axon, and the muscle cell is a neuromuscular junction called the ________________ ________________. When the nerve impulse reaches the end of the axon, it releases a chemical called ________________. This chemical diffuses across the junction and attaches to the cell membrane, the ________________. This action makes the membrane temporarily permeable to ________________. The muscle cell now has excessive _positive ions, which upsets the electrical condition; this electrical upset causes a(n) ________________ ________________.

Skeletal muscle contraction begins with the action potential that travels along the ________________ of the muscle fiber, from one end of the cell to the other. This energy source results in the ________________ of the muscle cells.

When the action potential is ended, the muscle cell relaxes and returns to its ________________ length.

Lactic acid is a product of muscle contraction that is changed back to ________________ and other substances with the help of oxygen. Sometimes when there is too much muscle activity and not enough of an oxygen supply (anaerobic), a buildup of ________________ ________________ will occur in the blood. This condition results in muscle ________________ and ________________. A person needs to stop, rest, and take in enough oxygen to complete the catabolism of lactic acid and relieve the muscle ________________.

E. Make the following statements about muscle tone accurate by circling the correct word.

1. Muscles are (always, sometimes, never) in a state of partial contraction.
2. In an isometric contraction, the tension in a muscle (decreases, increases, stays the same), and the muscle (does, does not) shorten.
3. In an isotonic muscle contraction, the muscle (does, does not) shorten.
4. When muscles are flaccid, they are (weak, strong).
5. In atrophy, the muscle (increases, decreases) in size from disuse.
6. In hypertrophy, the size of the muscle (shrinks, enlarges).

F. Muscles are named by location, size, number of origins, location of origins and insertions, and action. Match the muscles in Column A with the clues given in Column B.

Column A	Column B
________ 1. frontalis	a. action flexor
________ 2. gluteus maximus	b. direction of fibers
________ 3. triceps brachii	c. raises the body
________ 4. sternocleidomastoid	d. location
________ 5. flexor carpi ulnaris	e. number of heads of origin
	f. location of origin and insertion
	g. size or shape

G. Label the following two diagrams of the principal skeletal muscles, both anterior and posterior views. Color muscles that are massaged in massage therapy brown.

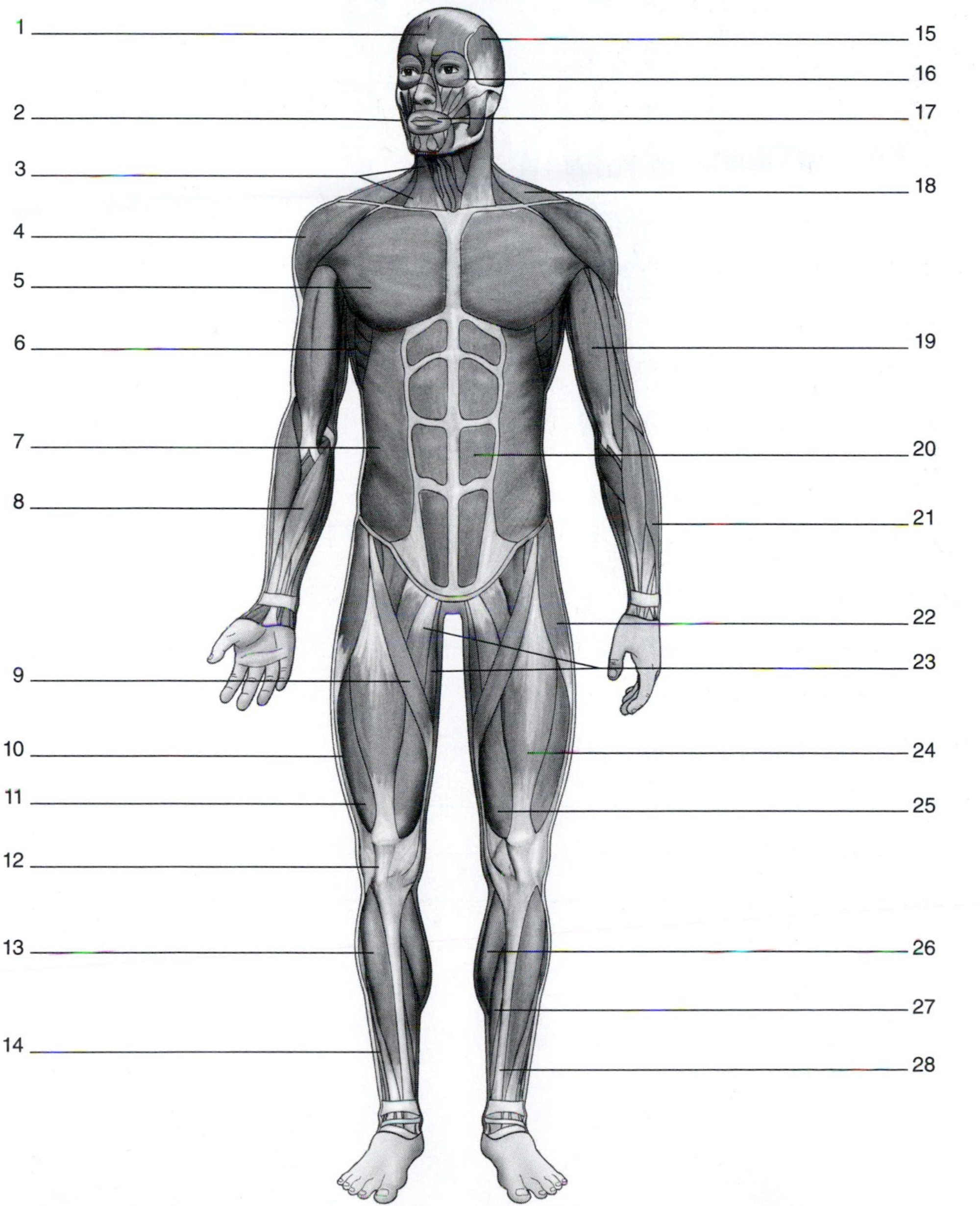

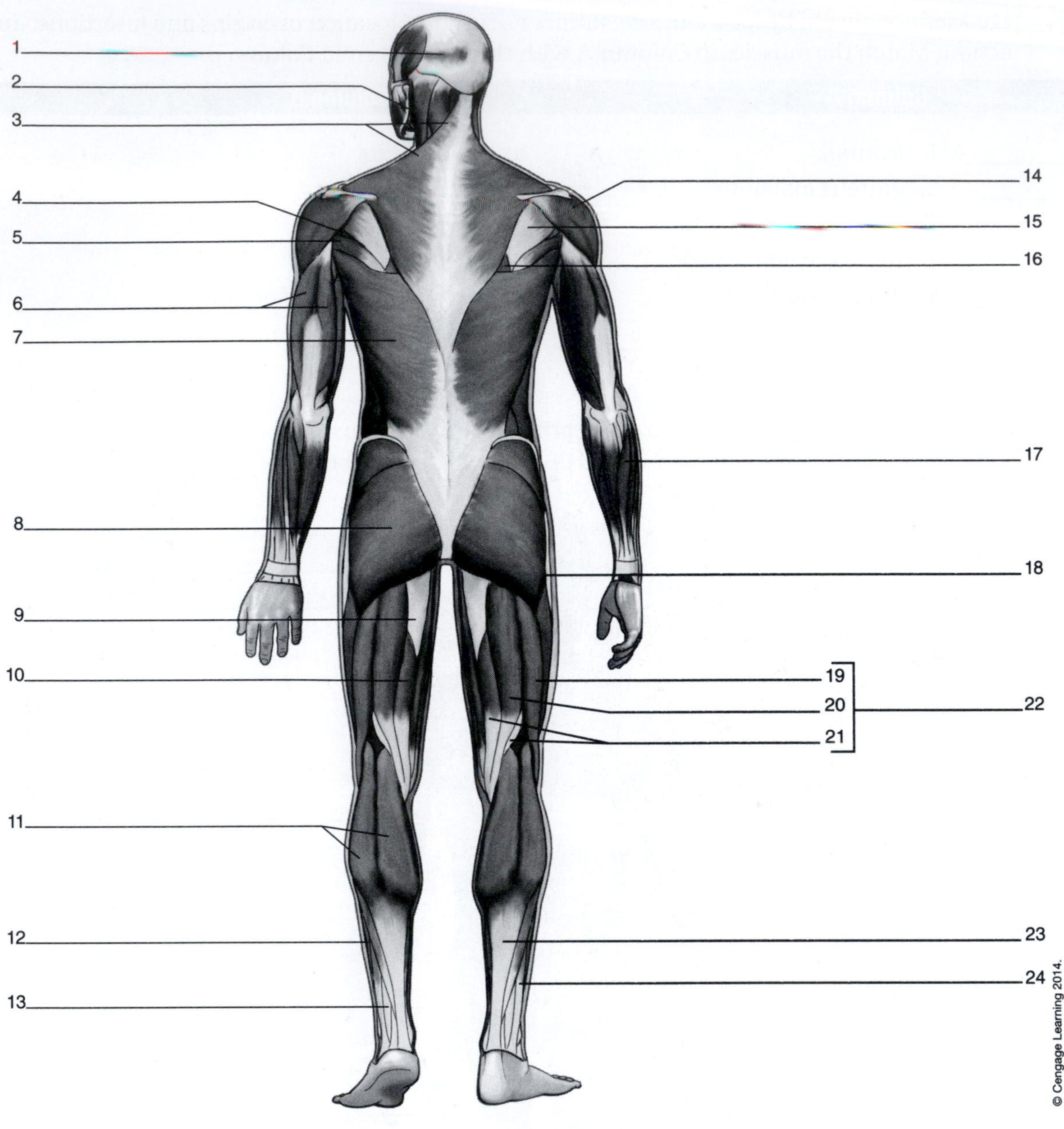

H. List the factors that affect a muscle contraction.

I. Label the muscles of the head and neck. Color all muscles named for location red.

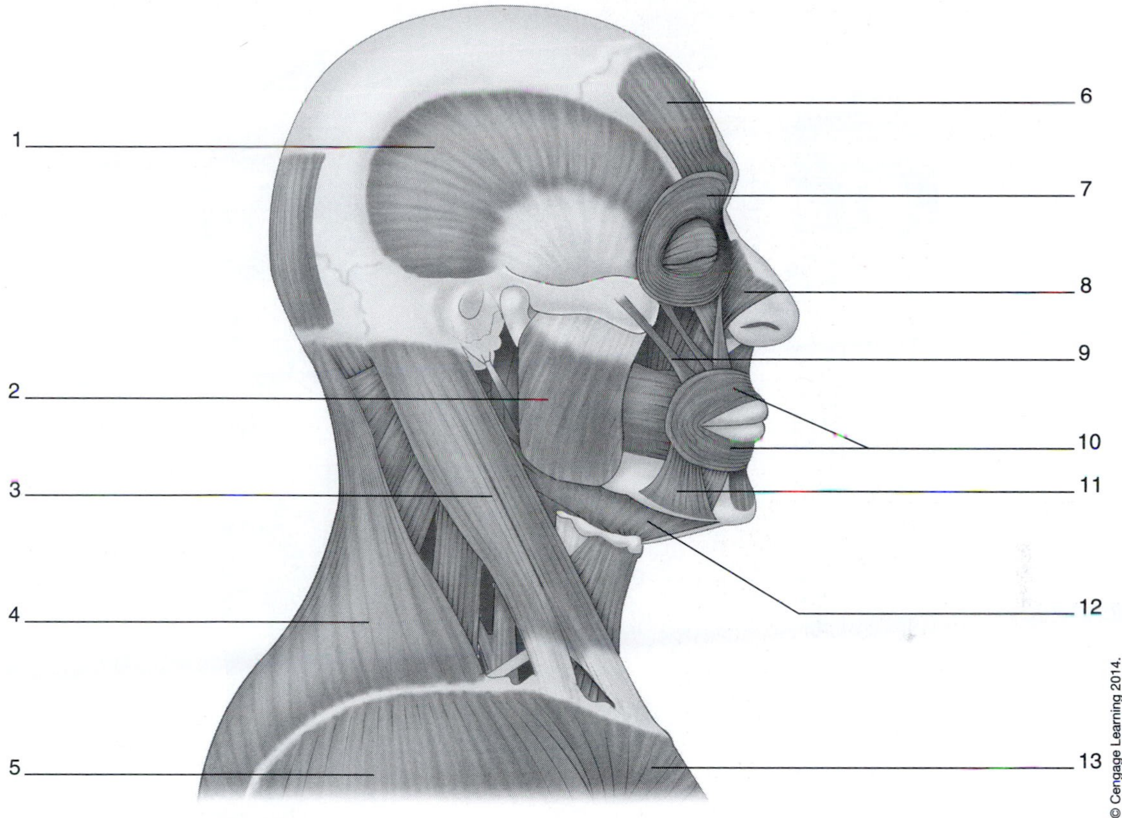

J. Answer the following riddles by naming the muscle.

WHO AM I?

1. I sit over the eyebrows and wait and see if you have a surprise in store for me. ____________________
2. The movie picture gave me a fright I responded with horror to the sight. ____________________
3. A smiling face is where to begin then I can help you laugh and grin. ____________________
4. I protect a delicate structure and faster than a wink, if anything comes near it I quickly blink. ____________________
5. This muscle structure opens wide, so food and drink can get inside. ____________________

K. Label the following diagram and complete the table.

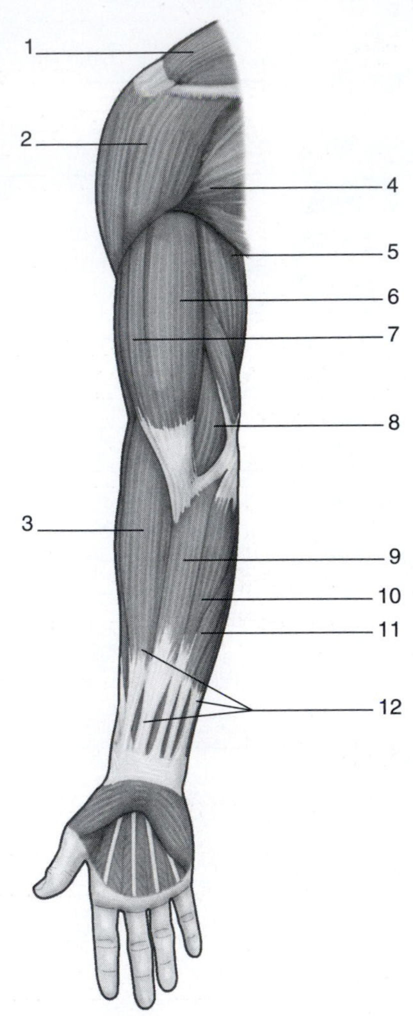

Anterior view

13
14
15
16
17
18
19
20
21
22

Posterior view

1. ____________________
2. ____________________
3. ____________________
4. ____________________
5. ____________________
6. ____________________
7. ____________________
8. ____________________
9. ____________________
10. ____________________
11. ____________________
12. ____________________
13. ____________________
14. ____________________
15. ____________________
16. ____________________
17. ____________________
18. ____________________
19. ____________________
20. ____________________
21. ____________________
22. ____________________

Representative Muscles of the Upper Extremities

MUSCLE	LOCATION	FUNCTION
Trapezius	A large triangular muscle located on the upper surface of the back	______ ______
Deltoid	______ ______	Abducts the upper arm
Pectoralis major	Anterior part of the chest	______ ______
______	Anterior chest	Moves scapula forward and helps to raise the arm
Biceps brachii	Upper arm to radius	______
Triceps brachii	______	Extends the lower arm
______ ______	Extends from the anterior and posterior forearm to the hand	Moves the hand
Extensor and flexor digitorium	______ ______	

L. Doing sit-ups can help get the abdomen into shape. Do a sit-up, and feel the muscles tighten. Label the following diagram with the muscles of the trunk.

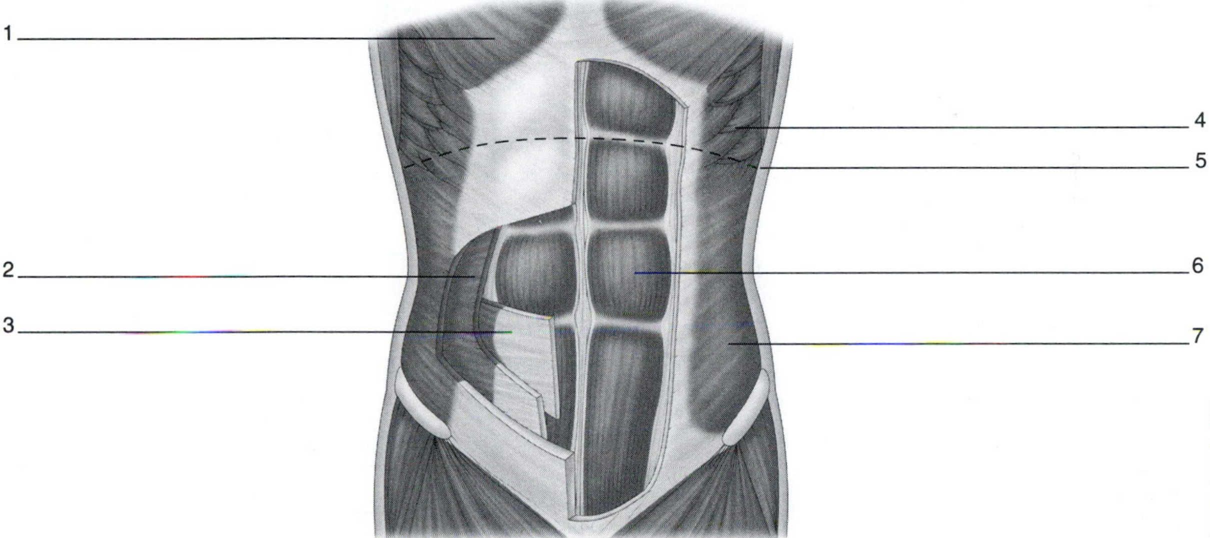

M. Mark each statement as either true or false. Correct the false statements.

______ 1. The diaphragm is a dome-shaped muscle that separates the thoracic and pelvic cavities.

______ 2. The intercostals are found between the ribs and help us breathe.

______ 3. The external oblique flexes the spinal column and compresses the abdominal cavity.

______ 4. The rectus abdominus is used when doing sit-ups. It compresses the abdomen.

______ 5. The internal oblique extends the spinal column and compresses the abdomen.

N. Label the following muscles of the lower extremity view.

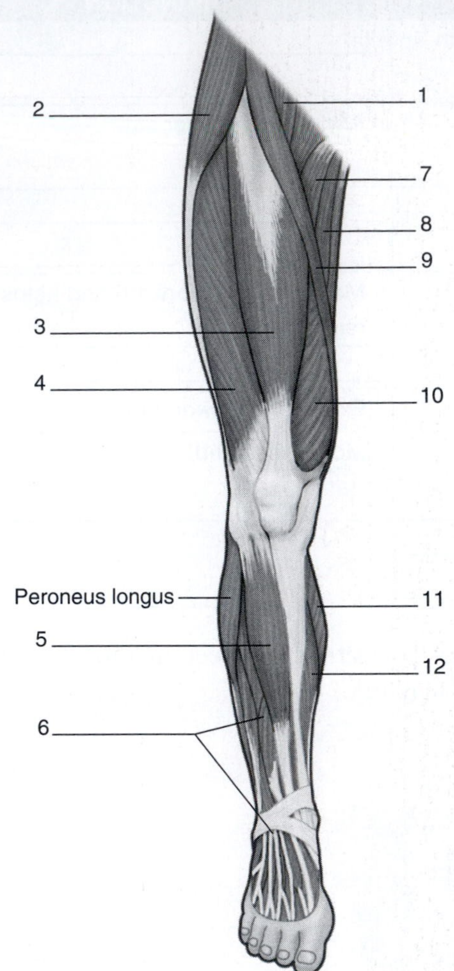

Anterior view

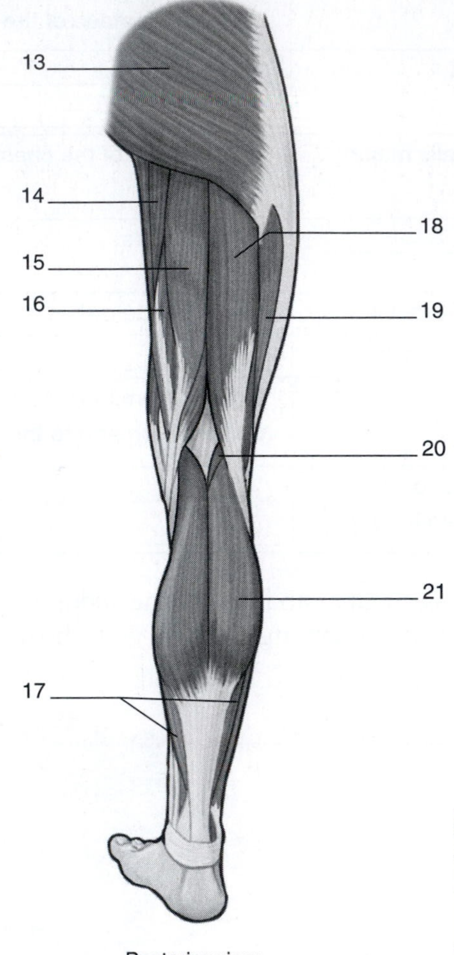

Posterior view

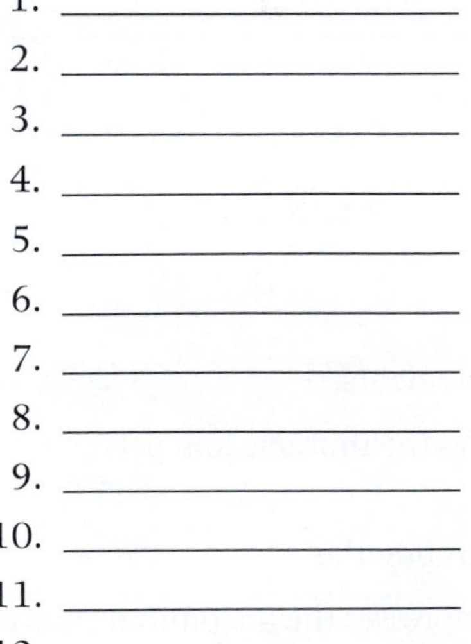

1. ____________________
2. ____________________
3. ____________________
4. ____________________
5. ____________________
6. ____________________
7. ____________________
8. ____________________
9. ____________________
10. ____________________
11. ____________________
12. ____________________
13. ____________________
14. ____________________
15. ____________________
16. ____________________
17. ____________________
18. ____________________
19. ____________________
20. ____________________
21. ____________________

O. Match the muscle function in Column B with the correct lower extremity in Column A.

Column A	Column B
_______ 1. gluteus maximus	a. extends the foot
_______ 2. gluteus medius	b. dorsiflexes the foot
_______ 3. tensor fasciae	c. supports the arches
_______ 4. rectus femoris	d. extends the femur
_______ 5. sartorius	e. abducts and rotates the thigh
_______ 6. tibialis anterior	f. extends the lower leg
_______ 7. gastrocnemius	g. flexes and rotates the thigh and leg
_______ 8. soleus	h. medially rotates the thigh
_______ 9. peroneus	i. points toe and flexes the lower leg

P. Select the letter of the choice that best completes each statement.

1. If you weigh 160 pounds, about how much weight is muscle?
   a. 60 pounds
   b. 70 pounds
   c. 80 pounds
   d. 90 pounds
2. Intercalated disks are found on the ______ muscle.
   a. striated
   b. nonstriated voluntary
   c. nonstriated involuntary
   d. cardiac
3. The characteristic of a muscle to be stretched is known as
   a. contractility.
   b. extensibility.
   c. elasticity.
   d. excitability.
4. Muscles that produce movement in a single direction are
   a. prime movers.
   b. antagonists.
   c. synergists.
   d. obliques.
5. A motor unit is a motor neuron (nerve cell) plus ________ of the muscle fibers it stimulates.
   a. one-half
   b. one-third
   c. three-fourths
   d. all

6. During a muscle contraction, the muscle cell membrane becomes temporarily permeable to
   a. acetylcholine.
   b. sodium.
   c. ATP.
   d. calcium.
7. Muscles are named in a variety of ways; the muscles on the sides of the head are named according to their
   a. size.
   b. location.
   c. action.
   d. location of origin.
8. The muscles that make up the hamstrings are the
   a. semitendinosus, biceps femoris, and semimembranous.
   b. gluteus maximus, semitendinosus, and biceps femoris.
   c. semitendinosus, gracilis, and semimembranous.
   d. semitendinosus, biceps femoris, and adductor magnus.
9. A single muscle contraction is called a(n)
   a. twitch.
   b. spasm.
   c. contraction.
   d. all or none law.
10. A __________ is a tear in the muscle.
   a. strain
   b. sprain
   c. spasm
   d. fracture

Q. List at least three effects of training on muscle efficiency.

____

____

____

R. Name the major muscle that would probably be worked in massage therapy for the following areas:

1. upper back ______________________________
2. lower back ______________________________
3. shoulder ______________________________
4. forearm ______________________________
5. chest ______________________________

6. buttock ______
7. anterior thigh ______
8. posterior thigh ______
9. lateral and proximal thigh ______
10. posterior leg ______
11. medial thigh ______
12. lateral leg ______

S. List one way to prevent each of the following conditions:

1. excess body fat ______
2. tetanus ______
3. muscle atrophy ______
4. shin splints ______
5. flaccid muscles ______

T. Describe a treatment for each of the following conditions:

1. insomnia ______
2. fibromyalgia ______
3. tennis elbow ______
4. tortocollis ______
5. rotator cuff injury ______
6. muscle fatigue ______

U. Circle the correctly spelled word in each of the following statements.

1. Chiropractors' approach to health care is (holistic, wholistic).
2. The term used to describe muscle pain is (mylagia, myalgia).
3. Plantar fascilitis is an (inflammation, inflamation) of the plantar fascia on the (sole, soul) of the foot.
4. A hiatal hernia occurs when the stomach is pushed through the (diaphram, diaphragm).
5. Tetanus is an (infectious, infectous) disease characterized by continuous spasms of (voluntery, voluntary) muscle.
6. Muscular (dystrophy, distrophy) is a group of diseases in which the muscle cells deteriorate.

7. Lateral epicondylitis, also referred to as tennis elbow, occurs at the bony (prominince, prominence) on the sides of the elbow.
8. Progressive muscular weakness and (paralysis, paralyses) are symptoms of myasthenia gravis.
9. Rapid blinking of the eyes is a type of (distonia, dystonia).
10. The most common (compliant, complaint) in rotator cuff injury is an (aching, acking) in the top and front of the shoulder.

V. Match the muscle system interactions in Column A with the correct body system in Column B.

Column A	Column B
________ 1. intercostal muscles assist breathing	a. integumentary
________ 2. skeletal muscle creates pressure on the vessels to return fluid to heart	b. skeletal
________ 3. moves eggs from ovary to oviduct	c. nervous
________ 4. muscles that show emotion	d. endocrine
________ 5. moves blood into capillaries	e. circulatory
________ 6. aid in control of body temperature	f. lymphatic
________ 7. responsible for taking in and chewing food	g. respiratory
________ 8. stores calcium necessary for muscle contraction	h. digestive
________ 9. growth hormone that affects skeletal growth	i. urinary
________ 10. forms voluntary sphincter to eliminate waste products	j. reproductive

APPLYING THEORY TO PRACTICE

1. In your own words, describe what happens during a skeletal muscle contraction. How fast does it occur?

____

____

____

____

2. If you want to get into shape, try this exercise routine. Stretch your arms up over your head. What muscles are you using?

____

For the buttocks and thighs, bring your right leg up and stretch it way out. Now do the same with the left leg. What group of muscles are you using?

____

To get physically fit you must exercise every day. Take the stairs, climb a hill, or walk a mile or two.

3. a. As a massage therapist, how would you explain the benefits of massage?

b. The following terms are used in the practice of massage: Swedish massage, deep tissue, effleurage, reflexology, acupressure, shiatsu, sports massage. Explain each term.

4. Mr. Che has been a house painter for over 30 years. He visits his doctor because of the constant pain he gets when he raises his right arm over his head.
   a. What diagnosis do you think the doctor will make?

   b. What is the cause of this condition?

   c. How is this condition treated?

5. Alycia is going to participate in a telethon on Labor Day. To prepare for this she must know the following information to answer the questions of people calling in:
   - What is muscular dystrophy?
   - What is the cause of this disease?

- What is the treatment for this disease?

___

___

___

- What is the prognosis?

___

___

6. Letisha plays tennis at least twice a week. Lately she has been experiencing pain in her right elbow. The doctor diagnoses the condition as tennis elbow. Describe what occurs in this condition. Name other activities that may cause tennis elbow. What treatment will the doctor prescribe for Letisha?

___

___

___

7. Eli is an active 70-year-old who exercises at least 2 hours each day. He relates to his chiropractor that lately he seems to get tired after exercise and has less energy. As the chiropractor, explain to Eli what changes are occurring in the muscle system as he gets older.

___

___

___

8. Kieran enjoys sports. A career that seems appealing to him is in sports medicine. On Career Day, he plans to give a presentation on sports medicine/athletic training. What information should he include in the presentation?

___

___

___

___

SURF THE NET

For additional information and interactive exercises, use the following key words:

- types of muscle
- muscle contractions and nervous system
- skeletal muscles
- diseases and conditions of the muscle system—strain, sprain, hernia, myasthenia gravis, muscular dystrophy, and recreation injuries
- benefits of exercise
- benefits of massage

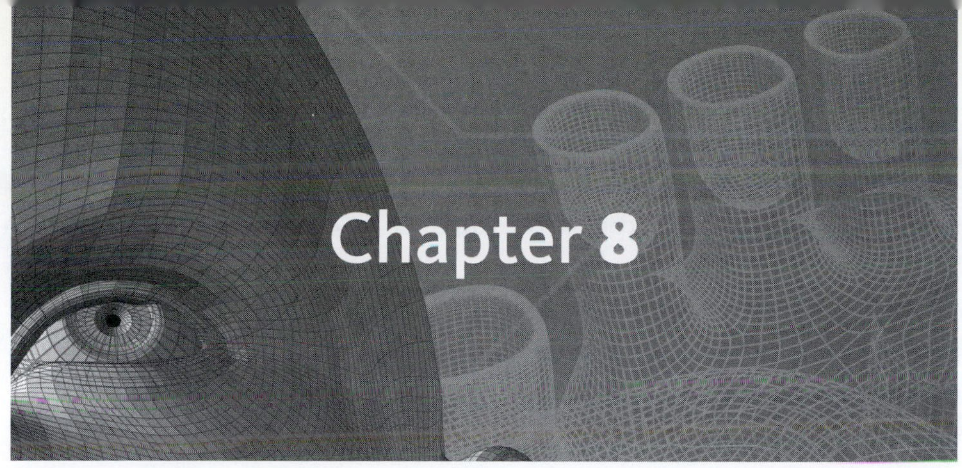

Central Nervous System

OVERVIEW

The **central nervous system** consists of the brain, spinal cord, and nerves; its chief function is to coordinate and integrate body activities. The brain is the seat of intellect and reasoning.

Divisions of the Nervous System

The nervous system is divided into three parts:

Central: brain and spinal cord

Peripheral: cranial and spinal nerves

Autonomic: peripheral nerves and ganglia, sympathetic and parasympathetic division

Neuron. The structural and functional unit of the nervous system, the neuron has extensions of its cytoplasm called processes or fibers. These fibers are *dendrites*, which carry messages to the cell body, and *axons*, which carry messages away from the cell body.

Axons are covered with a *myelin sheath* called *neurilemma.* The myelin sheath speeds up an impulse as it travels along the axon; it also produces myelin, which protects the axon.

Neuroglia. Another type of nerve cell that insulates, supports, and protects the neuron is the neuroglia.

Characteristics of the Neuron

Irritability is the ability to react when stimulated.

Conductivity is the ability to transmit a stimulus to another point.

Types of Neurons

Sensory or *afferent* neurons carry impulses to the spinal cord and brain.

Motor or *efferent* neurons carry impulses away from the brain and spinal cord to muscles and glands.

Associate, connecting, or *internuncial* neurons carry impulses from one neuron to another.

Function of a Nerve Cell. A nerve cell carries impulses by creating electric charges in a process known as *membrane excitability*.

Normal resting potential is negative inside the cell, positive outside the cell.
Depolarization is positive inside the cell, negative outside the cell.
Repolarization is negative inside, positive outside.

Refer to the textbook for further information on membrane excitability.

Synapse

A message or impulse going from the axon of one cell to the dendrite of the next cell is called a synapse. The space between is referred to as the *synaptic cleft*. The axon releases a neurotransmitter and the message jumps across the synaptic cleft from one cell to the next.

Effects of Aging on the Nervous System

There is a general slowing of nerve conduction due to a decrease in the number of functioning neurons along with the degeneration of existing nerves.

The Brain

The **brain** is in the cranial cavity and is protected by the skull and meninges. It is divided into white and gray matter. The **meninges** are the three membranous coverings of the brain and spinal cord:

Dura mater—outer covering of brain and spinal cord
Arachnoid—middle layer
Pia mater—inner covering of the brain and spinal cavity

The **ventricles** of the brain are four lined cavities within the brain that contain the choroid plexus, a rich network of blood vessels that help form the cerebrospinal fluid.

The **cerebrospinal fluid** acts as a shock absorber and a source of nutrients for the brain and spinal cord. A diagnostic test of the cerebrospinal fluid is called *lumbar puncture*.

Parts of the Brain. The **cerebrum** is the largest and highest part of the brain; it is a layer of gray matter that covers the upper and lower surfaces and is divided into two hemispheres. Each hemisphere is divided into frontal, parietal, occipital, temporal and limbic lobes, (the limbic lobe may be referred to as limbic system)

The functions of the **cerebral lobe** are as follows:

The *frontal lobe* is the motor area that controls voluntary muscles; the right hemisphere controls the left side of the body, and the left hemisphere controls the right side of the body. The speech area is located in the left hemisphere.
The *parietal lobe* is the sensory area that receives and interprets messages from the pain, touch, heat, and cold receptors and helps in determining distances, sizes, and shapes.
The *occipital lobe* is the visual area controlling eyesight.
The *temporal lobe* holds the auditory and olfactory areas.
The *limbic lobe* influences instinctive behaviors that relate to survival.

The **diencephalon** is located between the cerebrum and midbrain parts.
The **thalamus** is a relay station for incoming and outgoing nerve impulses.

The **hypothalamus** is the "brain" of the brain, and performs autonomic nervous system control. It is part of the limbic system (emotional control) and stimulates the pituitary to secrete hormones.

The **cerebellum** is located between the cerebrum and behind the pons; it coordinates skeletal muscle activity.

The **brainstem** is made up of the pons, midbrain, and medulla.

The **pons** is a two-way conductive pathway for nerve impulses between the cerebrum, cerebellum, and other areas; it is the center for respiratory control.

The **midbrain** contains the nuclei for the reflex center, which involves vision and hearing.

The **medulla** is the passageway between the brain and spinal cord; it contains the nuclei for vital functions, including heart rate and rate and depth of respiration. The medulla is the center for swallowing and vomiting and a vasoconstrictor for blood pressure regulation.

The Spinal Cord

The **spinal cord** begins at the foramen magnum and continues to the second lumbar vertebra. It functions as a reflex center and conductive pathway to and from the brain. It is made up of 31 segments, each one giving rise to a pair of spinal nerves.

Disorders of the Central Nervous System

Meningitis is inflammation of the lining of the brain and spinal cord.

Encephalitis is inflammation of the brain.

Epilepsy is a seizure disorder of the brain; seizures may be grand mal or petit mal.

Cerebral palsy is a disturbance in voluntary muscular activity caused by brain damage; its main characteristic is spastic paralysis.

Poliomyelitis is rarely seen in the United States; it is a disease of nerve pathways that causes paralysis.

Hydrocephalus is an increased volume of cerebrospinal fluid in the ventricles of the brain.

Parkinson's disease shows symptoms of shuffling gait and trembling; it may be caused by a decrease of the neurotransmitter dopamine.

Multiple sclerosis is when the myelin sheath around the axon is destroyed, slowing the nerve impulses; a loss of muscle coordination occurs.

Essential tremors is a nerve disorder causing tremors in a person who is moving or trying to move.

West Nile Virus is a mosquito-borne virus that may cause encephalitis or meningitis in the elderly.

Alzheimer's disease is a progressive disease of mental deterioration that occurs in three stages.

Brain tumors may develop in any area of the brain.

Central nervous system injuries include the following:

A *hematoma* is a localized mass of blood collection; it may occur in the spaces between the meninges.

A *concussion* is the result of a severe blow to the head; types are coup and contrecoup injury.

Spinal cord injury occurs when the spinal cord is injured at any level. The site and type of injury determines if paralysis will occur.

ACTIVITIES

A. Answer the following questions.

1. List the major functions of the central nervous system.

____

____

____

____

2. Compare the roles of the nervous system and the endocrine system in coordinating and integrating body activities.

____

____

____

____

B. Perform the following activities regarding the neuron.

1. Label the following diagram of a neuron.

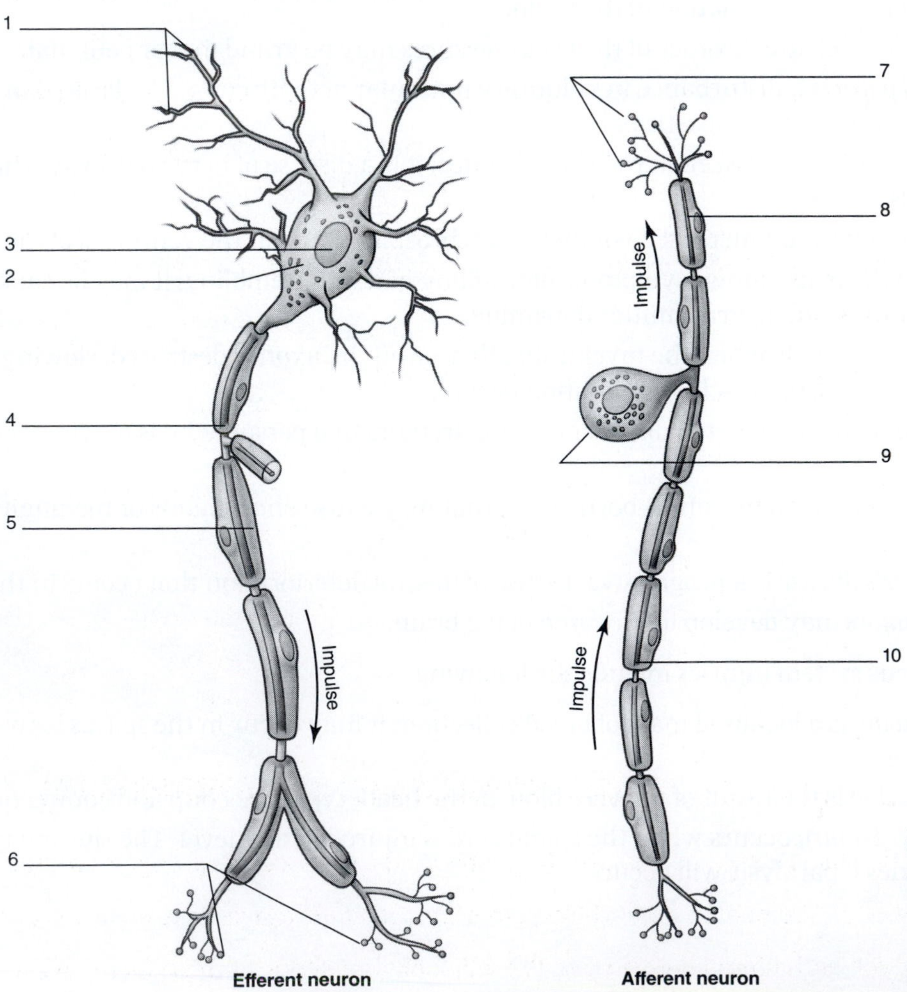

2. What are the roles of the axon and dendrite?

____

____

C. Circle the correct word or words in each of the following statements.

1. (Associative neurons, Efferent neurons) carry impulses from the sensory neurons to the motor neurons.
2. The extension of the neuron that carries the messages away from the nerve cell body is the (axon, dendrite).
3. The type of nervous tissue that insulates and supports the nerve is called "nerve glue" or (neuroglia, neuron).
4. (Conductivity, Irritability) is the ability of a neuron to react to stimuli.
5. Neurons that carry messages to the brain and spinal cord are (afferent, efferent) neurons.
6. A fatty substance called (neurogoglia, myelin sheath) protects the axon.
7. The extensions of the neuron that take messages to the cell body are called (axons, dendrites).
8. The two main communication systems of the body are the nervous system and the (endocrine, circulatory) system.
9. The myelin sheath (speeds up, slows down) an impulse as it travels along the axon.
10. Neurons that carry messages from the brain and spinal cord are called motor or (afferent, efferent) neurons.

D. Using the following words and symbols, complete the story on nerve functions.

action potential	ions	polarized
adjacent	K^+	positive
channels	large	potassium
cytoplasm	lower	receptors
depolarize	minute	repolarization
electrical	Na^+	restores
excitability	negative	reversed
extracellular	open	sodium-potassium
gated	opposite	small
higher	outside	stimuli

A STORY OF HOW A NERVE CELL FUNCTIONS (NERVES-R-US)

In our day-to-day lives we do not stop to think about all the processes going on in that magnificent machine, the body. The heart pumps, blood circulates, and air moves in and out. We jog, talk, reason, and carry out activities of daily living. We will look at just one of these incredible functions.

To understand how impulses (________________) are carried along nerves, we need to know about membrane ________________. Think of the nerve cell membrane as an envelope around the ________________ with lots of openings or ________________. Some of these channels are open and allow ________________ to move (leak) back and forth inside and ________________ during cell activity. Some of these openings are closed and ________________ only on special occasions. These closed channels are called ________________. Another special channel is called the sodium-potassium pump. It maintains the flow of ions from areas of ________________ concentration to ________________ concentration and serves to restore the cytoplasm and the ________________ fluid to their original states. You may think you have a lot to worry about, but think about the special channel. We have leaky ones that allow ions to flow in and out; we have gated channels that are open only on special occasions, and we have the sodium-potassium pump.

When the nerve cell is just hanging out, resting, the ions of ________________ (potassium) and ________________ (sodium) are where they are supposed to be. Inside the nerve cell are ________________ amounts of K^+ and ________________ amounts of Na^+. The ________________ is true in the extracellular fluid, which has more Na^+ ions than K^+ ions.

During this time, some K^+ cells sneak out through the membrane, which then makes the inside of the nerve cell more ________________. Now we have a situation where the environment inside of the cell is more negative than the environment outside of the cell. This state of affairs is called resting membrane potential, and the membrane is said to be ________________.

This is where the fun begins! A sensory receptor picks up a message, a stimulus such as a sound, and the stimulus energy is converted to a(n) ________________ signal. If it is strong enough, it will ________________ a portion of the cell membrane. This is the special occasion that causes those gated channels to open, initiating the ________________ ________________. The sodium ions in the extracellular fluid line up and march through the gated channel into the cytoplasm. Now the inside of the cell is more ________________. The membrane potential is reversed, and the gates close to additional sodium ions.

Well, just wait a minute. There are too many ions here, so the special potassium gates open and large amounts of potassium leave the cytoplasm of the cell, which results in the ________________ of the membrane. To restore order to this mess, the ________________-________________ pump gets into the act and ________________ the original concentrations of sodium and potassium ions. A simpler way of saying all this is that upon stimulation, a nerve cell goes from resting potential to depolarization and then to repolarization and back to resting potential.

Although this action occurs in just one part of the cell membrane, it spreads to ________________ membrane regions, continuing away from the original site of the stimulation, and sending messages over the nerves. Your nervous system is an electrical conduction system; sometimes we use such phrases as "sparks are flying." This could really be true. It is hard to imagine that this cycle is completed millions of times in a minute.

E. In the following statements, circle the item that makes each statement correct.

1. A nerve cell has (one, two, three) axon(s).
2. Dendrites carry messages (from, to) the cell body.
3. A (synapse, synaptic) cleft is the area where messages go from the axon of one cell to the dendrite of another.
4. An impulse travels along a (dendrite, axon) to the end where the neurotransmitter is released.
5. The neurotransmitter between muscle cells and nerve cells is (epinephrine, acetylcholine).

F. Match the words in Column A with the related items in Column B.

	Column A	Column B
________	1. central nervous system	a. ganglia and peripheral nerves
________	2. peripheral nervous system	b. 12 pairs
________	3. autonomic nervous system	c. cranial and spinal nerves
________	4. cranial nerves	d. 31 pairs
________	5. spinal nerves	e. brain and spinal cord

G. Label the parts of the brain in the following diagram.

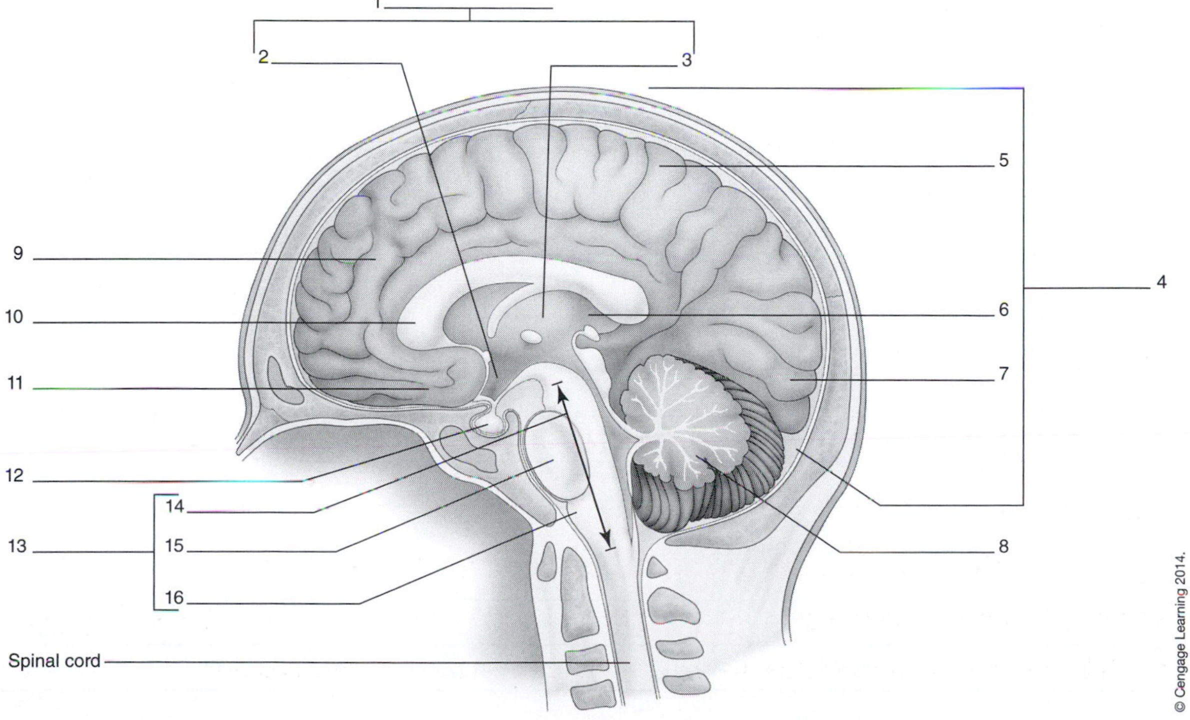

H. Describe in detail each of the three meninges, including their roles.

I. a. Describe how cerebrospinal fluid is formed.

b. What is the function of cerebrospinal fluid?

c. Describe the pathway of cerebrospinal fluid.

J. Answer the following questions.

1. Describe the role of the choroid plexus in the blood–brain barrier.

2. What is the result of an inflammation of the cranial meninges?

3. What is a lumbar puncture? What is the purpose of a lumbar puncture?

K. Compare the difference between each of the following.

1. sulci and gyri

2. cerebral parietal lobe and occipital lobe

3. hippocampus and parahippocampus

____

____

____

4. thalamus and hypothalamus

____

____

____

5. pons and medulla

____

____

____

L. Match the descriptions in Column B with the terms in Column A.

	Column A	Column B
________	1. peripheral nervous system	a. network of blood vessels of the pia mater
________	2. limbic system	b. convolution of the cerebrum
________	3. longitudinal fissure	c. cavities filled with cerebrospinal fluid
________	4. dura mater	d. cranial and spinal nerves
________	5. corpus callosum	e. conscious thought and responses
________	6. choroid plexus	f. inner lining of the brain
________	7. gyri	g. unconscious thought
________	8. cerebral ventricles	h. thalamus and hypothalamus
________	9. diencephalon	i. outer covering of the brain
________	10. cerebral cortex	j. band of axonal fibers in cerebrum
		k. divides the cerebrum into two hemispheres
		l. occipital lobe

M. Label and color the lobes of the cerebrum. Color the occipital green, the frontal blue, the temporal orange, and the parietal yellow. Next list the functions of each lobe of the cerebrum. Include the limbic lobe (not pictured in diagram)

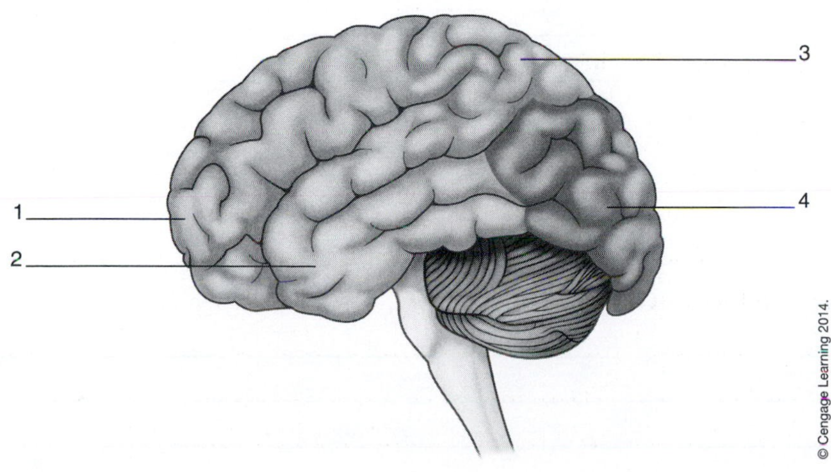

Functions:

____

____

____

____

Limbic Lobe: ____

N. Mark the underlined words in the following statements either true or false. Correct the false statements.

________ 1. The thalamus receives indirect nerve impulses and relays them to the cortex.

________ 2. In the medial hypothalamus is the "feeding center," which is stimulated by hunger.

________ 3. Damage to the thalamus of the brain may result in a total loss of consciousness.

________ 4. Information relating to skeletal muscle activity is carried to the cerebellum from sensory receptors in the outer ear, eye, and proprioceptors of the skeletal muscle.

________ 5. The cerebellum is responsible for coordination of muscle movements; raising the hand to the face requires the synchronized action of 50 or more muscles.

________ 6. The brainstem consists of the midbrain, pons, and medulla oblongata.

________ 7. The brainstem provides a pathway for ascending and descending tracts.

________ 8. The medulla oblongata contains the nuclei for the heart rate and the reflex center for vision and hearing.

________ 9. The spinal cord begins at the foramen magnum of the parietal bone.

________ 10. The spinal cord functions as a reflex center and a conduction pathway to and from the brain.

O. Answer the following questions about the hypothalamus.

1. The hypothalamus is considered the "brain" of the brain. Where is it located?

____

____

2. How are the following systems of the body affected by the hypothalamus?

a. Autonomic nervous system

____

____

____

b. Circulatory system

____

____

____

c. Digestive system

____

____

____

d. Endocrine system

____

____

____

e. Urinary system

____

____

____

f. Reproductive system

____

____

3. How does the hypothalamus affect our emotional states?

____

____

____

P. The limbic system encircles the top of the ________________.
The limbic system influences ________________ and ________________ behaviors.
This behavior is modified by the ________________.
A part of the limbic system is the ________________ bulb, which explains why the sense of ________________ is associated with emotions.

Q. Select the letter of the choice that best completes each statement.

1. In Parkinson's disease, a person exhibits a shuffling gait, tremors, and muscular rigidity. This disease is thought to be caused by a decrease in
   a. acetylcholine.
   b. dopamine.
   c. adrenalin.
   d. epinephrine.
2. The nerve cell sheaths are destroyed in
   a. epilepsy.
   b. cerebral palsy.
   c. meningitis.
   d. multiple sclerosis.
3. An inflammation of the brain is known as
   a. meningitis.
   b. encephalitis.
   c. poliomyelitis.
   d. osteomyelitis.

4. Epilepsy is characterized by recurring and excessive discharge of neuron activity. Seizures are said to be the result of
   a. spontaneous, uncontrolled cycles of electrical activity.
   b. deliberate, uncontrolled cycles of electrical activity.
   c. spontaneous, controlled cycles of electrical activity.
   d. uncontrolled cycles of electrical activity.
5. A bypass or shunt operation that diverts the cerebrospinal fluid is treatment for
   a. meningitis.
   b. hydrocephalus.
   c. encephalitis.
   d. cerebral palsy.
6. In multiple sclerosis, a symptom called nystagmus is
   a. seeing a halo around a light.
   b. a cataract.
   c. tremorous movement of the eye.
   d. double vision.
7. Cerebral palsy is a disturbance in voluntary muscle action. The most pronounced symptom is spastic paralysis that involves
   a. both arms.
   b. the arms and legs on one side of the body.
   c. both legs.
   d. the arms and legs on both sides of the body.
8. An injury to the spinal cord at the C-2 level may result in
   a. no paralysis.
   b. paraplegia.
   c. death.
   d. quadriplegia.
9. Mild cognitive impairment is usually a symptom of the ________ stage of Alzheimer's disease.
   a. preclinical
   b. middle
   c. third
   d. fourth
10. A subdural hematoma is a collection of blood between the ______________ of the brain.
   a. skull and dura mater layer
   b. dura mater and arachnoid layer
   c. arachnoid and pia mater layer
   d. dura mater and pia mater layer

R. List at least two symptoms and one treatment for the following:

1. Meningitis

____

____

2. Epilepsy

____

____

3. Essential tremors

____

____

4. Parkinson's disease

____

____

5. Brain tumor

____

____

S. Find the following words in the word search that relate to the central nervous system.

arachnoid
axon
cerebellum
cerebrum
dendrite
gyri
medulla
meninges
neuron
pons
synapse

j	n	d	a	c	j	d	o	w	m	g
s	s	o	i	c	d	d	x	u	y	n
e	y	g	x	o	f	n	l	r	p	e
g	n	f	v	a	n	l	i	q	t	u
n	a	j	k	e	e	h	g	j	l	r
i	p	v	q	b	e	m	c	a	d	o
n	s	u	e	f	e	f	s	a	c	n
e	e	r	x	g	h	b	b	n	r	k
m	e	m	e	d	u	l	l	a	o	a
c	d	e	t	i	r	d	n	e	d	p
p	o	l	m	u	r	b	e	r	e	c

APPLYING THEORY TO PRACTICE

1. Recall your earliest memory. How old were you, and why is the memory significant? Is there a correlation between what we remember and other significant events? Why are commercials repeated over and over?

2. A sign reads "Fresh-baked cookies." What parts of the brain and limbic system recall the appearance, taste, and smell of cookies?

3. Nichole is a nurse clinician with a specialty in gerontology. She is asked to speak at a conference on aging. Her topic will be "Hints to Stay Mentally Health as You Age." What information will Nichole include in her presentation?

4. Cathy has been complaining of double vision and generalized muscle weakness. Her doctor made a diagnosis of multiple sclerosis. Cathy tells you that the symptoms have disappeared and the doctor must have been mistaken in her diagnosis. Explain to her what is happening and what will happen to her in the years ahead.

5. Alzheimer's disease is a constant worry as people age. At a seminar on aging, Kayla is asked to give a presentation on Alzheimer's disease.

   The following issues must be addressed:

   - The changes that occur in the brain with Alzheimer's disease

   - The cause of the disease

- The new guidelines regarding the stages of the disease

  ____

  ____

- The symptoms that occur with each stage

  ____

  ____

- How the disease is treated

  ____

  ____

6. Perform the following nerve impulse calculations: If a nerve impulse travels at 120 meters per second, how many seconds would it take a nerve impulse to travel 900 meters? To travel 360 meters? 1200 meters? 460 meters?
   a. 900 meters ____________
   b. 360 meters ____________
   c. 1200 meters ____________
   d. 460 meters ____________

7. While playing football, Christopher collides with another player. He gets up after a minute or two and seems groggy. When the EMTs arrive, their concern is that Christopher may have a concussion. What are the signs and treatment for a concussion?

   ____

   ____

   ____

8. Dominick is preparing for his final exams to qualify for his EEG certification. He is complaining of a headache, which feels like a dull squeezing pain. What type of headache does Dominick have? Name the other types of headache.

   ____

   ____

   ____

9. You observe that your neighbor, Mr. Roland, seems to have some trouble walking, and you notice his hand trembling. His wife knows you are in the health care field and asks for your opinion. You advise her to take Mr. Roland to see the doctor. What do Mr. Roland's symptoms indicate, and how is it treated? What other diagnosis is possible?

   ____

   ____

   ____

   ____

10. Many spinal cord injuries result from automobile accidents, diving, sports injuries, home injuries, and falls that compress the vertebrae.

    a. What would be the result of the injury if it involved the L-3 vertebrae?

    ____

    ____

    ____

    b. How can spinal cord injuries be prevented?

    ____

    ____

SURF THE NET

For additional information and interactive exercises, use the following key words:

- central nervous system
- memory process
- nerve cell function
- parts of the brain—cerebrum, cerebellum, thalamus, hypothalamus, pons, medulla
- functions of the lobes of the brain
- spinal cord
- diseases of the central nervous system—epilepsy, cerebral palsy, meningitis, essential tremors, multiple sclerosis, Alzheimer's, brain tumor, concussion, spinal cord injuries

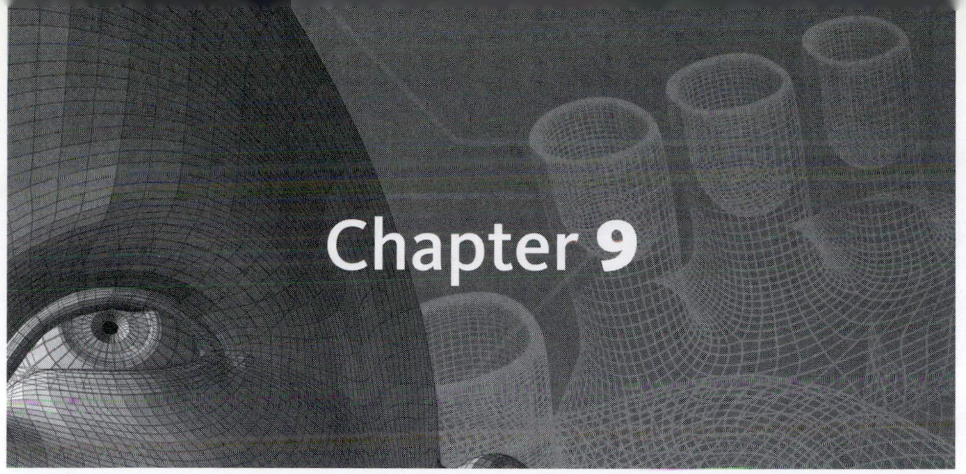

Peripheral and Autonomic Nervous System

OVERVIEW

The **peripheral nervous system** includes all the nerves of the body (cranial and spinal). A specialized part of the peripheral system is the autonomic nervous system.

Peripheral Nervous System

Functions of the peripheral nervous system include:

Controlling the automatic or involuntary activities of the body
Acting as the reflex center of the body

Nerves

A **nerve** is a bundle of nerve fibers, either *sensory* or *motor*. If it contains both types of fibers it is called a *mixed* nerve. A sensory or afferent nerve carries impulses from the sense organs to the brain or spinal cord; a motor or efferent nerve carries impulses from the brain and spinal cord to the muscles or glands.

Cranial Nerves

Cranial nerves begin in areas of the brain and are concerned mainly with the action of the head and neck, except for the vagus nerve. There are 12 pairs.

Spinal Nerves

Spinal nerves originate at the spinal cord and go through the openings on the vertebrae; they carry messages to and from the spinal cord, brain, and all parts of the body; there are 31 pairs.

A *plexus* is a network of spinal nerves and veins in a particular part of the body.

Autonomic Nervous System

The autonomic nervous system includes nerves, ganglia, and plexus; its function is to control the involuntary activities of the body. It has two divisions, the sympathetic and parasympathetic. The autonomic nervous system is strongly influenced by emotions.

The *sympathetic division* is often referred to as the fight-or-flight system. It stimulates the heart, stomach, small intestines, blood vessels, sweat glands, iris of the eye, and bladder.

The *parasympathetic division* has the opposite effect—to maintain a balance. The most active in this division are the vagus and pelvic nerves.

Reflex Arc. The **reflex arc** is the simplest type of nervous response; it involves both stimulus and response and is involuntary (reflex).

A *stimulus* is any change in the environment that causes a response.

Receptors are special structures that pick up stimuli.

Effectors are muscles that react to a stimulus.

The **reflex arc** is the pathway of a reflex action; it involves sensory, connecting, and motor neurons.

Biofeedback helps people learn how to manipulate physiological responses through mental activity.

Disorders of the Peripheral Nervous System

Neuritis is inflammation of a nerve or nerve trunk; symptoms may include pain and paresthesia, which is a tingling, burning, or crawling sensation of the skin.

Sciatica is a type of neuritis that affects the sciatic nerve; pain radiates through the buttocks and behind the knee to the foot.

Neuralgia is a sudden and severe, sharp, stabbing pain along the pathway of a nerve; types are named according to the nerve affected.

Trigeminal neuralgia involves the fifth cranial nerve; it has sudden onset, with spasms of pain in the cheek and jaw; it is also known as tic douloureux.

Shingles or *herpes zoster* is an acute viral infection, usually on one side of the body, affecting the intercostal nerves.

Carpal tunnel syndrome affects the median nerve and flexor tendons that attach to the bones of the wrist.

Bell's palsy is a condition that involves the seventh cranial nerve; the patient exhibits stroke-like characteristics on one side of the face.

Peripheral neuropathy describes damage to the peripheral nerves, usually involves multiple nerves, and is frequently caused by diabetes.

ACTIVITIES

A. Use Figure 9-2 (Divisions of the nervous system) to answer the following questions regarding these divisions.

a. What nerve pairs make up the peripheral nervous system?

____

____

b. Name the two divisions (subcategories) of the peripheral nervous system.

____

____

c. Name the division of the system that conducts impulses to and from the brain and spinal cord to the skeletal muscles.

____

____

d. Name the division that is sometimes called the automatic system, and name and list the functions of its subdivisions.

____

____

B. Select the word or words from the following list that best describe each statement.

acetycholine	efferent nerve	peripheral NS
afferent nerve	facial nerve	sensory nerve
autonomic nervous system	nerve	spinal nerve
central nervous system	norepinephrine	vagus
cranial nerves	optic nerve	plexus

1. The parasympathetic nervous system uses the neurotransmitter ____________________.
2. This structure consists of a bundle of nerve fibers enclosed by connective tissue. ____________________
3. A specialized part of the peripheral nervous system that controls the involuntary activities of the vital organs. ____________________
4. Spinal nerves may form a network with adjacent spinal nerves and veins; this is known as a(n) ____________________.
5. The name of this nerve may give you a clue about how it functions. ____________________
6. The nerve carrying impulses from the sense organs to the brain and spinal cord. ____________________
7. A nerve that carries only sensory fibers. ____________________
8. This cranial nerve affects the smooth muscle of the stomach. ____________________
9. This system includes the brain and spinal cord. ____________________
10. This group of nerves contains mixed nerves. ____________________

C. Complete the following table of the cranial nerves.

NUMBER	NAME	FUNCTION
I	Olfactory	
II		Vision, eyesight
III	Oculomotor	
	Trochlear	Movement of eye muscle
V	Trigeminal	
	Abducens	Movement of eye muscle
VII	Facial	
	Vestibulocochlear (auditory)	Hearing and balance
IX		Movement of throat muscles
X	Vagus	
	Accessory	Movement of neck muscles
XII	Hypoglossal	

D. Complete the riddles, giving the correct name and Roman numberal of the cranial nerves.

WHO AM I?

What is that, what did I hear?
I affect your balance and your ear.

Nerve name and number ______________________, ___________

I can make your eyes roll and other tricks.
Sometimes one or another of my pairs get me in a fix.

Nerve name and number ______________________, ___________

I hit the palate and places inside your mouth;
even difficult words I help you pronounce.

Nerve name and number ______________________, ___________

I turn your head about, going to and fro.
There are times I do not know which way you want to go.

Nerve name and number ______________________, ___________

When you have a cold, I do not do well;
a running nose really affects my sense of smell.

Nerve name and number ______________________, ___________

Medicine really does not have a good taste;
I swallow it down quickly in great haste.

Nerve name and number ______________________, ____________

They say it takes many muscles to cry and to smile,
yet there is only one pair of me to weep and beguile.

Nerve name and number ______________________, ____________

In this group I am quite out of place;
my action does not affect your head or your face.

Nerve name and number ______________________, ____________

E. Label the diagram of the spinal nerve plexus and name one major nerve in each plexus.

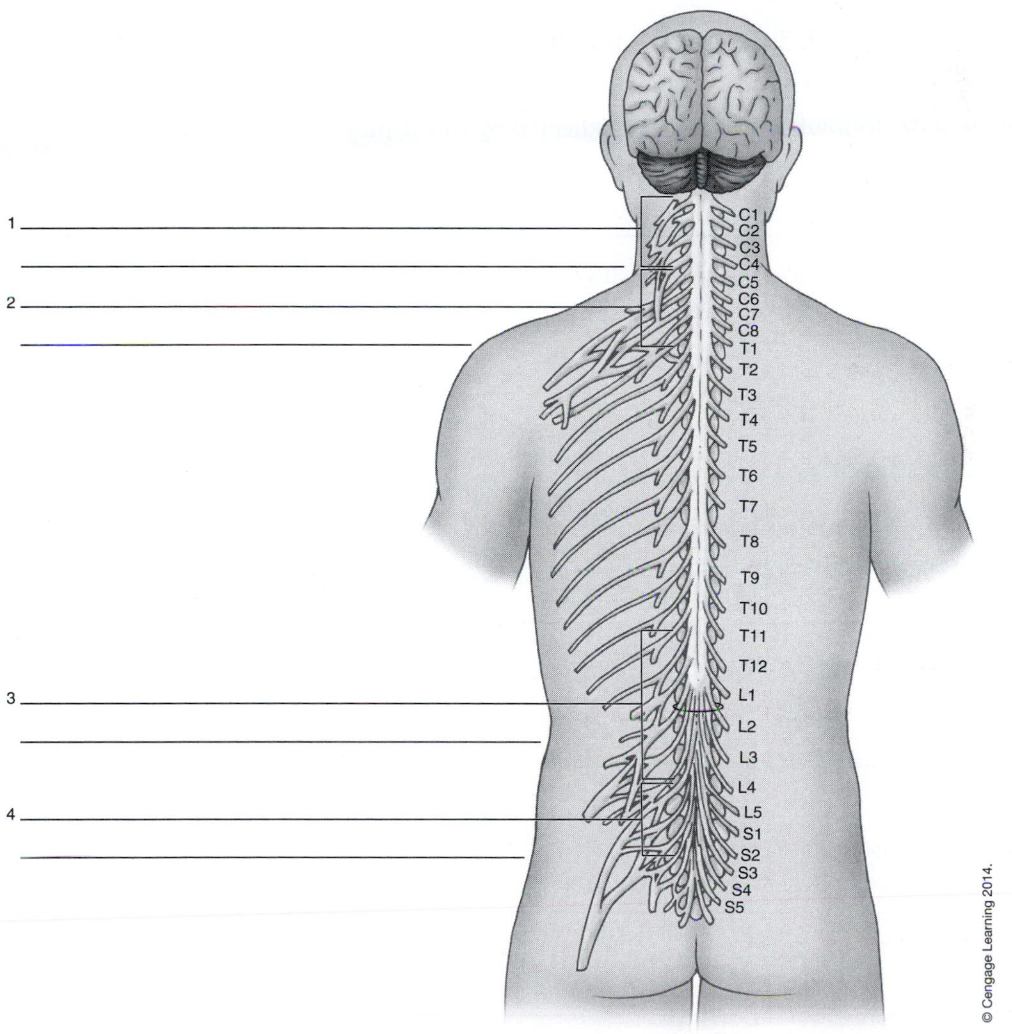

F. Match the following plexus names with the descriptions.

Brachial (B)
Cervical (C)
Lumbar (L)
Sacral (S)

_________ 1. Supplies nerves to scalp, neck, and part of shoulder and chest

_________ 2. Contains the origin of the phrenic nerve that influences respiration

_________ 3. Forms the median, radial, and axillary nerves

_________ 4. Supplies motor movement to the buttocks, anterior leg, and thighs

_________ 5. Femoral nerve is part of this plexus

_________ 6. Provides the entire nerve supply for the arm

_________ 7. Forms the sciatic nerve

G. John Smith, age 19, dove off the dock into the water and broke his neck at the area of the brachial plexus.

1. How will the following functions be affected by this injury?

   Speaking and understanding words

   ____

   Bending his elbow and making a fist with his fingers

   ____

   Breathing

   ____

   Hearing and seeing

   ____

   Picking up his right leg

   ____

   Bladder and bowel function

   ____

   Chewing his food and swallowing

   ____

   Writing a note

   ____

2. What emotional support will John need to cope with this injury?

   ____

   ____

3. Name some devices that may be helpful to him.

____

____

H. Answer the following questions.

1. Name the two divisions of the autonomic nervous system.

____

____

2. List the organs affected by the autonomic nervous system.

____

3. Why is the sympathetic nervous system referred to as the fight-or-flight system?

____

____

4. What other body system is directly connected to the sympathetic nervous system?

____

I. Mark the underlined word in the following statements either true or false. Correct any false statements.

________ 1. Some reflex arcs are preceded by a stimulus.

________ 2. A simple reflex involves a sensory and motor neuron.

________ 3. Tapping the knee to demonstrate a reflex is a method of checking the condition of the muscular and nervous systems.

________ 4. The reflex arc is conscious and involuntary.

________ 5. Reflex actions are automatic reactions controlled by the brain.

J. Select the letter of the choice that best completes the statement.

1. The peripheral nervous system consists of
   a. peripheral nerves and the brain.
   b. peripheral nerves and the spinal cord.
   c. the peripheral and sensory nerves.
   d. the brain and sensory nerves.

2. The vagus nerve is also known as cranial nerve ____.
   a. V
   b. X
   c. VIII
   d. IV

3. The lumbar plexus includes which of the following nerves?
   a. Femoral and obturator
   b. Phrenic
   c. Axillary, median, and radial
   d. Sciatic
4. A cranial nerve that carries only sensory fibers is the ______________ nerve.
   a. olfactory
   b. oculomotor
   c. trigeminal
   d. glossopharyngeal
5. The autonomic nervous system carries impulses to all
   a. skeletal muscles.
   b. striated muscle.
   c. smooth muscle.
   d. voluntary muscle.
6. A simple reflex is one that has only a(n) ________ neuron.
   a. sensory
   b. afferent
   c. efferent
   d. sensory and motor
7. The term *tic douloureux* refers to
   a. trigeminal neuralgia.
   b. Bell's palsy.
   c. neuralgia.
   d. sciatica.
8. In the patient with alcoholism, neuritis usually occurs because of a lack of
   a. vitamin A.
   b. vitamin B.
   c. vitamin C.
   d. vitamin D.
9. The pain due to sciatica radiates
   a. into the right hip.
   b. into the left hip.
   c. through the buttock and down the front of the leg.
   d. through the buttock and behind the knee.
10. The virus that causes shingles also causes
    a. chickenpox.
    b. measles.
    c. mumps.
    d. hepatitis B.

K. Circle the correct word or words in each of the following statements.

1. (Noritis, Neuritis) is an inflammation of a nerve or nerve track in which the patient experiences (paresthesia, parathesia).
2. Treatment for sciatica includes hot or cold packs and (physiotherapy, physotherapy).
3. A sudden severe pain along the pathway of a nerve is (neuralagia, neuralgia).
4. A condition that involves the fifth (cranial, crenial) nerve is trigeminal (neuralagia, neuralgia).
5. In Bell's palsy, the patient must do (whisling, whistling) exercises to prevent atrophy of the cheek muscle.
6. Bell's palsy affects the (facial, facile) nerve; the mouth droops and the eyelid does not close (properley, properly).
7. Shingles is an acute viral nerve infection characterized by a one-sided inflammation of a (cutaneous, cutanous) nerve.
8. Carpal tunnel syndrome may be caused by repetitive movements in which swelling or (edemma, edema) develops around the carpal tunnel.
9. The diagnostic test for carpal tunnel syndrome is an (electramyograph, electromyograph).
10. The causes of neuritis may be infectious, chemical, or chronic alcoholism. The pain can be (relieved, releived) by (analgesics, anolgesics).

L. Quiz—Mark the underlined word in the statement true or false. Correct the false statements.

1. ________ The cranial nerves consist of <u>24</u> pairs that begin in areas of the brain.
2. ________ The phrenic nerve is located in the <u>lumbar</u> plexus.
3. ________ The <u>brachial</u> nerve stimulates the hand and wrist.
4. ________ <u>Parathesia</u> is a tingling, burning, and crawling sensation of the skin.
5. ________ Trigeminal neuralgia is a condition that affects the <u>third</u> cranial nerve.
6. ________ <u>Bell's palsy</u> is a condition that affects only one side of the face.
7. ________ The sciatic nerve is located in the <u>brachial</u> plexus.
8. ________ <u>Biofeedback</u> enhances relaxation for tense muscles.
9. ________ <u>Peripheral neuropathy</u> may occur as a result of diabetes.
10. ________ Treatment for peripheral neuropathy includes soaking the hands or feet for <u>30</u> minutes at least twice a day.

M. Define the following terms and then use them in the crossword puzzle. Definition blanks indicate the number of letters in the answer.

1. Cranial nerve III affects the movement of the
   Answer: _ _ _
2. Cranial nerve II
   Answer: _ _ _ _ _
3. Olfactory nerve does this
   Answer: _ _ _ _ _
4. Efferent nerve may also be known as
   Answer: _ _ _ _ _
5. Spinal nerves and vein network
   Answer: _ _ _ _ _ _
6. Plexus for L4–5 S1–2
   Answer: _ _ _ _ _ _
7. Cranial nerve V function
   Answer: _ _ _ _ _ _ _
8. Nerve cell bodies
   Answer: _ _ _ _ _ _ _
9. Stimulates the diaphragm
   Answer: _ _ _ _ _ _ _
10. Largest nerve in body
    Answer: _ _ _ _ _ _ _
11. Picks up stimuli
    Answer: _ _ _ _ _ _ _ _ _
12. System that controls involuntary activities
    Answer: _ _ _ _ _ _ _ _ _ _
13. Painkiller
    Answer: _ _ _ _ _ _ _ _ _
14. Simplest nervous response
    Answer: _ _ _ _ _ _ _ _ _
15. Cranial nerve IV
    Answer: _ _ _ _ _ _ _ _ _
16. Both afferent and efferent fibers
    Answer: _ _ _ _ _ _ _ _ _ _
17. Motor nerve also known as
    Answer: _ _ _ _ _ _ _ _ _
    _ _ _ _
18. Records muscle electric activity
    Answer: _ _ _ _ _ _ _ _ _
    _ _ _ _ _ _
19. System that slows the heartbeat
    Answer: _ _ _ _ _ _ _ _ _
    _ _ _ _ _ _
20. Involved with hearing and balance
    Answer: _ _ _ _ _ _ _ _ _
    _ _ _ _ _ _ _ _ _
21. Condition that affects median nerve and flexor tendons
    Answer: _ _ _ _ _ _ _ _ _
    _ _ _ _ _ _ _ _ _
    _ _

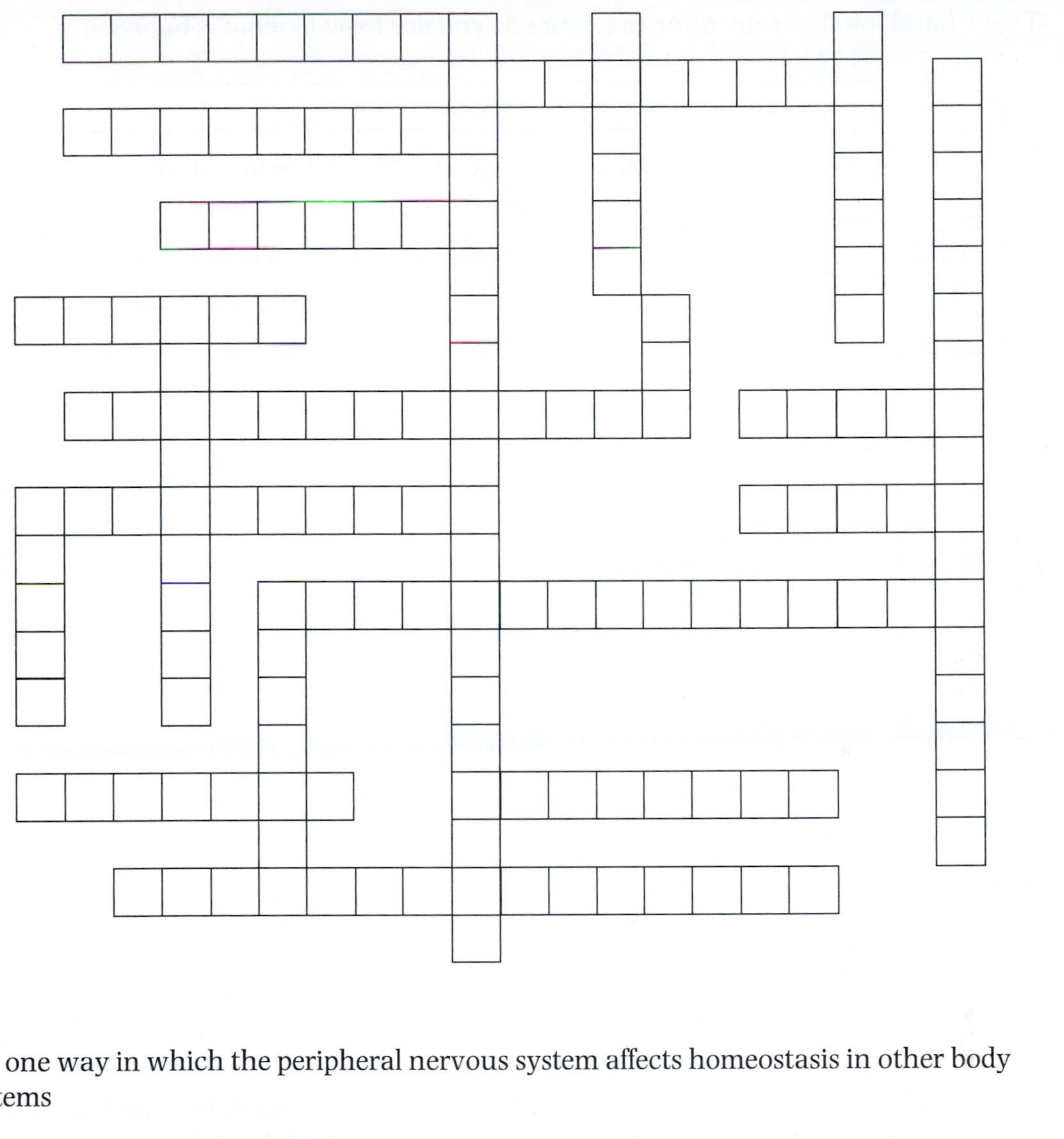

N. List one way in which the peripheral nervous system affects homeostasis in other body systems

____

____

____

APPLYING THEORY TO PRACTICE

1. When frightened, your sympathetic nervous system reacts. Describe your reaction. How does this affect your body systems? Name one relaxation technique to reduce stress.

____

____

____

____

____

2. If your hand touches something hot, what do you do? Explain what is happening.

3. A patient visits the doctor's office because when she awoke, her mouth was sagging on one side and her eyelid was drooping. How would you explain this condition and treatments for it?

4. Carolyn has been under a great deal of stress because of job responsibilities. She does not want to use medication that may interfere with her job duties. Carolyn has heard about biofeedback and comes to the health clinic to ask the medical assistant for more information.

   Explain to Carolyn what biofeedback is.

   Describe how the method is used.

   Describe the benefits of biofeedback to Carolyn.

5. Scotty, age 42, works at a local lumber yard. One day while at work he experienced difficulty in walking, which was accompanied by pain radiating through his left buttock into his left knee. What diagnosis was made at the company's health maintenance organization (HMO)? What causes this condition? Describe the treatment.

6. Victoria has been experiencing a sudden sharp pain on the side of her face that occurs when she is eating. This pain lasts only a few seconds. Victoria visits her dentist because she thinks it may be a problem with her teeth. The dentist tells her that her teeth are fine. The dentist tells her the pain is from what condition? Explain the condition, its symptoms, and its treatment to Victoria.

7. Mr. Vincent is 50 and has had type I diabetes for about 5 years. He has developed pain and tingling in his feet. At the HMO, the doctor tells Mr. Vincent that he has peripheral neuropathy. As the health educator at the HMO, you must talk to Mr. Vincent about his condition and how he can obtain relief from his symptoms. What information would you provide?

____

____

____

____

____

____

____

SURF THE NET

For additional information and interactive exercises, use the following key words:

- peripheral nervous system, somatic division and automatic division
- cranial nerves, spinal nerves
- reflex arc
- biofeedback
- diseases of the peripheral nervous system; cause, treatment, and lasting effects for sciatica, neuralgia, Bell's palsy, trigeminal neuralgia, shingles, peripheral neuropathy, carpal tunnel syndrome, neuralgia

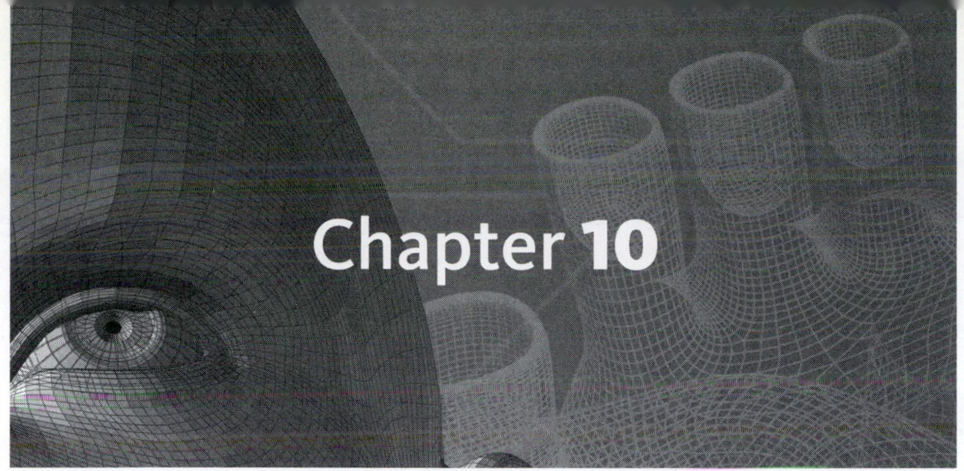

Special Senses

OVERVIEW

Special senses are organs and sensory receptors associated with touch, vision, hearing, taste, and smell.

Sensory Receptors

Sensory receptors are specialized structures found all over the body. A receptor site is stimulated and the impulse is taken to the brain, interpreted, and referred back to the sense. This is called projection of the sensation.

Eye

The eye is a sphere protected by the orbital socket of the skull, eyebrows, eyelids, and eyelashes. The eyes are bathed in tears produced by lacrimal glands. The three layers of the eye are the sclera, choroid, and retina.

Sclera. The **sclera** is a white fibrous capsule that maintains the shape of the eye; *extrinsic muscles* responsible for moving the eye are attached to the outside of sclera (see Table 10-1 in textbook).

The *cornea* is the circular, clear area in the anterior center of the sclera; it is transparent to let light rays pass through it and is avascular.

Choroid. The **choroid** is the middle layer of eye, containing blood vessels and nonreflective dark pigment.

The *pupil* is the circular opening in front of the choroid layer.

The *iris* is the colored part of the eye. The *intrinsic muscles* of the iris react to the amount of light; *sphincter pupillae muscles* contract the eye in bright light, and *dilator pupillae muscles* dilate the pupils in dim light.

The *lens* is the crystalline and elastic structure that forms a biconvex shape. The function is to refract or bend light as it passes through. The *suspensory ligaments* hold the lens in place.

Chambers are the areas where the lens is situated, between the anterior and posterior chambers of the eye. The anterior chamber is filled with *aqueous humor*; the posterior chamber is filled with *vitreous humor*. Both substances maintain the shape of the eyeball and refract light.

Retina. The **retina** is the innermost, or third, light-sensitive layer. It contains special cells, the *rods* and *cones.*

Rod cells are sensitive to dim light. Cone cells are sensitive to bright light and are responsible for color vision. Within the yellow disk on the retina (macula lutea) is the *fovea centralis,* which contains the cones for color vision.

The *optic disk,* or blind spot, is the area where the nerve fibers from the retina gather to form the optic nerve; no rods or cones are present.

Pathway of Vision

Images in light "hit" the cornea, then the pupil, lens, retina, optic nerve, and, finally, the occipital lobe of the brain for interpretation.

Eye Disorders

Conjunctivitis is a contagious inflammation of the conjunctival membrane; it is commonly known as pink eye.

Glaucoma is excessive interocular pressure that results in damage to the retina and optic nerve.

A *cataract* is a gradual cloudiness of the lens of the eye.

Macular degeneration is a thinning of the retina area; there is a loss of sharp, central vision.

A *detached retina* occurs when vitreous fluid contracts as it ages, pulling on the retina and causing a tear.

Diabetic retinopathy is caused by changes in the blood vessels in the retina; it is the leading cause of blindness in American adults.

A *sty* is a tiny abscess at the base of the eyelid; it can be very painful.

Eye Injuries. Objects may become embedded in the eye; patch both eyes and get medical attention.

Corneal abrasion—cornea injured; scarring may be the result.

Eye irritations—many causes.

Night blindness—rod cells are affected, making it difficult to see at night.

Color blindness—inability to distinguish colors.

Eyestrain—experienced as burning, tightness, or sharp or dull pain in the eye, usually caused when viewing something for too long.

Vision Defects. Visual problems of the eye include the following:

Presbyopia—lenses lose their elasticity; loss of ability to focus on objects close at hand.

Hyperopia—farsightedness; focal point beyond retina.

Myopia—nearsightedness; focal point in front of retina.

Astigmatism—irregular curvature of cornea or lens.

Strabismus—crossed eyes; muscles of the eyeball do not coordinate their action.

Amblyopia—dimness of vision.

Diplopia—blurred vision.

The Ear

The ear is a special sense organ adapted to pick up sound waves to send to the auditory center of the brain. The ear is also responsible for balance and equilibrium. It has three parts: outer, middle, and inner ear.

The *outer* or *external ear*, the *pinna*, collects sound waves and directs them to the middle ear.

The *middle ear* is separated from the outer ear by the tympanic membrane; it contains the eustachian tube, which connects the ear to the throat.

The *inner ear* contains the *cochlea* and *semicircular canals*. The cochlea is a spiral-shaped structure containing the organ of hearing (organ of Corti); it picks up sound waves and sends them to the auditory nerve and then to the brain. Semicircular canals are special structures that send impulses regarding balance to the brain.

Pathway of Hearing

Sound moves from the auditory canal to the tympanic membrane, then to the ear bones, the cochlear duct, the organ of Corti, the auditory nerve, and the brain.

Pathway of Equilibrium

A movement of the head reaches receptors in the semicircular canals. The impulse moves to the vestibular nerve and finally to the cerebellum.

Ear Disorders

Otitis media is inflammation of the middle ear.

Otosclerosis is a chronic, progressive disease in which the stirrup becomes spongy and then hardens, resulting in hearing loss.

Tinnitus is ringing or buzzing in the ear.

Presbycusis is deafness due to aging.

Meniére's disease affects the semicircular canals, causing vertigo.

Hearing loss can result from exposure to loud noise, conductive loss, and sensorineural damage.

Sense of Smell/Nose

The nose detects about 10,000 smells; a specialized patch of tissue called the olfactory epithelium has the receptors that send stimuli to the olfactory nerve, which relays them to the limbic system, thalamus, and frontal cortex.

Disorders of the Nose

Rhinitis is inflammation of the lining of the nose.

Nasal polyps are growths in the nasal cavity.

A *deviated nasal septum* is a bend in the cartilage of the nose; it may result in a blockage of the air passage.

Sense of Taste/The Tongue

The tongue is a mass of muscle tissue that has structures called *papillae*, which contain the taste buds. All taste buds can detect all five sensations: umami, sweet, salty, sour, and bitter.

Tongue Disorders

Injury—may occur when the tongue is bitten.

Discoloration—may indicate a disease process (e.g., a pale tongue = anemia).

Infection—may result from tongue piercing.

Cancer—most oral cancers grow on the side of the tongue or on the floor of the mouth.

Burning mouth syndrome—cause is unknown; feels as if the mouth was burned by a drink that was too hot.

The Effects of Aging on the Sensory System

The loss of sensory nerves may lead to a loss of independence and social isolation. There may be a loss of sensory receptors, vision, hearing, smell, and taste.

ACTIVITIES

A. Label the diagram of the external view of the eye. State how the eye is protected by the following structures.

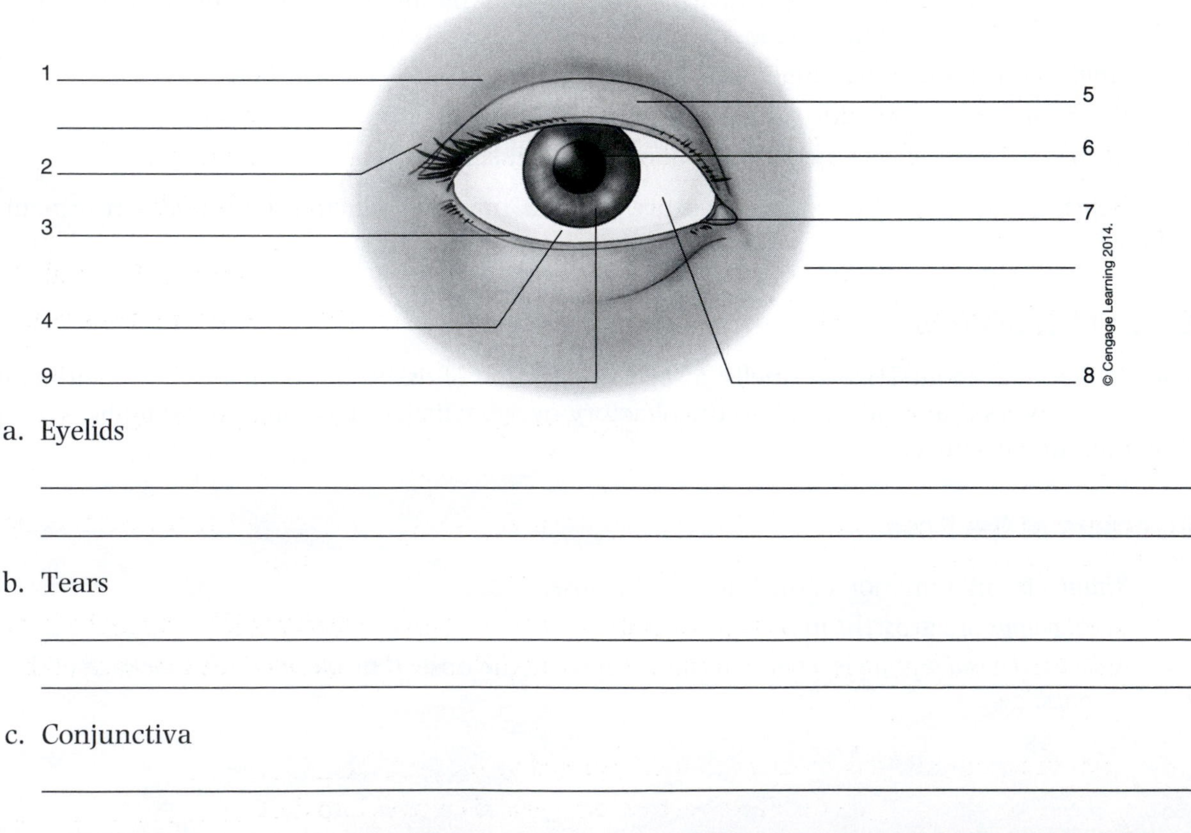

a. Eyelids

____

____

b. Tears

____

____

c. Conjunctiva

____

____

B. Complete the following activities related to the eye muscles.

1. Label and color the diagram of the eye muscles. Color the eye muscle that turns the eye upward brown, downward orange, and toward the nose green.

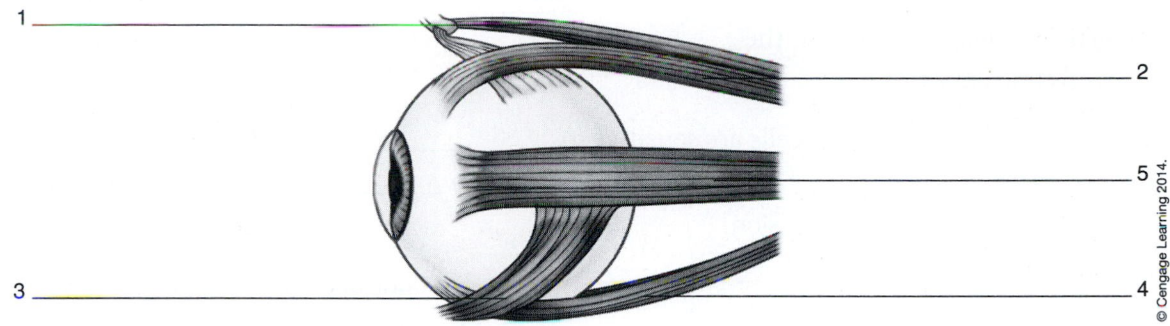

2. How does the name of the eye muscle relate to its action?

____

____

C. Complete the sentences using words from the following list. Words may only be used once.

avascular	cornea	optic
biconvex	dim	projection
blind spot	extrinsic	pupil
bright	intrinsic	retina
choroid	iris	rod
color	lacrimal duct	sclera
cone	lacrimal gland	spherical
constrict	lens	temperature
contract	opaque	transparent

1. The sensory receptors for touch, pain, ____________________, and pressure are found all over the body. The sensation takes place in the brain and is referred back to sensory organs, a characteristic known as the ____________________ of sensation.

2. In the anterior center of the outer layer of the eye is a circular clear area called the ____________________, which is ____________________.

3. The structure located behind the pupil is the ____________________, which has an anterior and posterior convex surface forming a(n) ____________________ lens.

4. The ____________________ layer that contains blood vessels has a circular opening in front called the ____________________, which is surrounded by the colored muscular layer, the ____________________.

5. The eye is continuously bathed in a fluid secreted by the ____________________ ____________________, which flows across the eye and empties into the ____________________.

6. The movement of the eye is controlled by ____________ muscles that are attached to the white of the eye, or the ____________.

7. Stimulated by a bright light, intrinsic muscles ____________ and ____________ the pupil.

8. The third layer of the eye, the ____________, contains special cells known as the rods and cones.

9. ____________ cells are sensitive to ____________ light, whereas ____________ cells are sensitive to ____________ light and ____________ vision.

10. The ____________ ____________, or optic disk, is where the nerve fibers from the retina gather to form the ____________ nerve; there are no rods or cones present.

D. Label the diagram of the eye.

E. Match the following descriptions with the names of the structures in the previous diagram.

a. Opening in the choroid coat ____________

b. Clear area in the anterior surface of the sclera ____________

c. Watery fluid in the anterior chamber of the eye ____________

d. Have the intrinsic muscles that control the amount of light entering the pupil ____________

e. Contains the cones for color vision ____________

f. Nonreflective pigment preventing light reflection ____________

g. Tough, fibrous capsule ____________

h. Jellylike substance that gives the eyeball its shape and refracts light ____________

i. Holds the lens in place ____________________

j. Does not extend to the anterior surface of the eye ____________________

F. Look at an object. Now label the diagram and use it to illustrate the pathway of vision.

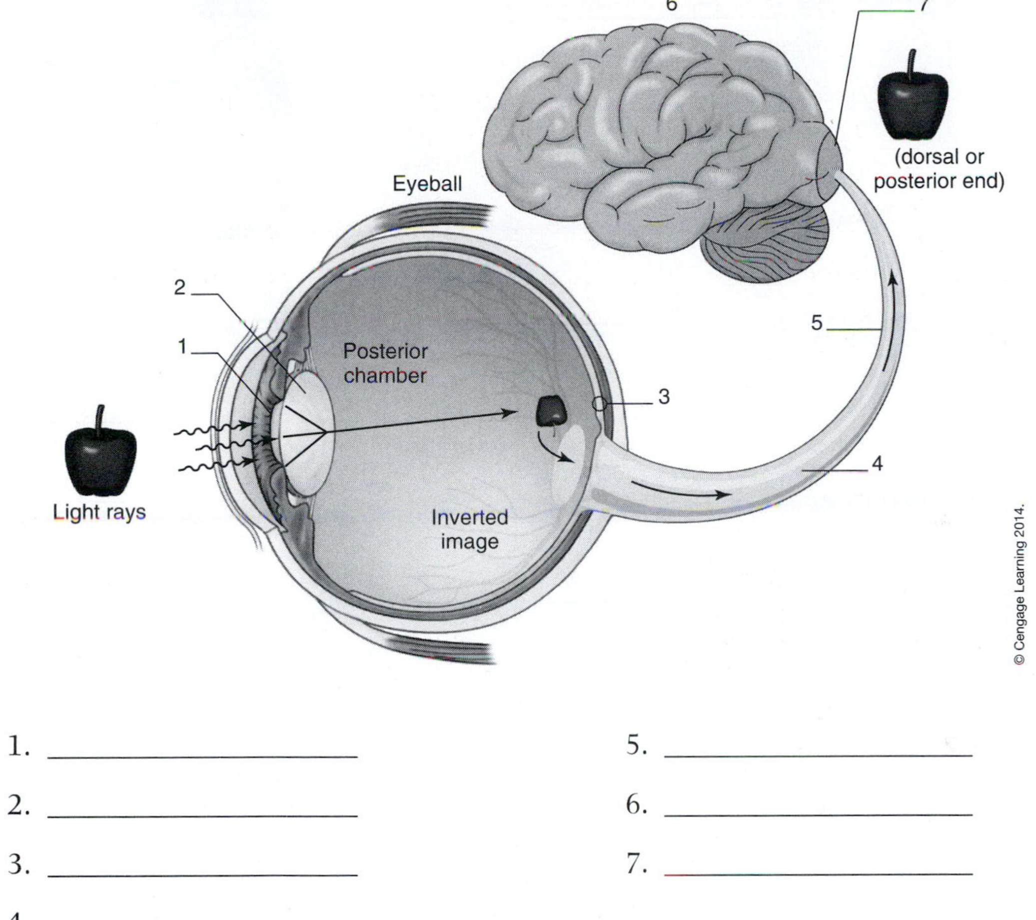

1. ____________________
2. ____________________
3. ____________________
4. ____________________
5. ____________________
6. ____________________
7. ____________________

G. Match the disorders in Column B with the correct descriptions in Column A.

	Column A	Column B
________	1. double vision	a. eyestrain
________	2. focal point behind retina	b. myopia
________	3. lenses lose their elasticity	c. presbyopia
________	4. watery, blurry vision	d. strabismus
________	5. rod cells are affected	e. color blindness
________	6. dimness of vision	f. night blindness
________	7. irregular curvature of the lens	g. diplopia
________	8. focal point in front of the retina	h. amblyopia
________	9. cones are affected	i. astigmatism
________	10. muscles do not coordinate their activity	j. hyperopia

H. Label the diagram of the ear.

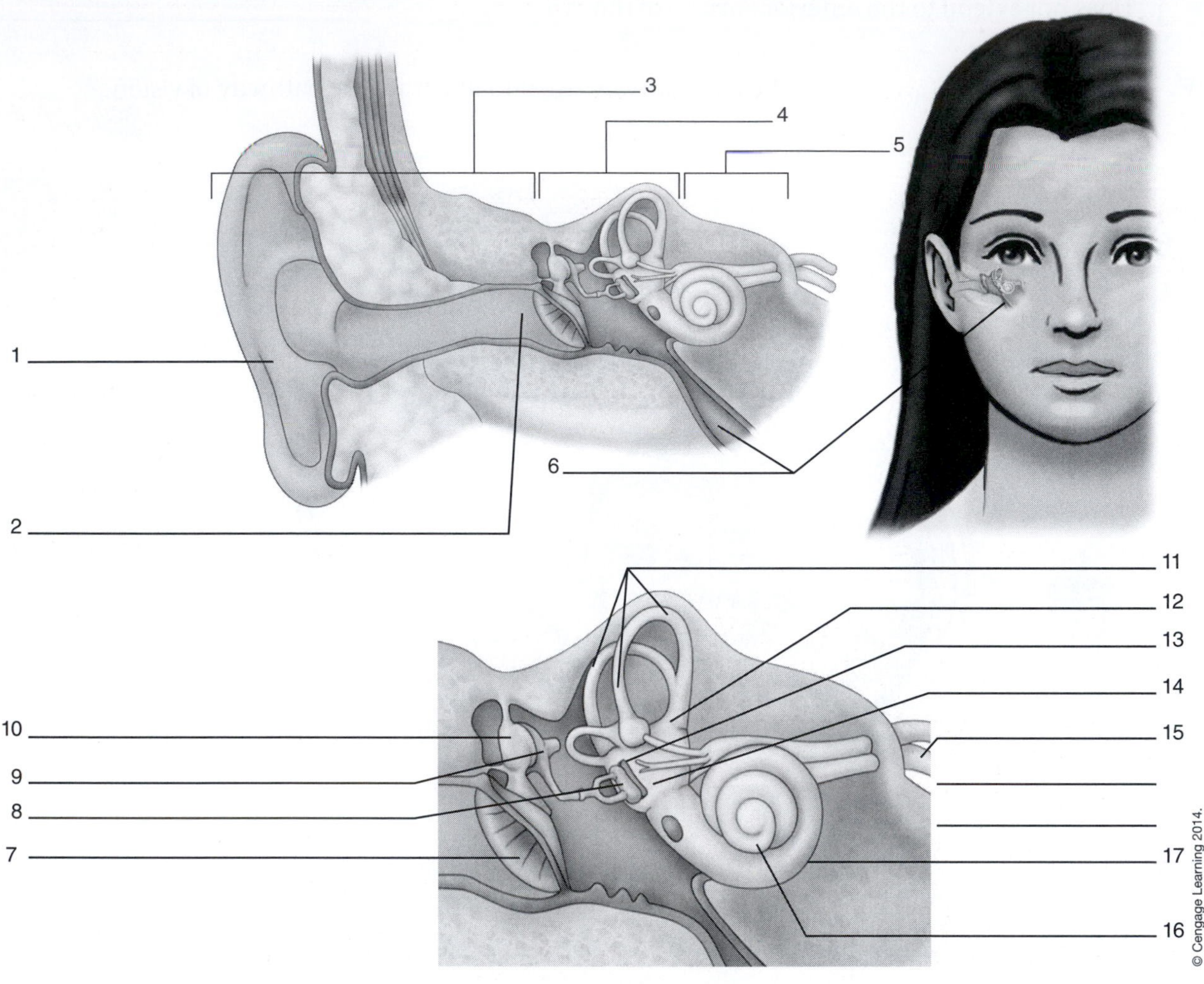

I. Using the previous diagram, answer the following questions.

1. What lines the auditory canal, and what is its function?

___

___

___

2. Name the structure between the outer and middle ear.

___

3. What is the purpose of the eustachian tube?

___

___

___

4. What are the functions of the hammer (malleus), anvil (incus), and stirrup (stapes)?

____

____

____

5. What is the function of the cells of the organ of Corti?

____

____

____

6. What is the function of the semicircular canal?

____

____

____

J. Use the diagram of the ear to describe the pathway of hearing and explain the function of each structure.

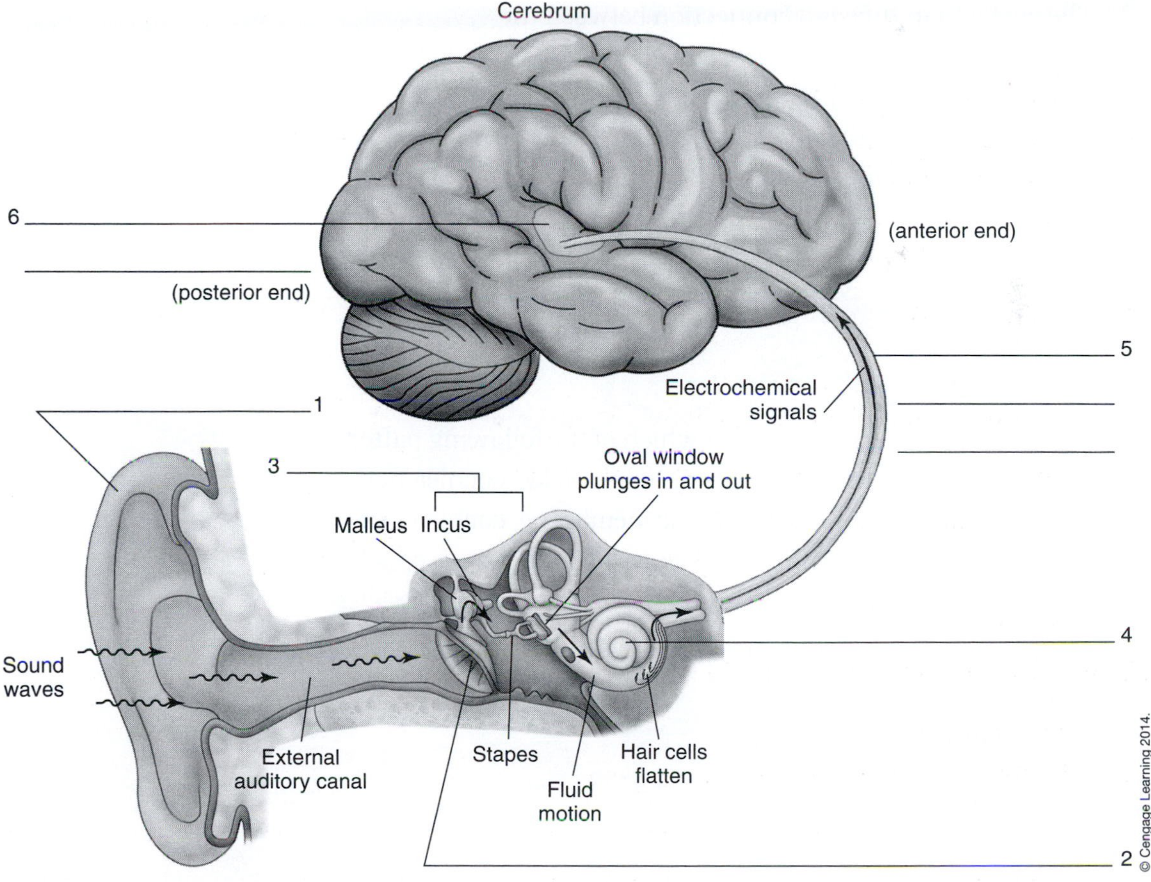

K. Explain the pathway of equilibrium.

____

____

____

L. Select the letter of the choice that best completes the statement.

1. The ear is adapted to pick up sound waves and transmit them to the auditory center of the brain located in the ______________ lobe.
   a. frontal
   b. temporal
   c. occipital
   d. parietal
2. The ear is also involved with equilibrium; the receptors for equilibrium are found in the
   a. organ of Corti.
   b. middle ear.
   c. semicircular canals.
   d. outer ear.
3. The eustachian tube is a connection between the
   a. outer ear and the pharynx.
   b. inner ear and the pharynx.
   c. middle ear and the pharynx.
   d. inner ear and the larynx.
4. The structure of the inner ear is known as the
   a. auditory canal.
   b. pinna.
   c. ear ossicle.
   d. labyrinth.
5. Sound waves are transmitted in which of the following patterns?
   a. Outer ear, tympanic membrane, ear ossicles, cochlea nerve
   b. Outer ear, ear ossicles, tympanic membrane, cochlea nerve
   c. Outer ear, tympanic membrane, cochlea nerve, ear ossicles
   d. Outer ear, cochlea nerve, tympanic membrane, ear ossicles
6. A myringotomy is a procedure done to relieve the symptoms of
   a. otosclerosis.
   b. otitis media.
   c. tinnitus.
   d. presbycusis.

7. Sound is measured in decibels (dB); more than 90 dB for 8 hours may damage your hearing. Ninety dB is about the level of sound of
   a. the scream of a jet engine.
   b. a shotgun blast.
   c. busy city traffic.
   d. the buzz of a chain saw.
8. The main symptom of Meniére's disease is
   a. vertigo.
   b. buildup of fluid.
   c. partial deafness.
   d. complete deafness.
9. A nasal strip across the nose may alleviate the symptoms of
   a. a deviated nasal septum.
   b. rhinitis.
   c. nasal polyps.
   d. sneezing.
10. The physician who diagnoses and treats eye disease is called an
   a. optometrist.
   b. optician.
   c. ophthalmologist.
   d. audiologist.

M. Underline the correct word in each of the following statements.

1. The nerve cells of the nose are located on a patch of tissue called the olfactory (epithelium, epethilium).
2. Growths in the nasal cavity are known as (nasal polups, nasal polyps).
3. "Hairiness" in the tongue may appear after (antebiotic, antibiotic) treatment.
4. The taste buds are located on structures of the tongue called (papillae, papila).
5. The (umami, unami) taste sensation is responsible for the (savory, savery) taste of food.
6. The sour taste sensation guides the intake of fruits to meet the body's need for (vitamen, vitamin) C.
7. The bitter taste sensation protects us by detecting spoiled food and (poisens, poisons).
8. The sweet taste sensation guides the intake of sugar to meet the body's need for (carbohydrates, carbohydretes).
9. The salty taste sensation guides the intake of foods that meet the body's need for (neccesary, necessary) minerals.
10. Infections on the tongue may be caused by tongue (piercing, peiricing).

N. Use the following words to complete the story on the senses.

astigmatism	presbyopia
hearing	sharp
lenses	smells
nose	taste buds
pain	vision
presbycusis	wax

COMING TO THE SENSES: EFFECTS OF AGING

Once upon a time I could see far and near.
Everything I heard was crisp, loud, and clear.

Now that aging has approached,
I have to ask, "What's that?" as I search and grope.

My eyes have developed ____________________;
images no longer fall ____________________ and clear on my cones and rods.

I now need bifocal ____________________ to see life's smiles and nods.
The bright side of this comes as the mirror I face
does not show wrinkles appearing, the lines of aging grace.
____________________ now causes some eyestrain;
special glasses will relieve the blurred ____________________ and ____________________.

Did you say something? I didn't quite hear.
Then again, it may be that I have ____________________ in my ear.
My hearing loss also could be due to a ____________________ state;
a(n) ____________________ aid helps keep my listening skills up to date.
Even though my ____________________ seems to have gotten a little longer,
the ____________________ do not seem to be any stronger.
There is one sense I truly miss the most:
My fading ____________________ ____________________ cannot tell crackers from toast.

The positive side to the fading of the senses you will learn;
I will tell you all about it when my memory returns.

APPLYING THEORY TO PRACTICE

1. Teachers must be alert for an eye condition known as pinkeye. What is the medical term for this condition? What instructions should the school nurse give to parents if a child has this condition?

2. Emary is a geriatric nurse practitioner and is asked to give a talk at the senior community center about eye and ear conditions that occur with aging. Emary will include discussion of glaucoma, cataracts, macular degeneration, detached retina, presbycusis, and deafness in her presentation. Describe the latest methods of treating these conditions.

3. Working in a computer lab at school, Kieran's eyes feel gritty and burn. What do you think is the cause? How can Kieran prevent this problem?

4. Adriana has been diabetic for over 20 years. She worries about going blind. She heard that the number one cause of blindness is diabetic retinopathy. She asks you, the health educator at the diabetes clinic, whether it can be prevented and how it is treated.

5. Bryan is an EMT, so he knows about emergency procedures. How would he treat the following conditions?
   a. glass in the eye
   b. chemicals in the eye

6. Jamal has had chronic ear infections for the past 3 years. The usual antibiotic treatment is not effective. What condition does Jamal have and what will be the course of treatment?

7. Leslie has chronic sleeping problems, and her husband complains that she snores loudly. What may be the cause of this problem? Can you suggest a treatment for Leslie?

8. Burning mouth syndrome is a problem that may occur as one ages.
   a. Explain this condition or psychological factors that may be involved.
   b. Who is affected by it?
   c. What is the treatment?

SURF THE NET

For additional information and interactive exercises, use the following key words:

- eye—pathway of vision
- diseases of the eye—glaucoma, cataract, macular degeneration, detached retina, diabetic neuropathy
- vision disorders and treatment—presbyopia, myopia, hyperopia, strabismus, diplopia, astigmatism
- ear—pathway of hearing, equilibrium
- diseases of the ear and treatment—otitis media, otosclerosis, presbycusis, deafness, and Meniere's disease
- Types and benefits of hearing aids
- Loud noises and deafness
- Nose—structure and function
- Tongue—structure and function
- Effects of aging on the senses

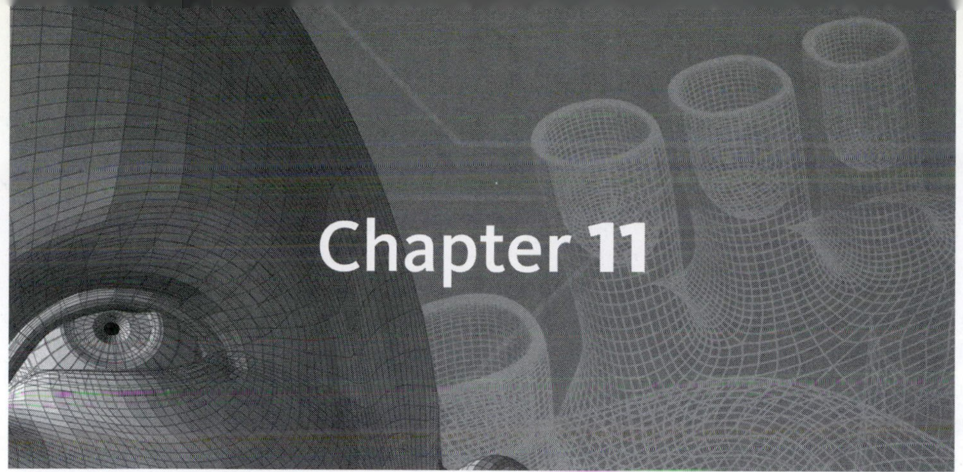

Endocrine System

OVERVIEW

Glandular systems secrete chemical substances, or hormones, that coordinate and direct the activities of target cells and organs. There are two types of systems: exocrine and endocrine.

Exocrine gland secretions go through a duct before reaching their target organs. Their functions are discussed in the chapters involving the systems in which they function.

Endocrine gland, or ductless gland, secretions go directly into the bloodstream.

Hormones

Hormones are chemical messengers with specialized functions in regulating the activities of specific cells, organs, or both. The classes of hormones are based on their chemical composition, as follows: amines, derived from one amino acid; peptides, derived from many amino acids; and steroids, converted from the parent composition cholesterol.

Other hormones produced in the body include prostaglandins and neurohormones.

Prostaglandins. **Prostaglandins** secrete hormones in tissues throughout the body; their activity depends on which tissue secretes them.

Function of the Endocrine System

Endocrine glands are ductless glands; hormones are secreted directly into the bloodstream. Glands include the *pituitary, thyroid, parathyroid, thymus, adrenal, pancreas, gonads,* and *pineal.*

Hormonal Control

Hormonal control is governed by a negative feedback system; it is under the control of the nervous system.

Negative feedback occurs when there is a drop in the level of the hormone in the blood; this triggers a chain of events that occurs to increase the amount of hormone in the blood.

Pituitary Gland

The **pituitary gland**, or hypophysis, is located in the sphenoid bone and has an anterior and posterior portion. It is called the master gland because it controls the activities of other endocrine glands. It has two lobes.

The **posterior lobe** stores *oxytocin* and *ADH*, which are manufactured in the hypothalamus.

The **anterior lobe** secretes *GH* (growth), *TSH* (thyroid), *ACTH* (adrenal), *FSH* (ovary and testes), *LH* (ovary), *PR* (mammary gland), and *ICSH* (testes).

The **intermediate lobe** consists of only a few cells that produce melanocyte-stimulating hormone, which stimulates the melanin cells in the skin.

Thyroid and Parathyroid Glands

The thyroid and parathyroid glands are located in the neck, close to the cricoid cartilage of the larynx (Adam's apple).

The **thyroid gland** is located in the anterior portion of the neck; the thyroid cells are stimulated by TSH of the pituitary to produce T_3, T_4, and calcitonin. $\mathbf{T_3}$ **and** $\mathbf{T_4}$ function as *thyroxine*, which controls the rate of metabolism and how cells utilize oxygen, stimulates protein synthesis, stimulates the breakdown of liver glycogen, and stimulates the cellular breakdown of glucose. **Calcitonin** controls the calcium ion concentration in the blood by lowering the blood calcium level.

There are four **parathyroid glands;** they are located on the posterior side of the thyroid and produce *parathormone*, which controls the calcium ion concentration in the blood by raising the blood calcium level.

Thymus Gland

The **thymus gland** is posterior to the sternum and secretes many hormones, one of which is thymosin. **Thymosin** stimulates lymph cells to produce T-lymphocytes, which produce antibodies against certain diseases.

Adrenal Glands

The **adrenal glands** are located over the top of the kidneys and are divided into two parts, the cortex and medulla. The adrenal cortex produces:

Mineral corticoids—mainly *aldosterone*, which affects the kidney tubule and plays an important role in electrolyte and water balance.

Glucocorticoids—mainly *cortisol* and *cortisone*, which increase the amount of glucose in the blood.

Androgen—a male sex hormone responsible for male characteristics.

The adrenal medulla responds to the sympathetic nervous system and produces epinephrine (adrenaline) and norepinephrine.

Gonads

Gonads or **sex glands** include the ovaries in the female and testes in the male. *Ovaries* secrete estrogen and progesterone necessary for ovulation and female sex characteristics. *Testes* have cells that produce sperm and the testosterone essential for the male sex characteristics.

Pancreas

The **pancreas** is posterior to the stomach and produces insulin and glucagon. *Insulin* promotes the utilization of glucose in the cells; it is important in protein and fat metabolism. *Glucagon* increases the blood level of glucose.

Pineal Gland

The **pineal gland** is a pinecone-shaped organ attached to the third ventricle; it produces melatonin, which causes body temperature to drop.

The Effects of Aging on the Endocrine System

The production of hormones is reduced as the body ages.

Disorders of the Endocrine System

Most endocrine system disorders occur because of oversecretion (hyperfunction) or undersecretion (hypofunction) of hormones.

HYPERFUNCTION	HYPOFUNCTION
PITUITARY DISORDERS	
Gigantism: an overgrowth of long bones that occurs in childhood	Dwarfism: occurs in children; body has normal proportions and intelligence is normal
Acromegaly: overdevelopment of bones of the face in adults	Diabetes insipidus: a decrease of ADH, causing an excessive loss of water
THYROID DISORDERS	
Hyperthyroidism: increase in thyroxine; symptoms include hypertension, tachycardia, goiter, and exophthalmos	Hypothyroidism: decrease in thyroxine, which slows metabolic processes Myxedema: severe form of hypothyroidism that slows body processes to critical condition; occurs in adults Cretinism: occurs in children; slows mental and physical development
PARATHYROID DISORDERS	
Kidney stones and bone deformity	Severely diminished calcium levels, which lead to tetany
ADRENAL DISORDERS	
Cushing's syndrome: includes hypertension, muscular weakness, and "moon" face	*Addison's* disease: symptoms are bronze skin and electrolyte imbalance
PANCREAS DISORDERS	
Unknown	Diabetes mellitus: hypofunction of the islets of Langerhans, which produce insulin

Diabetes Mellitus. *Diabetes mellitus* is of two types:

Type I—no insulin is produced; occurs mostly in juveniles.

Type II—small or inadequate amounts of insulin produced; occurs mainly in adults.

Because of the lack of insulin in diabetes mellitus, cells are unable to obtain glucose, resulting in hyperglycemia. For oxidation to occur, the body must oxidize fats, causing a buildup of ketone bodies, leading to ketoacidotic coma. Patients must be familiar with signs of hypoglycemia and hyperglycemia.

Treatment for type I diabetes is insulin, exercise, and diet control. Treatment for type II is oral hypoglycemic agents, exercise, and diet control.

ACTIVITIES

A. Answer the following questions.

1. Two systems are responsible for coordination of body activities. They are the ____________________ and the ____________________.
2. Glands that make secretions are composed of ____________________ tissue.
3. Compare the endocrine and exocrine glands.

____

____

____

____

B. Select the letter of the choice that best completes the statement.

1. The type of hormone derived from a single amino acid is called a(n)
   a. peptide.
   b. amine.
   c. steroid.
   d. prostaglandin.
2. ___________ is a hormone produced in the adipose tissue.
   a. Leptin
   b. Thyroid
   c. Mineralcorticoid
   d. Ghrelin
3. Hormones converted from cholesterol are
   a. steroids.
   b. peptides.
   c. neurohormones.
   d. amines.

4. Hormones secreted by the hypothalamus that influence the secretions of pituitary are
   a. prostaglandins.
   b. steroids.
   c. neurohormones.
   d. ghrelins.
5. Hormones that consist of three or more amino acids are:
   a. steroids.
   b. peptides.
   c. amines.
   d. prostaglandins.
6. Leptins act in the hypothalamus to
   a. increase the appetite.
   b. influence the secretions of the pituitary.
   c. suppress the appetite.
   d. induce labor.
7. Insulin is found in the pancreas and is a type of
   a. amine.
   b. peptide.
   c. steroid.
   d. neurohormone.
8. The activity of __________ depends on the type of tissue that secretes them.
   a. prostaglandins
   b. amines
   c. peptides
   d. steroids
9. Estrogen is considered to be a type of
   a. steroid.
   b. leptin.
   c. peptide.
   d. prostaglandin.
10. An appetite stimulant produced by the stomach is
    a. mineralcorticoid.
    b. insulin.
    c. ghrelin.
    d. leptin.

C. Label the glands of the endocrine system.

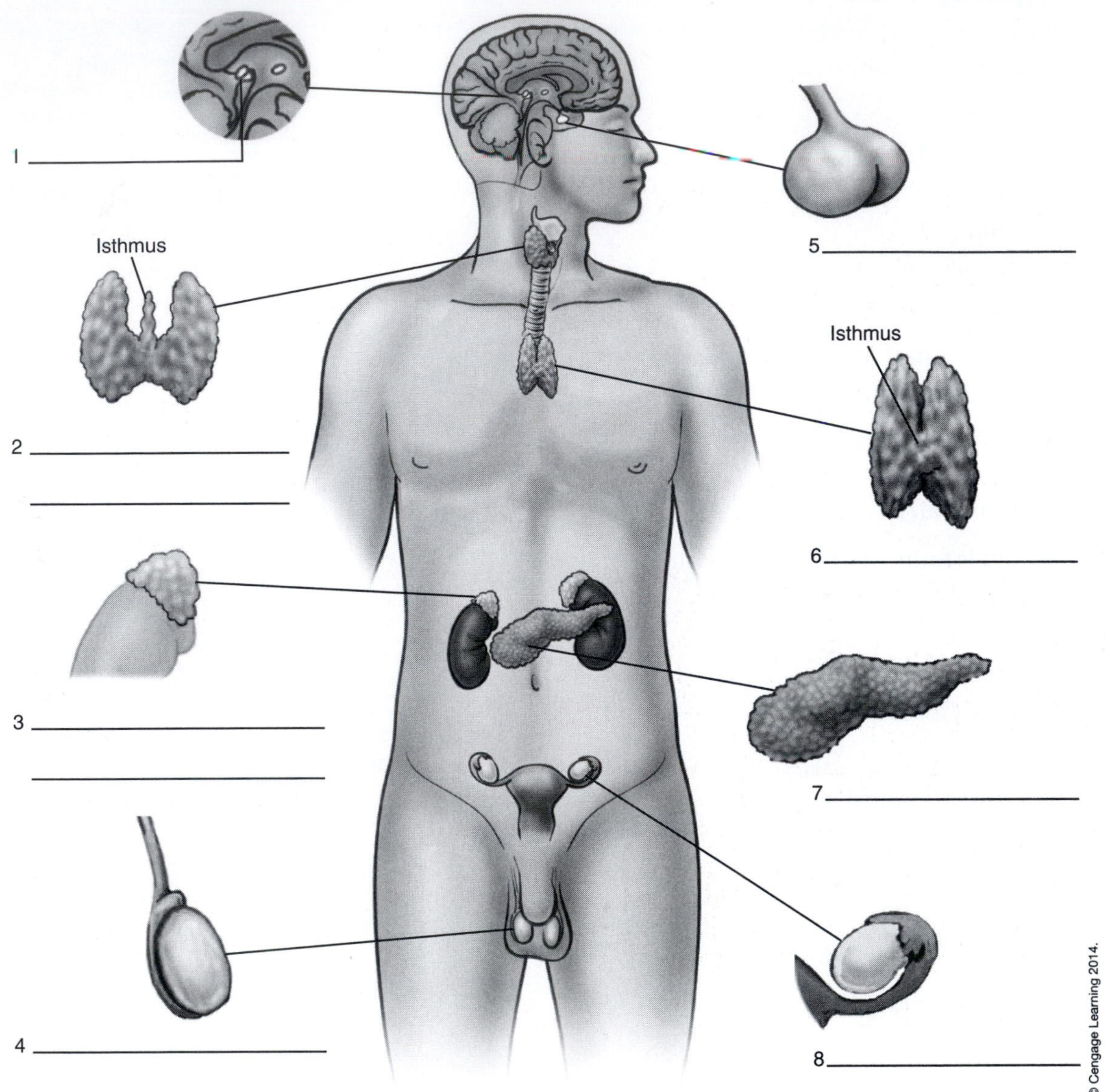

D. 1. Complete the diagram of the anterior pituitary, the hormones produced, and the organs affected by these hormones.

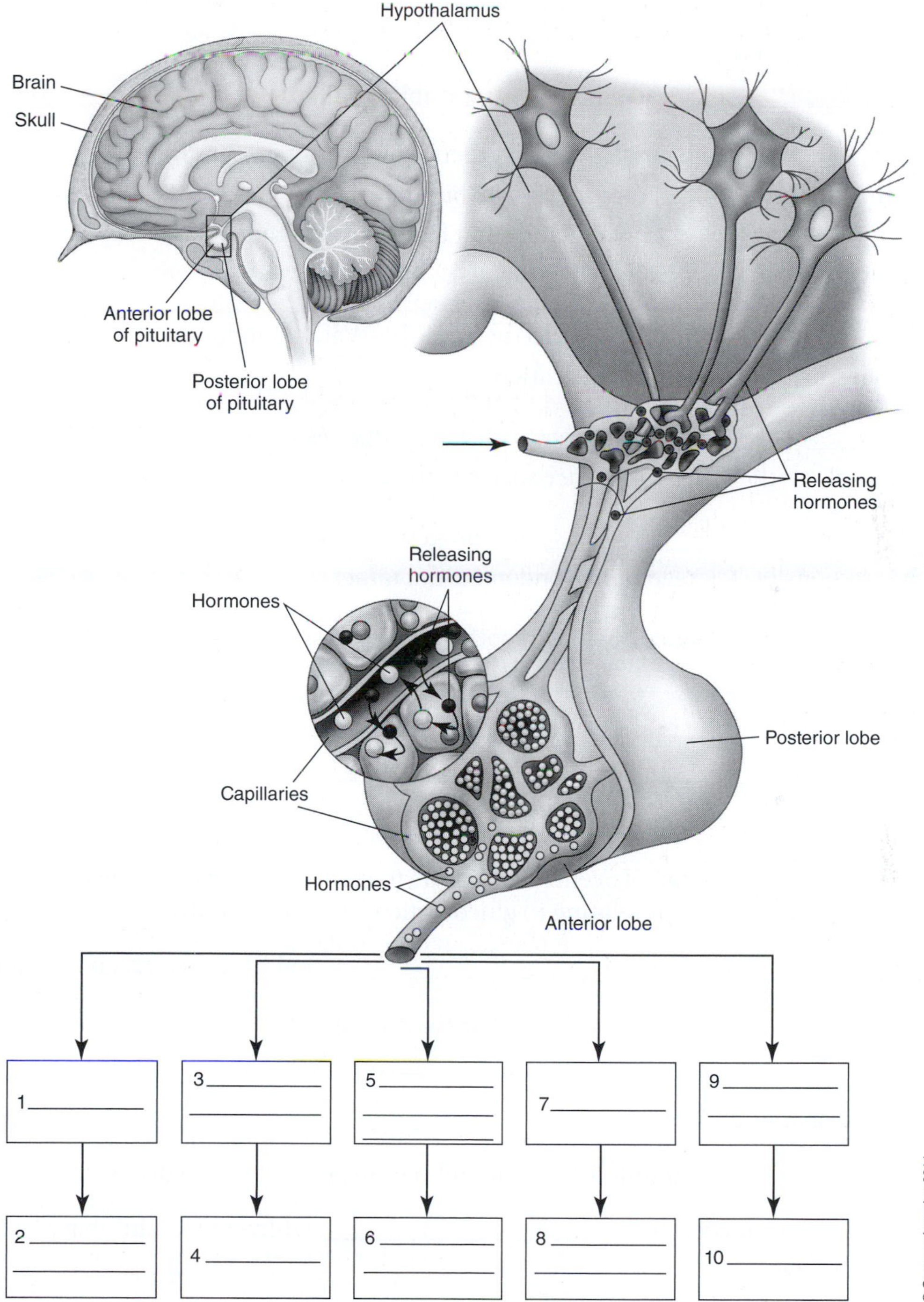

2. Describe the interaction between the hypothalamus and the anterior pituitary.

____

____

____

E. In this exercise, fill in the blanks with the acronyms for the hormones of the pituitary gland.

THE ALPHABET SOUP RHYME

Whether you are short or tall,
the ____________________ hormone is responsible for all.

____________________ helps the cells to produce testosterone,
which changes boys' voices from soprano to baritone.
____________________ works on glands that have a neat perch;
they sit over the kidneys and watch the waterworks.

The ____________________ belongs to the Save-the-Water foundation;
when doing its job it prevents dehydration.

____________________ stimulates the ovary to produce estrogen;
it also stimulates the testes to produce sperm in men.

The hormone ____________________ gets progesterone into the act,
which is responsible for keeping the endometrium intact.

F. Name the hormones produced by the hypothalamus and stored in the posterior pituitary lobe.

____

____

____

____

G. Negative feedback is a chain of events that occurs to maintain the blood level of a hormone. Complete the following steps relating to glucocorticoid secretion control.

1. The blood level of glucocorticoid ____________________ and triggers a chain reaction.
2. The ____________________ of the brain gets the message and sends a releasing factor for ____________________ to the ____________________ gland.
3. The gland responds and releases ____________________.
4. ____________________ stimulates the adrenal cells to produce glucocorticoid.
5. The blood level of glucocorticoid ____________________, which in turn inhibits the releasing factor in the brain.

H. Mark the underlined word in the statement true or false. Correct the false statements.

1. ____________________ To form hormones of the <u>parathyroid</u> gland, iodine is needed.
2. ____________________ The <u>thymus</u> gland is part of the lymphatic and endocrine system.
3. ____________________ The hormone of the <u>thyroid</u> is needed for the conversion of glycogen from sources other than sugar.

4. ______________________ Parathormone is produced by the <u>parathyroid</u> gland.

5. ______________________ How cells use glucose and oxygen to produce heat and energy is affected by the secretion of the <u>parathyroid</u> gland.

6. ______________________ This hormone produced by the <u>parathyroid</u> gland decreases calcium levels in the blood.

7. ______________________ The lymphoid cells responsible for T-lymphocytes are influenced by the hormone produced by the <u>thymus</u> gland.

8. ______________________ Calcitonin is produced by the <u>thyroid</u> gland.

9. ______________________ This secretion of the <u>parathyroid</u> gland helps in protein synthesis.

10. ______________________ The <u>parathyroid</u> gland is located posterior to the sternum.

I. Label the following diagram regarding the effects of parathormone and calcitonin on calcium concentration in the blood.

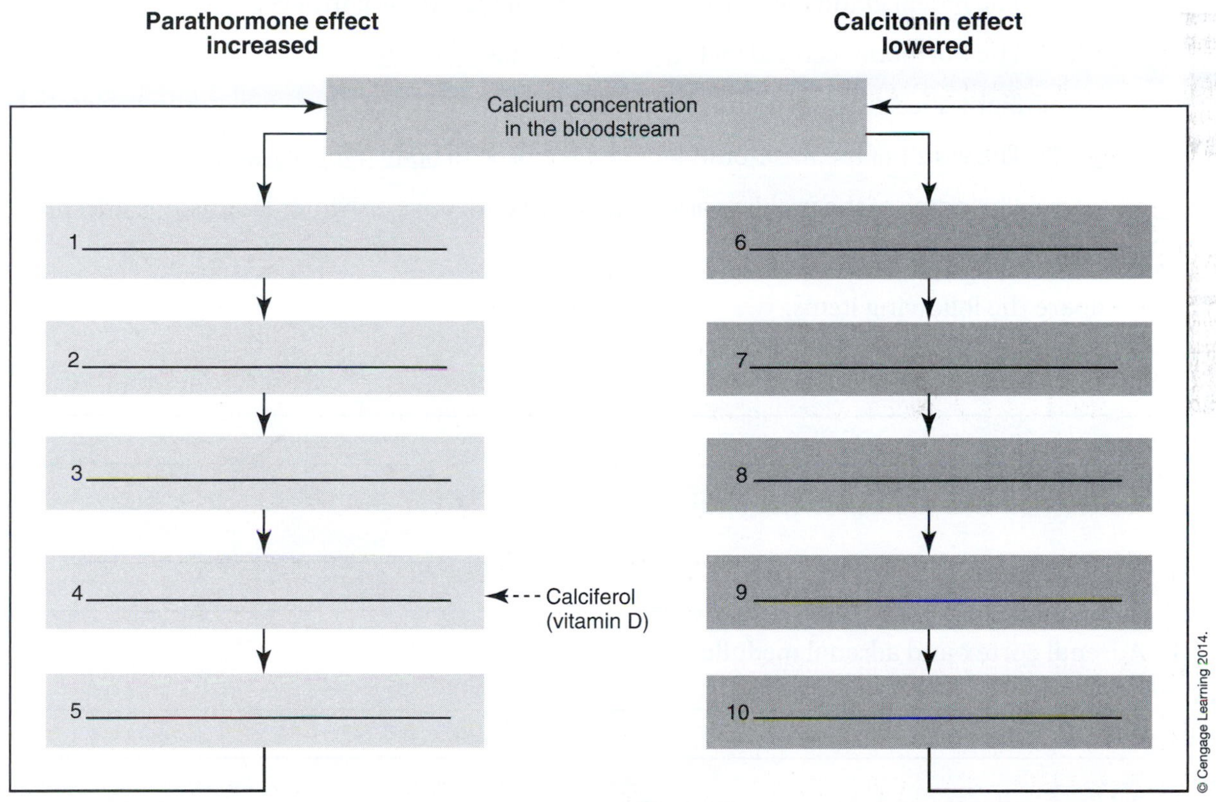

J. Answer the following questions about the adrenal glands.

1. The adrenal glands are located on top of the kidneys. Name the two parts of each gland.

____

2. Name and describe the functions of the hormones of the adrenal cortex.

a. ____

____

b. ____

____

c. ____

____

3. Next to each statement, write whether it is an effect of **epinephrine** or **norepinephrine** secreted by the adrenal medulla.
   a. Dilatation of the iris ______________
   b. Vasoconstriction of the muscles ______________
   c. Increase in heart rate ______________
   d. Rise in blood pressure, both systolic and diastolic ______________
   e. Increase in blood flow to muscles ______________
   f. Slight effect on cardiac output ______________

K. Mark the underlined word or words in the following statements either true or false. Correct any false statements.

________ 1. The pineal gland reacts to the amount of light entering the eye.

________ 2. The hormone secreted by the pineal gland is melanin.

________ 3. Light affects the secretion of the pineal; when it is dark, more melatonin is secreted.

________ 4. The result of the melatonin secreted is a drop in body temperature.

________ 5. The name of the problem associated with dark days or winter is sunshine affective disorder.

L. Compare the following items.

1. Myxedema and cretinism

____

____

2. Anterior pituitary and posterior pituitary

____

____

3. Adrenal cortex and adrenal medulla

____

____

4. Addison's disease and Cushing's syndrome

____

____

5. Type I diabetes and type II diabetes

____

____

6. Short stature and cretinism

____

____

M. Circle the correctly spelled words in each of the following statements.

1. Hypersecretion of the pituitary increases GH, which leads to (gigantism, gigiantism), an overgrowth of long bones.
2. In (diabetes insipidus, diabetes insepidus), there is a decrease of ADH, and a person will complain of (polydypsia, polydipia).
3. An increase of GH in adults is called (acromegaly, acramegaly) and results in an overgrowth of the bones of the face, hands, and feet.
4. Hypofunction of the pituitary leads to short stature, in which growth of the long bones is (abnormally, abnormaly) decreased.
5. The body of a person with short stature is of normal (porportion, proportion) and (intelligence, intellegence) is normal.

N. Complete the following word puzzle relating to hyperthyroidism by using the word clues given.

Puzzle	Clues
_ _ _ _ h _ _ _ _ _ _ _	1. bulging of the eyeballs
_ _ y _ _ _ _ _ _	2. secretion of the thyroid gland
_ _ _ _ p _ _ _ _ _ _ _	3. increase in sudoriferous gland activity
_ _ _ _ e _ _ _ _ _ _	4. these become fast growing and rougher
_ _ r _ _ _ _ _ _ _ _ _	5. person may also suffer from this
_ _ _ _ _ t _ _ _ _ _ _	6. increased blood pressure
_ _ _ h _ _ _ _ _ _ _	7. increased heart rate
_ _ _ _ y _ _ _ _ _ _ _ _ _ _ _	8. medication used to treat disease
_ r _ _ _ _ _	9. this may develop with disease
_ _ _ _ o _ _ _ _ _	10. sugar in the urine
_ _ _ i _ _ _ _ _ _ _	11. the type of iodine used in the test
_ _ _ _ _ _ d _ _ _ _ _ _	12. another name for hyperthyroidism
_ _ i _ _ _	13. enlargement of the thyroid
_ _ _ _ s _ _ _ _ _ _ _ _	14. the cause of hyperthyroidism
_ _ _ _ _ m _ _ _	15. goal is to reduce the activity of the thyroid gland

O. Select the letter of the choice that best completes the statement.

1. In severe hypothyroidism in adults, the condition is known as
   a. Graves' disease.
   b. myxedema.
   c. cretinism.
   d. Addison's disease.

2. Hypothyroidism symptoms include all of the following, *except*
   a. dry, brittle hair.
   b. sweaty and clammy skin.
   c. constipation.
   d. muscle cramps.

3. Hyperfunction of the parathyroid leads to
   a. kidney stones.
   b. tetany.
   c. spasms of the respiratory muscles.
   d. decreased calcium blood levels.

4. Hyperfunction of the parathyroid causes the bones to
   a. develop arthritic changes.
   b. become more flexible.
   c. become brittle.
   d. shorten.

5. Hypofunction of the parathyroid leads to ________.
   a. myxedema
   b. goiter
   c. tetany
   d. exophthalmos

P. Write **C** if the following conditions refer to Cushing's syndrome or **A** if they refer to Addison's disease.

________ 1. Hypersecretion of adrenal cortex

________ 2. Decrease in sodium level in blood

________ 3. Bronze skin

________ 4. "Moon" face

________ 5. Low blood pressure

________ 6. Hyposecretion of adrenal cortex

________ 7. Electrolyte imbalance

________ 8. Hirsutism

________ 9. Hypoglycemia

________ 10. Obesity

________ 11. More frequent in women

________ 12. Redistribution of body fat

Q. What is the reason for the symptoms of polyuria, polydypsia, and polyphagia in type I diabetes mellitus?

____

____

____

____

____

____

R. State whether the following pertains to hypoglycemia or hyperglycemia.

1. skin is flushed, dry, and hot ______________
2. breath has no odor ______________
3. onset is slow ______________
4. pale, moist skin ______________
5. blood sugar over 150 ______________
6. onset is sudden ______________
7. person is drowsy, lethargic, and weak ______________
8. person is nervous, trembling, and confused ______________
9. breath has fruity odor ______________
10. blood sugar below 80 ______________

S. Find the following words related to the endocrine system.

acromegaly
ACTH
Addison's disease
adrenal
adrenalin
androgen
calcitonin
cretinism
Cushing's syndrome
diabetes insipidus
diabetes mellitus
dwarfism
estrogen
exocrine
FSH
GH
gigantism
glucagon
goiter
gonads
hormones
hyperthyroidism
hypothyroidism
ICSH
insulin
LH
melatonin
myxedema
norepinephrine
oxytocin
pancreas
parathormone
parathyroid
pineal
pituitary
PR
progesterone
prostaglandin
testosterone
thymus
thyroid
thyroxin
TSH

d h S a i T g p r o g e s t e r o n e g s a t

i y a l n n e o O b W H R K H S T e o u d h p

a p G m r d s m i i O E Z M d p s n m r y t a

b e n f e N r u o t E X O k z a a y e r G H r

e r i J x d z o l r e J y M e d h n o G H N a

t t d h o P e p g i d r c s s t a i t s o u t

e h n n c R q x l e n n i r m l d y l W r Z h

s y a L r y s l y C n d y c e e a a s D m D o

m r l U i A O h q m s a d s a t l E i w o s r

e o g l n l G p W ' c e g i s l i a O Z n H m

l i a a e v F y n r E i P d o g c n t E e T o

l d t e H F n o o s g e w K o r n i i o s C n

i i s n S B s m n a f a x x t n y i t s n A e

t s o i F i e i n B r r y h Y s e h h o m i a

u m r p d g l t y f H t y c q Y a g t s n c n

s P p d a a i r i n o r B h A K y e o a u i o

s K A l n s a s o c o b w F z y h K r r r C n

L H y e m t m g i x c v Z X I E U K k c t a Z

H M r n i W a n i B r Q R i o H S C l K n s p

L d c u E c w n e n o r e t s o t s e t A a e

a J t G u n o r e p i n e p h r i n e m d E p

i i J l F u i O m s i d i o r y h t o p y h c

p E g d i a b e t e s i n s i p i d u s k u q

APPLYING THEORY TO PRACTICE

1. It is difficult to imagine that a pea-sized organ affects so many body activities. If a person had a tumor of the pituitary causing hypersecretion of hormones, what would be the result?

2. a. Carolyn has thyroid cancer and is having a thyroidectomy done. Why is there a vial of calcium gluconate at the bedside?

   b. After surgery, Carolyn will have to take thyroxine. What is one of the most important things to remember about this medication?

3. a. A classroom discussion develops regarding the number of people who will be diagnosed with diabetes mellitus in the next 20 years. The teacher divides the class in two. One group states that more people will be affected; give the rationale. The other group says less; give the rationale.

____

____

____

b. What are some of the latest advances in the treatment of diabetes?

____

____

____

c. What is the goal of diabetes treatment?

____

____

4. What is the most serious complication of hypofunction of the parathyroid gland?

____

____

____

____

5. Dan comes to the HMO office complaining of weakness, weight loss, and vomiting. Lauren, the medical assistant, notices that Dan's skin appears bronzed. Name the condition Dan may be diagnosed as having. How is this condition treated?

____

____

6. Nichole, age 14, wants to become an expert swimmer. She hears about using steroids to make her stronger. What advice should the health care professional give Nichole regarding the use of steroids?

____

____

7. Victoria states that because she has so much stress in her job she is having problems sleeping and remembering things. How does stress affect one's mental and physical state? What role does hormonal imbalance play in our physical and mental health?

____

____

____

____

8. Your aunt tells you the doctor has diagnosed her with type II diabetes. She is 70 years old and has always exercised and kept her weight in line with recommended weight charts. The doctor tells her the reason for her condition has something to do with hormonal changes occurring at her age.

   Explain to your aunt how the endocrine system is affected with age.

   ____
   ____
   ____
   ____

9. The endocrine system helps to coordinate and integrate body functions through hormones and maintain homeostasis. How does the endocrine system interact with other body systems to maintain homeostasis?

   ____
   ____
   ____
   ____
   ____
   ____
   ____
   ____
   ____

SURF THE NET

For additional information and interactive exercises, use the following key words:

- endocrine system—glands and hormones
- hormonal control—negative feedback
- structure, function, and hormones secreted—pituitary, thyroid, parathyroid, adrenal, pancreas, thymus, gonads
- fight-or-flight response
- disorders of endocrine system—gigantism, acromegaly, dwarfism, Graves' disease, cretinism, myxedema, tetany, Cushing's syndrome, Addison's disease
- steroid use and abuse
- diabetes mellitus—types, occurrence, treatment, complications, and prognosis

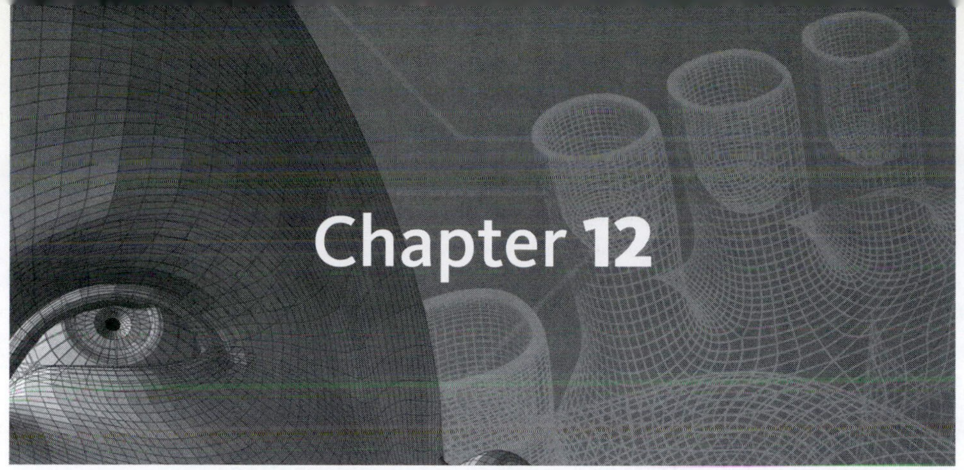

Blood

OVERVIEW

The major function of **blood** is to transport fluid, carrying nutrients and waste products, throughout the body. It also aids in the distribution of heat, helps regulate acid–base balance, fights infection, and produces clots to prevent excessive bleeding.

Blood Composition

Blood is made of plasma, red blood cells (erythrocytes), white blood cells (leukocytes), and thrombocytes (platelets).

Blood Plasma

Blood plasma is a straw-colored fluid containing 92% water and the following *plasma proteins:*

Fibrinogen is necessary for blood clotting.
Albumin maintains osmotic pressure.
Globulin synthesizes antibodies (gamma globulin).
Prothrombin helps to coagulate blood.

Blood also contains the following:

Nutrients: glucose, fatty acids, cholesterol, and amino acids
Electrolytes: sodium, chloride, and potassium
Other material: hormones, vitamins, enzymes, and metabolic waste products

Formation of Blood Cells

Red blood cells, or erythrocytes, are biconcave cells that have no nucleus and contain hemoglobin. **Hemoglobin** is made from heme (iron) and globin (protein) and carries oxygen and carbon dioxide. **Erythropoiesis** is the manufacture of red blood cells that occurs in the bone marrow. **Hemolysis** is the rupture or bursting of red blood cells. The *normal red blood cell count* is 4.5 to 6.2 million in men and 4.2 to 5.4 million in women.

White Blood Cells

White blood cells, or leukocytes, protect against infection and injury. The two types of leukocytes are granulocytes and agranulocytes.

Granulocytes have cytoplasmic granules; the three types are neutrophils, eosinophils, and basophils.

Neutrophils perform phagocytosis (engulf and digest harmful substances).

Eosinophils perform phagocytosis and increase in allergic reactions.

Basophils perform phagocytosis and increase during inflammation.

Agranulocytes have no granules in the cytoplasm; the two types are monocytes and lymphocytes.

Monocytes aid in phagocytosis.

Lymphocytes synthesize and release antibodies formed by the lymph nodes, the B-lymphocytes formed in bone marrow, and the T-lymphocytes formed in the thymus gland.

Leukocyte count is normally 3,200 to 9,800 cells. Leukocytes help protect the body against infection by (1) phagocytosis and destruction of bacteria, (2) synthesis of antibody molecules, (3) cleaning up of cellular remnants after inflammation, and (4) walling off the infected area.

Inflammation

Inflammation occurs when tissues are subjected to physical or chemical trauma or are invaded by pathogenic organisms. The process includes basophils releasing histamine, which is responsible for the increased permeability of the blood vessels, which then allows large amounts of white blood cells through the capillaries to phagocytize and bring antibodies to the site.

The result of inflammation is pus (a fluid filled with dead and live bacteria), white blood cells, and plasma. If the damage is below the skin, an *abscess* may form; if it is above the skin, an *ulcer* may form.

Thrombocytes (Blood Platelets)

Thrombocytes, or platelets, are not true cells but pieces of large megakaryocyte cells that help in blood clotting.

Coagulation, or **blood clotting,** is the process of forming a blood clot that depends on *platelets, thromboplastin, fibrinogen,* and *prothrombin.* Platelets and injured tissue release thromboplastin. The thromboplastin, calcium, and blood clotting factors change prothrombin to thrombin; finally, thrombin changes fibrinogen to fibrin (blood clot).

Thromboplastin also neutralizes the *anticoagulants* in the blood (antithromboplastin and antiprothrombin). *Clotting time* is the time it takes blood to clot (5 to 15 minutes).

Blood Types

Blood types are determined by the presence or absence of an *antigen* (anything that produces an antibody). They are classified as **O, A, B,** or **AB.** The plasma carries the antibodies for these antigens (i.e., a person with type A antigens has type B antibodies).

The **universal donor** is type O, because it carries no antigen; in an emergency, type O blood can be given to all patients.

The **universal recipient** is type AB. People with this type carry no antibodies in their plasma, so they can receive all four blood types.

Rh Factor

Rh factor is the presence of another antigen; if you have the antigen you are considered *Rh positive;* if you do not, you are considered *Rh negative.* This situation may present a problem in childbirth: An Rh-negative mother can produce an Rh-positive child, resulting in a condition known as *erythroblastosis fetalis.*

Disorders of the Blood

Anemia is a deficiency in the number or percentage of red blood cells and hemoglobin. Types of anemia include the following:

Hemorrhagic: due to loss of blood.

Iron deficiency: inadequate amount of iron in the diet; affects hemoglobin formation.

Pernicious: inadequate amount of vitamin B_{12} and intrinsic factor; affects the development of the red blood cells.

Aplastic: caused by suppression of the bone marrow by chemical agents, certain drugs, or radiation therapy.

Sickle cell: chronic blood disease inherited from both parents; causes abnormal shaping of the red blood cells, which then carry less oxygen and break easily.

Cooley's: caused by defect in hemoglobin formation.

Polycythemia occurs when too many red blood cells are being formed, causing a thickening in the blood with possible clot formation.

Embolism is a condition in which an embolus is carried by the bloodstream until it reaches an artery too small for passage. An *embolus* may be a blood clot, air, cancer cells, or any other substance foreign to the bloodstream.

Thrombosis is the formation of a blood clot in a blood vessel; it stays in the same place.

Hematoma describes a localized mass of blood in an organ, tissue, or space.

Hemophilia is an inherited disease in which there is a missing blood clotting factor; blood clots slowly or abnormally.

Thrombocytopenia is a decrease in the number of platelets.

Leukemia is a cancerous condition in which there is a great increase in the number of white blood cells.

Multiple myeloma is a malignant neoplasm of plasma cells.

Septicemia is the term used to describe pathogenic organisms or toxins in the blood.

ACTIVITIES

A. Select the letter of the choice that best completes the statement.

1. The liquid portion of blood called plasma contains water and other substances. The water makes up what percentage of the volume of plasma?
   a. 92%
   b. 53%
   c. 55%
   d. 43%

2. An average adult has ______________ of blood.
   a. 8 to 10 quarts
   b. 8 to 10 pints
   c. 6 to 8 pints
   d. 6 to 8 quarts
3. Blood does all of the following, *except*
   a. carry nutrients from the digestive tract to cells.
   b. secrete hormones.
   c. aid in the distribution of heat.
   d. regulate the acid–base balance.
4. The blood protein fibrinogen is necessary
   a. to maintain blood osmotic pressure.
   b. to carry oxygen and carbon dioxide.
   c. to destroy harmful bacteria.
   d. for blood clotting.
5. The plasma protein that maintains osmotic pressure and volume is
   a. fibrinogen.
   b. prothrombin.
   c. albumin.
   d. globulin.
6. The plasma protein responsible for the synthesis of antibodies is
   a. fibrinogen.
   b. prothrombin.
   c. gamma globulin.
   d. albumin.
7. The white blood cells include all of the following, *except*
   a. thrombocytes.
   b. lymphocytes.
   c. monocytes.
   d. polymorphonuclear leukocytes.
8. Vitamin K is necessary to synthesize ______________.
   a. albumin
   b. globulin
   c. prothrombin
   d. fibrinogen
9. Erythropoiesis is influenced by the hormone erythropoietin, which is secreted by the
   a. kidney.
   b. liver.
   c. spleen.
   d. heart.

10. The function of thrombocytes is to
    a. produce antibodies.
    b. carry oxygen and carbon dioxide.
    c. create a platelet plug.
    d. phagocytize pathogenic bacteria.

B. Using the following words, complete the story on the blood.

biconcave	erythropoiesis	hemoglobin	protein
blood vessel	flat	iron	recycle
carbon dioxide	folic acid	liver	red marrow
carbon monoxide	globin	lung	short
doughnut	hemacytoblast	nucleus	vitamin B_{12}
erythrocyte	heme	oxygen	

I AM THE RED BLOOD CELL

My manufacturing process goes by the fancy name of ____________. I originated from stem cells called ____________. When I am grown up I get my official name as a red blood cell or ____________.

I began life in a long bone structure, with white walls surrounding me; my special place of development is called ____________________.

Like any other teenager, as I grew, changes started to take place. First, I moved to another room in the house, called the ____________________ bones. Sometimes, for privacy, I crawled into another smaller boxlike structure called the ____________________ bones. I shed my ____________________ like teens shed baby fat and got a nice new shape, ____________________. Some people say I look good enough to eat with my ____________________ shape. To grow big and strong, I have a special food pyramid that includes plenty of ____________________, ____________________, cobalt, copper, and a great big helping of ____________________. I need this becausee my job description consists of two parts: an ironlike substance called ________________ and a(n) ________________ called ____________________.

Well, I finally graduated, and now I am armed with my job description, __________________, which sticks out all over me like pride. I am now ready to go to work.

I have applied for a job at the heart factory, in the circulation division, which means I will be working in these special tubes or ____________________ ____________________. My main function is to work as an escort service, picking up ____________________ from the __________, taking it first to the factory's pump division, then to cells, where it gets dropped off. My next stop is to pick up ____________________ ______________, which has been thrown out of a cell, take it back to the major distribution center, and then to the lungs, where it gets blown off.

On my next trip through the tubes, I spot the most attractive molecule, but I had better be careful. My mother has warned me against taking up with that molecule, ____________________ ____________________, because it will be a deadly combination.

I work very hard, but my days are numbered—usually I only last about 120 days and then they retire me to the ____________________ plant, the ____________________. I will not mind it too much because they recycle most of my parts and *I shall return.*

C. Label and color the cellular elements of the blood. Color erythrocytes red, granulocytes blue, and agranulocytes pink.

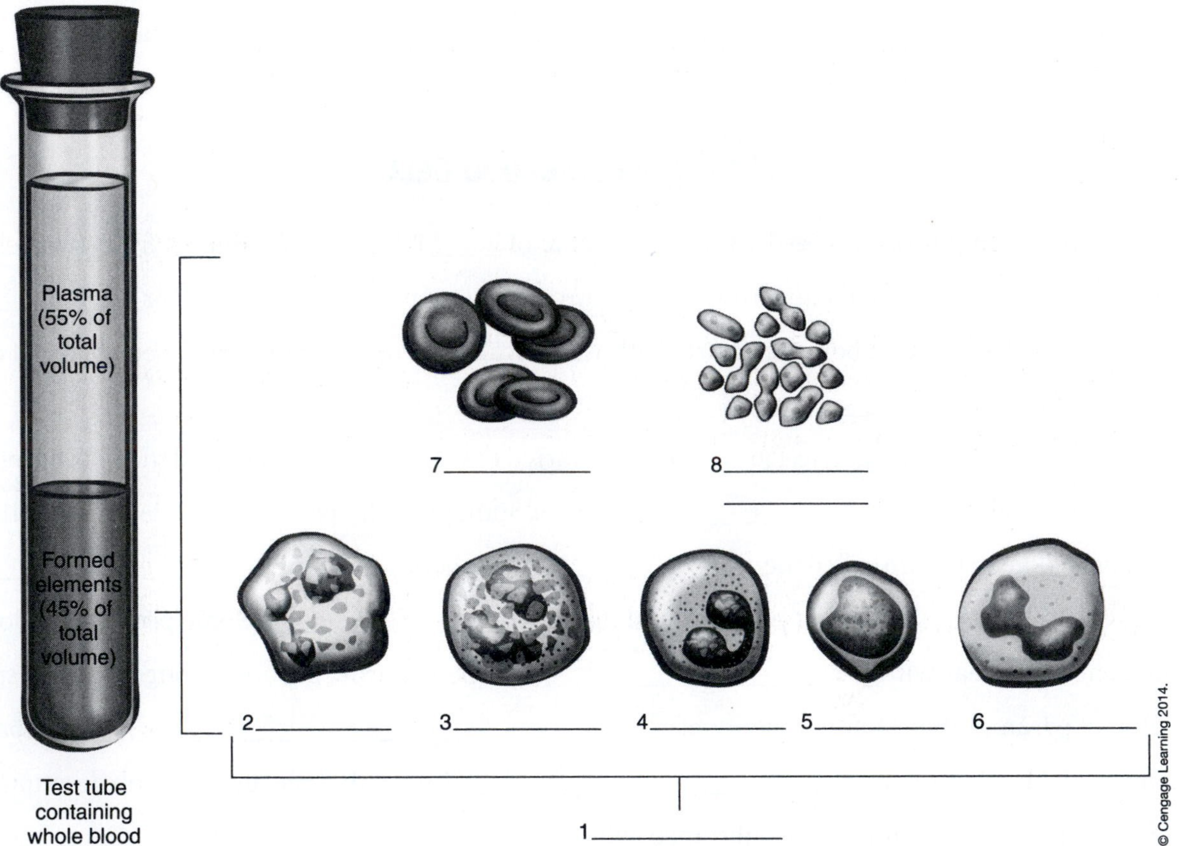

D. Using the following list of words, fill in the blanks with the name or action of the leukocytes. Words may be used more than once.

allergic
bacteria
basophil
diapedesis
eosinophil
heparin
histamine
infection
lymph
lymphocyte
monocyte
neutrophil
neutrophils
pathogenic
phagocytize
phil

THE LEUKOCYTE POEM

We are family, and we belong to the leukocyte tree.

The granulocytes workers are called ______________ and ______________________.
They are so busy at times, they work day and night.

Mono's job is to eat up _________________ and surround them with a wall.
____________________ performs an antibody reaction to slay ____________________,
the round, the short, and the tall.

It is a family tradition to have the young boy's name end in _____________________.
Their given names are ___________________, __________________,and __________________.

The _____________________ have many lobes and _____________________,
eating up bacteria and bringing them down to size.

Basophil produces _____________________ and _____________________,
which help fight _____________________, keeping wounds clean.

This blue lymphocyte named _____________________ pops up all over the place.
When you have a(n) _____________________ reaction he shows his face.

Most members of our granulocyte family have the ability to _____________________
through intercellular space, leaving not one _____________________ bacteria in place.

Now come, be our guest, and complete the following table to learn the rest.

E. Complete the following table on the characteristics and functions of the leukocytes.

Characteristics and Functions of the Leukocytes

LEUKOCYTE	WHERE FORMED	TYPE OF NUCLEUS	CYTOPLASM	FUNCTION
Agranular leukocytes 1. ______	3. ______	5. ______ Spherical ______: may be indented	Cytoplasm stains pale blue	7. ______
2. ______	4. ______	6. ______	Abundant cytoplasm	8. ______
Granular leukocytes a. ______	Formed in bone marrow from neutrophilic myelocytes	b. ______	Cytoplasm has a pink tinge with very fine granules	c. ______
d. ______	Formed in the bone marrow from eosinophilic myelocytes	Irregular shape with two lobes	Cytoplasm has a blue tinge with many coarse uniform round or oval bright-red granules	e. ______
f. ______ (mast cell)	Formed in the bone marrow from baso-philic myelocytes	g. ______	Cytoplasm has a mauve color with many large deep-purple granules	h. ______

F. Unscramble the letters to form the word that is the answer to the statement.

1. White blood cells with no granules in the cytoplasm — ENASOYCGAULTR
2. The ability to move through the intercellular spaces of the capillary walls to the surrounding tissue — EAISPEDIDS
3. A rupture or bursting of the red blood cell — YLEMOIHSS
4. Chemical produced by WBCs that increases blood flow to the injured area — ASIMITEHN
5. A decrease in the number of white blood cells — EAKLIUNEOP
6. Refers to stopping or controlling bleeding — ASSHETOMIS
7. Another term for a disease-causing microorganism — OCGPTEIHNA
8. A process that surrounds, engulfs, and digests harmful bacteria — OTCOIHGYASPS

9. A function of the blood that involves circulating antibodies to combat infection — IONCPERTOT

10. Blood test that measures the percentage of the volume of whole blood that is made up of red blood cells — TOCIMRTAEH

G. Answer the following questions regarding inflammation.

1. State the reasons for the process and symptoms of inflammation.

____

____

____

2. Describe the roles of the following in the process of inflammation.

   a. Histamine ____

   ____

   b. Fibrinogen ____

   ____

   c. Neutrophils ____

   ____

   d. Pyrogens ____

   ____

H. Match the statements in Column B with the words in Column A.

Column A	Column B
________ 1. pus	a. fever
________ 2. abscess	b. damaged area below epidermis
________ 3. pyrexia	c. normal white blood cell count
________ 4. leukocytosis	d. temperature control center
________ 5. leukopenia	e. phagocytosis
________ 6. ulcer	f. increase in number of neutrophils
________ 7. hypothalamus	g. liquid containing dead and live bacteria
	h. damaged area on epidermis
	i. decrease in number of white blood cells

I. Complete the statements by using the following words. Words may be used more than once.

blood clot	fibrin	prothrombin
blood clotting	fibrinogen	serum
calcium	injured tissue	thrombin
coagulation	liver	thromboplastin
crust		

1. A complicated and essential process that depends on thrombocytes is called ____________________ or ____________________.

2. Complete the following statements describing the blood clotting or coagulation process:
   a. Thromboplastin is released by ____________________ ____________________.
   b. Prothrombin is a plasma protein made in the ____________________.
   c. Thromboplastin and ____________________ ions react only in the presence of ____________________ to change ____________________ to ____________________.
   d. Thrombin changes ____________________ to ____________________.
   e. The ____________________ threads create a fine, meshlike network over the cut.
   f. The ____________________ network entraps red blood cells, platelets, and plasma, creating a ____________________ ____________________.
   g. At first, ____________________ oozes out of the cut; this dries and a ____________________ forms over the fibrin threads, completing the clotting process.

3. What is the role of thromboplastin with anticoagulants?

   ____

   ____

4. Where are prothrombin and fibrinogen manufactured?

   ____

   ____

J. Multiple choice: Blood tests are ordered by the physician to help diagnose diseases. Circle the normal test results in the following questions.

1. The average number of red blood cells in adult males is ____________ million.
   a. 4.5–7.2
   b. 5.4–6.2
   c. 4.5–6.2

2. The average adult white blood cell count is
   a. 5,000–9,000.
   b. 3,200–9,800.
   c. 9,000–10,000.

3. The average adult platelet count is
   a. 150,000–350,000.
   b. 250,000–450,000.
   c. 300,000–400,000.

4. The average adult coagulation time is ____________ minutes.
   a. 3–5
   b. 5–15
   c. 10–15

5. The average sedimentation rate for adult women is ___________ mm/hour.
   a. 0–20
   b. 10–20
   c. 15–25
6. The average hemoglobin amount for adult men is ___________ g/dl.
   a. 12–14
   b. 14–16
   c. 14–18
7. The average adult bleeding time is ___________ minutes.
   a. 1–3
   b. 3–5
   c. 5–7
8. The average hematocrit percent in an adult woman is
   a. 17%.
   b. 32%.
   c. 42%.
   d. 62%

K. Answer the following questions.

1. If the hemoglobin in an adult woman is 25% below normal, what is it?

   ____

2. If the platelet count is 0.20 below normal, what is it?

   ____

3. If the total number of white blood cells is 9,600, the percentage of the following groups is listed. How many of each type of WBC would there be?
   a. Lymphocytes 20%–59% ___________________
   b. Monocytes 5%–8% ___________________
   c. Granulocytes 60%–70% ___________________
4. Identify the four major blood groups.

   ____

   ____

5. How is blood type determined?

   ____

   ____

6. What is an agglutinin or antibody? Name the type of antibody for O, A, B, and AB blood.

   ____

   ____

7. What is the possible cause of death in a blood transfusion?

____

____

8. What is meant by the Rh factor?

____

____

9. Can a person with type A blood receive type O blood?

____

10. Define *universal donor* and *universal recipient.*

____

____

L. Complete the following table on blood types.

IF THE PATIENT'S BLOOD TYPE IS:	THE DONOR'S BLOOD TYPE MUST BE:
1.	O+, O−
O− (universal donor)	2.
A+	3.
4.	A−, O−
B+	B+, B−, O+, O−
5.	B−, O−
6.	AB+, AB−, A+, A−, B+, B−, O+, O−
AB−	7.

M. Circle the correctly spelled words in the following statements.

1. A decrease in the number of red blood cells and the amount of hemoglobin is called (anemia, anemea).
2. A drop in the number of red blood cells is characterized by (parlor, pallor), fatigue, (palpation, palpitation), and dyspnea.
3. A drop in hemoglobin means there is a deficiency of oxygen (transportaion, transportation) to the cells for oxidation.
4. Iron-deficiency anemia may be alleviated by intake of iron (supplyments, supplements) and green leafy (vegetables, vegtables).
5. The anemia caused by lack of vitamin B_{12} and/or the intrinsic factor is (pernicious, prenecious) anemia.
6. Polycythemia, a condition of too many red blood cells, causes (thickening, thickning) of the blood.

7. Embolus, a (foreign, foriegn) substance in the blood vessel, may be air, a blood clot, or another substance.
8. Thrombosis is the formation of blood clots, which may be caused by (mobility, immobility).
9. Hemophilia is a (heriditary, hereditary) disease that interferes with the blood clotting process.
10. (Septicemia, septecemia) is the presence of pathogenic organisms in the bloodstream.

N. Describe the disease and treatment for the following conditions:

a. Hemorrhagic anemia

____

____

b. Aplastic anemia

____

____

c. Polycythemia

____

____

d. Leukemia

____

____

e. Multiple myeloma

____

____

____

APPLYING THEORY TO PRACTICE

1. Safety experts advise people to have carbon monoxide detectors in their homes.
   a. What is the reason for this recommendation?

   ____

   b. What are the causes of carbon monoxide poisoning?

   ____

   ____

   c. What process occurs with carbon monoxide poisoning?

   ____

   ____

d. List the symptoms of carbon monoxide poisoning.

____

____

e. What safety rules should be followed to prevent carbon monoxide poisoning?

____

____

2. Mrs. Smith's baby is born with erythroblastosis fetalis. The mother is very upset. Explain the condition to her. Can this condition be prevented?

____

____

____

____

3. George has been tired, lethargic, and short of breath over the past few weeks. He decides to see his doctor. After an initial examination and blood test, the doctor's diagnosis is pernicious anemia. The doctor requests his office nurse, Kenneth, to explain pernicious anemia to George and discuss its cause and treatment.

____

____

____

____

4. In hemophilia, blood factor VIII is missing. How does this interfere with the clotting process?

____

____

5. Kyle is 6 years old and has been hospitalized with a sickle cell anemia episode. Kyle is listless and is complaining of severe pain in his knees. Kyle's parents are worried about his condition. Define sickle cell anemia. What is the cause of Kyle's pain? Explain to Kyle's parents the treatment options and the research currently being done.

____

____

____

____

6. Estelle, age 82, has been hospitalized for a fractured hip. What type of blood complication can occur because of the immobility?

____

____

7. What are some of the deciding factors that must be considered for a bone marrow transplant?

SURF THE NET

For additional information and interactive exercises, use the following key words:

- blood components and their function
- inflammation process
- blood clotting process
- blood types and incompatibility
- disorders of the blood—anemia, iron-deficiency anemia, pernicious anemia, aplastic anemia, Cooley's anemia, sickle cell anemia, polycythemia, embolism, thrombosis, multiple myeloma, septicemia
- bone marrow transplants
- Careers as clinical laboratory technicians and clinical laboratory technologists

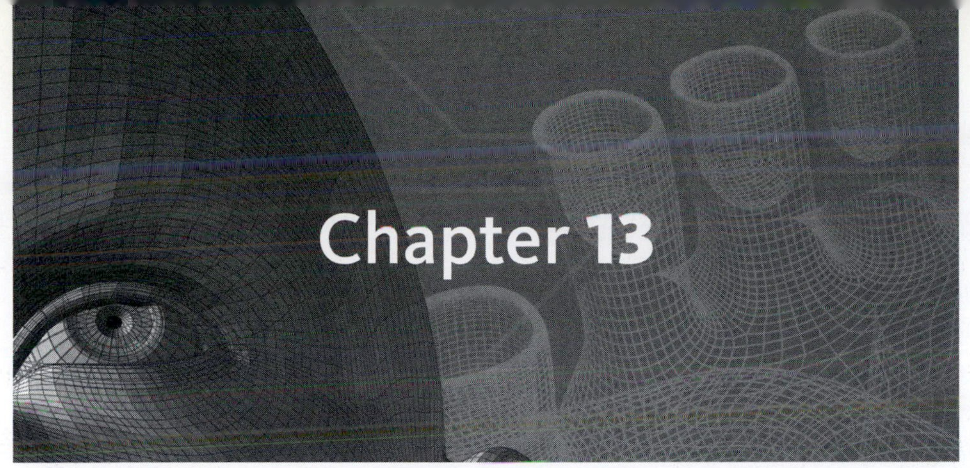

Heart

OVERVIEW

The circulatory system includes the heart, which pumps the blood to all parts of the body and carries away the waste products by means of arteries, capillaries, and veins.

Functions of the Circulatory System

The *heart* is the pump necessary to circulate blood to the body.

Arteries, veins, and *capillaries* are the structures that take blood from the heart to the cells and return blood from the cells back to the heart.

Blood carries oxygen, nutrients, and waste products.

The *lymph system* returns excess fluid from tissues to general circulation.

General, or *systemic,* circulation carries blood throughout the body. *Cardiopulmonary* circulation carries blood from the heart to the lungs and back to the heart.

Organs of the Circulatory System

The organs of the circulatory system include the heart, arteries, veins, capillaries, lymphatic system, and blood.

Structure of the Heart

The **heart** is a tough muscle, about the size of a fist, located in the thoracic cavity; the apex of the heart lies on the diaphragm and points toward the left side of the body.

The *structure* of the heart is a hollow, muscular, double pump, with the following layers:

Pericardium: fibrous, double outer layer that has pericardial fluid between the layers.

Myocardium: cardiac muscle tissue; the wall of the heart.

Endocardium: inner lining of the heart.

Septum: muscular wall that separates the heart into right and left sides.

Structures Leading to and from the Heart. The following passageways help circulate blood through the heart:

The *superior* and *inferior vena cava* are blood vessels that bring deoxygenated blood to the right atrium.

The *coronary sinus* opening takes blood from the heart muscle to the right atrium.

The *pulmonary artery* takes deoxygenated blood from the right ventricle to the lungs to exchange carbon dioxide for oxygen.

The *pulmonary vein* brings oxygenated blood from the lungs to the left atrium.

The *aorta* takes blood from the left ventricle to the body.

Chambers and Valves. The human heart is divided into four chambers. The four valves within the heart permit blood flow in one direction only.

Upper chambers: right and left atria or auricles.

Lower chambers: right and left ventricles.

Tricuspid valve: between the right atrium and right ventricle.

Bicuspid or *mitral valve:* between the left atrium and left ventricle.

Pulmonary semilunar valve: at the orifice of the pulmonary artery.

Aortic semilunar valve: at the orifice of the aorta.

Circulation/Physiology of the Heart. In the *right heart,* blood flows into the right atrium from the superior and inferior vena cava, through the tricuspid valve to the right ventricle, and through the pulmonary semilunar valve to the pulmonary artery, which takes blood to the lungs, where an exchange of gases—carbon dioxide for oxygen—takes place.

In the *left heart,* blood flows into the left atrium from the pulmonary veins, through the bicuspid valve to the left ventricle, and through the aortic semilunar valve to the aorta.

The *coronary artery* supplies blood to the heart muscle.

Heart Rate and Cardiac Output. The heart beats between 72 and 80 times per minute. The ventricles eject between 60 and 80 ml of blood with each beat; this is known as the stroke volume. The cardiac output is the total volume of blood ejected from the heart per minute.

Heart Sounds. The valves of the heart make a sound as they close, called the lubb-dupp sounds. The lubb sound is heard as the tricuspid and bicuspid valves close, and the dupp sound is heard as the semilunar valves close.

Conduction System of the Heart

The heart muscle is stimulated by specialized conducting cells in the right atrium known as the sinoatrial (SA) node, or pacemaker of the heart. The SA node sends an electrical impulse to the atrioventricular (AV) node, which sends an impulse to the conducting fibers in the septum known as the atrioventricular bundle. This impulse divides into a right and left branch, then subdivides into a network spreading through the ventricles called the Purkinje fibers. The electrical impulse continues to the apex of the heart.

The Effects of Aging on the Heart Muscle

With age, the heart muscle tissue is replaced with fibrous tissue and cardiac output decreases.

Prevention of Heart Disease. Heart disease is the number one leading cause of death in the United States. Steps to lower risk include prevention and control of cholesterol and triglyceride levels, prevention and control of high blood pressure, control of diabetes, maintaining a healthy weight, exercising regularly, and eating a nutritious diet.

Diseases of the Heart

Arrhythmia is any change or deviation from the normal heart rhythm.

Bradycardia is a slow heart rate, less than 60 beats per minute.

Tachycardia is a rapid heart rate, more than 100 beats per minute.

Murmurs are a gurgling or hissing sound that can indicate some type of defect in the valves of the heart.

Mitral valve prolapse is when the valves between the left atrium and the left ventricle do not close perfectly.

Diagnostic Tests for Heart and Circulatory Function. Tests done to determine the function of the heart and circulation include both noninvasive and invasive tests as well as blood tests. *Cardiac catheterization* is used to determine the patency of the coronary blood vessels and the efficiency of the structures of the heart.

Stress tests determine the physiological stress of vigorous exercise on the heart.

Infectious Diseases of the Heart. Infectious heart diseases are usually caused by bacteria or a virus.

Pericarditis is inflammation of the outer membrane of the heart.

Myocarditis is inflammation of the muscle of the heart.

Endocarditis is inflammation of the lining of the heart.

Rheumatic heart disease is the result of a strep infection; the antibodies formed to fight the strep infection attack the lining and valves of the heart, especially the bicuspid valve, which leads to scarring and the valve's inability to close properly.

Heart Disease. *Coronary artery disease* is the narrowing of the arteries that supply oxygen and nutrients to the heart. *Angina* is the most important symptom of this disease.

Angina pectoris is severe chest pain; it occurs when the heart does not receive an adequate oxygen supply.

Myocardial infarction (MI), or heart attack, is caused by a lack of blood supply to the myocardium, possibly due to a thrombus (blood clot).

Heart Failure. *Heart failure* occurs when the ventricles of the heart contract ineffectively and blood pools in the heart, leading to edema and ascites.

Congestive heart failure is similar to heart failure, but edema of the lower extremities also occurs.

Conduction Defects. *Conduction defects* occur when the electrical conduction of the heart is affected.

Heart block is the interruption of the AV node message from the SA node; there are three types: first-degree, second-degree, and third-degree (or complete) heart block.

Premature contractions occur when the heart sets up an ectopic beat; these may be premature atrial contractions, premature junctional contractions, or premature ventricular contractions. The premature ventricular contractions (PVCs) can be benign or deadly.

Fibrillation is when heart rhythm breaks down and muscle fibers contract without coordination; this disorder is life threatening and can be treated by a defibrillator.

For the **prevention** of heart disease, the National Institutes of Health states that lifestyle changes can reduce heart attacks.

Types of Heart Surgery

Angioplasty is a procedure that helps to open clogged vessels; it is also known as balloon angioplasty.

Coronary bypass is a detouring bypass to allow the blood supply to go around the blocked area of the coronary artery.

Heart transplants are done when an individual's heart can no longer function.

Cardiac stents are tiny webbed stainless steel devices that hold the arteries open after an angioplasty.

Transmyocardial laser revascularization (TMR) is used to puncture holes in the heart muscle to improve blood flow.

ACTIVITIES

A. Answer the following question.

1. List the functions of the circulatory system.

____

____

____

B. Select the letter of the choice that best completes the statement.

1. If the blood flow to the brain ceases for 5 to 10 seconds, the muscles will start to twitch convulsively within
   a. 1 minute.
   b. 15–20 seconds.
   c. 4–5 minutes.
   d. 6–9 minutes.

2. The average heart rate is ____________ beats per minute.
   a. 80–100
   b. 70–80
   c. 50–70
   d. 60–70

3. The recommended rate of chest compressions in cardiopulmonary resuscitation (CPR) is ______ per minute.
   a. 60
   b. 80
   c. 90
   d. 100

4. The heart is located in the thoracic cavity
   a. posterior to the sternum and superior to the diaphragm.
   b. posterior to the sternum and inferior to the diaphragm.
   c. anterior to the sternum and anterior to the vertebrae.
   d. inferior to the diaphragm and anterior to the vertebrae.

5. The heart pumps 5 quarts per minute. The amount of blood pumped in 1.5 hours is ______ quarts.
   a. 300
   b. 450
   c. 600
   d. 400

6. To listen to the heart sounds, place the stethoscope between the
   a. fifth and sixth ribs, middle of left clavicle.
   b. fifth and sixth ribs, middle of right clavicle.
   c. third and fourth ribs, middle of left clavicle.
   d. fourth and fifth ribs, middle of left clavicle.

7. The S_1 sound occurs when
   a. the tricuspid valve opens and the bicuspid valve closes.
   b. the semilunar valves close.
   c. the tricuspid valve closes and the bicuspid valve opens.
   d. both the tricuspid and bicuspid valves close.

8. The SA node sends an electrical impulse to the atria that causes them to
   a. rest.
   b. depolarize.
   c. repolarize.
   d. relax.

C. Follow the directions regarding each of the structures of the heart. Label the callouts according to the numbers.

1. Label and describe the layers of the heart.

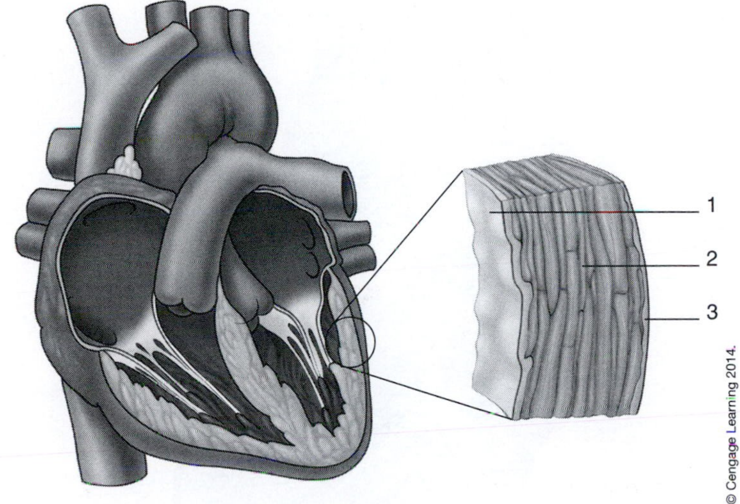

1. ______________________

2. ______________________

3. ______________________

2. Describe the double layer of fibrous tissue surrounding the heart. What is the name of the fluid between the two layers? What is the function of this fluid?

____

____

3. Label the chambers of the heart

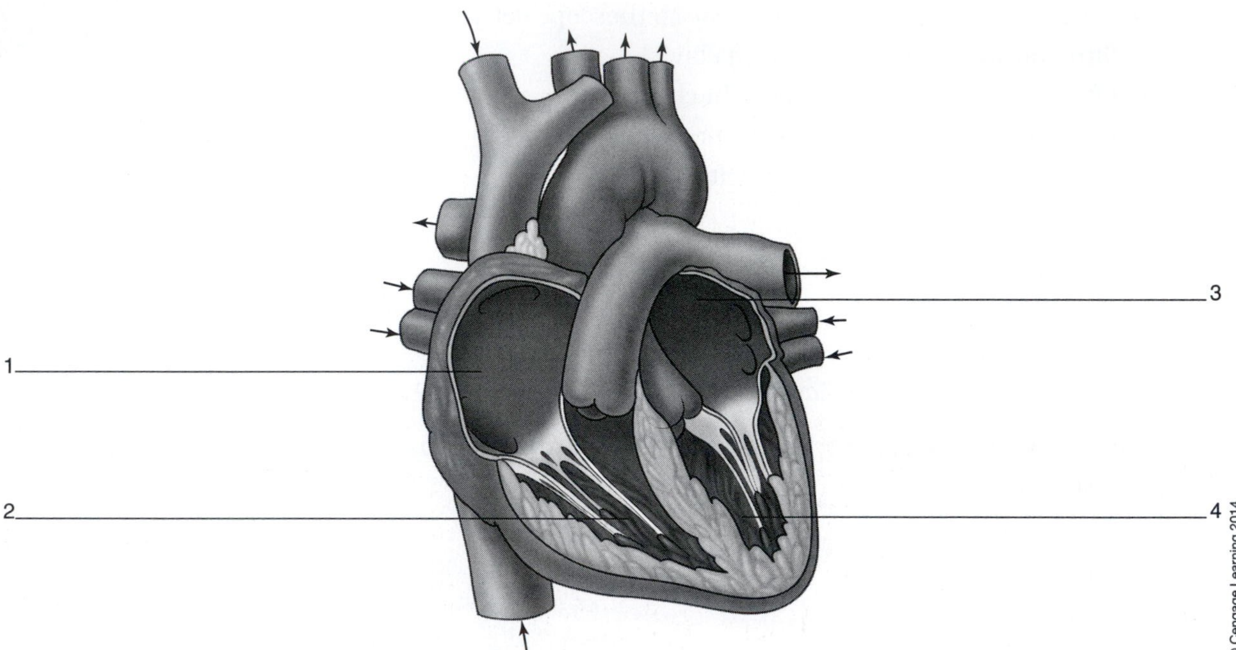

4. Label the structures leading to and from the heart.

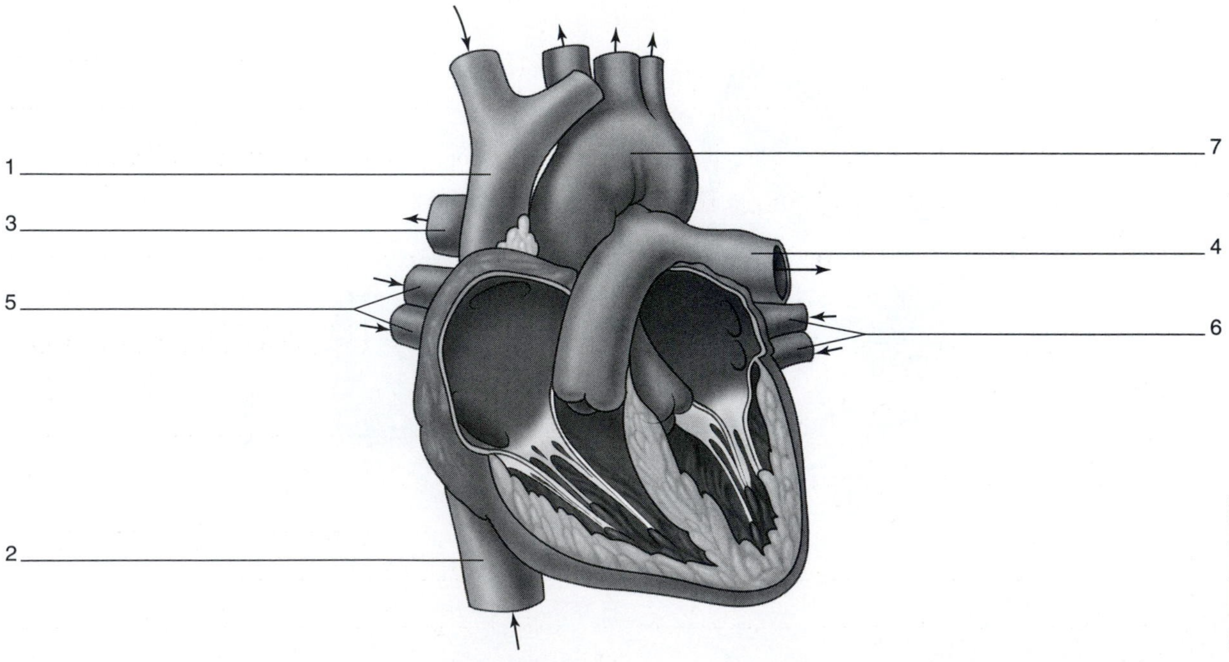

5. Where do these structures go to or come from?

____

____

____

____

6. Label the four valves of the heart and their locations.

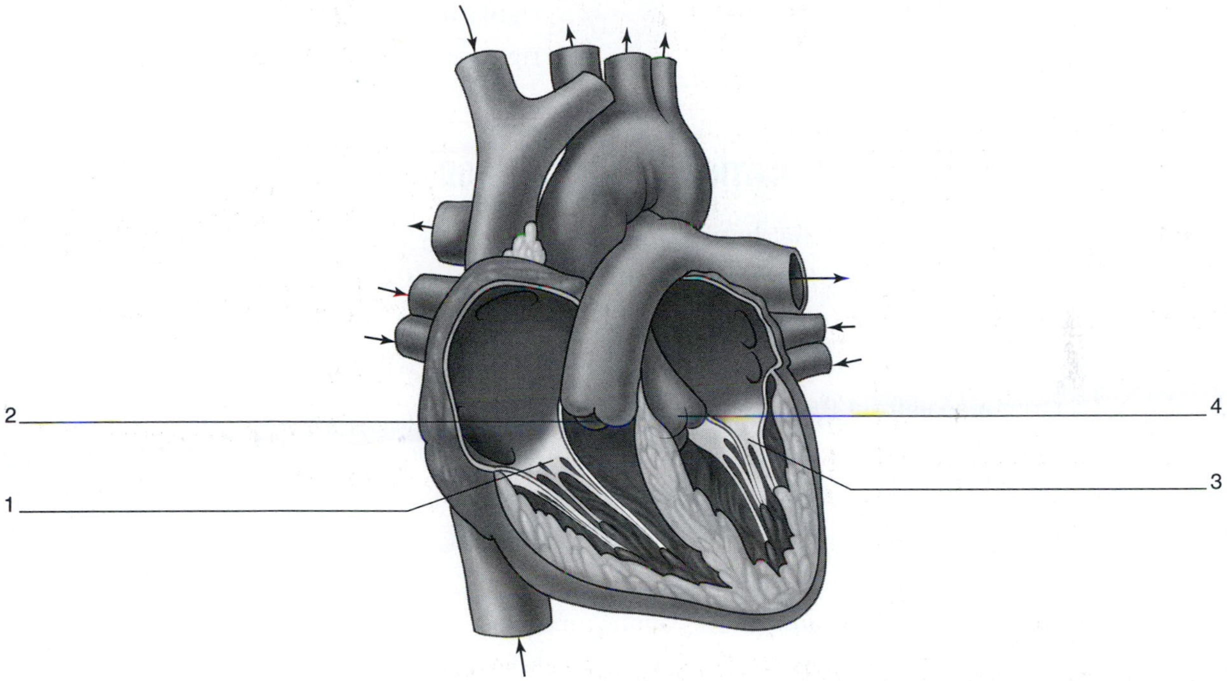

7. What is unique about the structures of the heart valves?

____

____

8. Name the structure that separates the heart into two halves. What is the major difference between the right heart and the left heart?

____

____

D. Using Figure 13-6 in your textbook as a guide, list the steps that take blood from the superior vena cava to the aorta.

____

____

____

____

____

____

____

E. Use the words in the following list to complete the story on circulation.

aorta	lung
aortic semilunar	miter
bicuspid valve	oxygen
carbon dioxide	pulmonary artery
descending aorta	pulmonary semilunar valve
inferior vena cava	pulmonary veins
left atrium	right atrium
left ventricle	right ventricle
liver	tricuspid valve

CIRCULATION OF A RED BLOOD CELL

I am tired. I am a red blood cell that has journeyed through this maze of blood vessels for the past 100 days. I am on my way back to the PUMP factory, carrying with me carbon dioxide thrown out as waste by a muscle cell.

I will be glad to get there to unload this baggage, and then I will pick up oxygen for one of my last trips. The major road from the **liver** is called the ____________ ____________ ____________, which goes to the right upper room, or ____________ ____________, at the factory. After getting dumped there, I feel the walls start to vibrate and close around me. I get pushed through a door marked ____________ ____________. I am now in the lower room called the ____________ ____________. Just as I get comfortable, I hear that same sound again, and these walls start to move from the other side, pushing me upward through another door, which looks like a half moon. This one is called the ____________ ____________ valve. Now I find myself pushed through the ____________ ____________ tunnel, which goes from the heart to a spongy-looking building complex with lots of wings; this is known as the ____________ factory.

When I arrive I am sent to a small chamber, and there I drop off my ____________ ____________. "Wait," the supervisor calls out. "You have to take this little fellow ____________ back to the PUMP factory with you." As I leave the buildings, I am pointed in the direction of a maze of four highways also known as the ____________ ____________. I am told that any of those roads will get me back to the PUMP factory.

I choose the least-crowded lane and land back at the PUMP factory on the left side of the building. I am now in the ____________ ____________ chamber. OH NO! It is happening all over again. The room starts to shake, the walls start closing in, and my little friend Oxy and I are pushed through a door marked ____________ valve. This one has a funny top to it; it looks like a bishop's ____________. Now, here I am, in the ____________ ____________, and before you know it the walls are pushing at me again. Up, up, and away through the ____________ ____________ valve. Oxy and I are in a bigger tunnel this time; it is called the ____________. At the end of this road is a curve with three major arteries coming off it; we will take the road going south, marked ____________ ____________.

This is my route back to the ____________________, taking Oxy along. I am so tired of getting pushed and shoved, I think I will just drop Oxy off and stay there and retire to the recycle plant.

Can you guess the name of the pump? ____________________

F. 1. Label the figure that illustrates the conduction system of the heart.

1 ____________________

2 ____________________

____________________ 3

____________________ 4

2. What is the cardiac cycle? The following sentences illustrate the actions that occur during the cardiac cycle. Complete the blanks using the words provided. Words may be used more than once.

aorta	contraction	pulmonary artery	semilunar
atria	closed	pulmonary veins	tricuspid
bicuspid	open	relax	ventricles

Depolarization

1. The SA node stimulates the ____________________ of both ____________________. Blood flows from the ____________________ into the ____________________. The ventricles are relaxed, the ____________________ valves are ____________________, and blood cannot enter the ____________________ ____________________ and ____________________.

2. The AV node receives the impulse from the SA node and stimulates the ____________________ of both ____________________, which pumps blood into the ____________________ ____________________ and ____________________. The atria are ____________________, and the ____________________ and ____________________ valves are closed.

Repolarization

3. Ventricles, ____________________, and semilunar valves are ____________________, which prevents blood from flowing back into the ____________________. The heart rests.

4. On an electrocardiogram:
   A. What action of the heart does the P wave and QRS wave represent?

   ____

   B. What action of the heart does the T wave represent?

   ____

   C. What information does an EKG give the physician?

   ____

G. Match the statements in Column B with the terms in Column A.

	Column A	Column B
________	1. arrhythmia	a. gurgling or hissing sound made by the valves
________	2. diuretic	b. difficulty in breathing
________	3. bradycardia	c. balloon surgery
________	4. murmur	d. pulse rate below 60 beats per minute
________	5. mitral valve prolapse	e. inflammation of the heart muscle
________	6. angioplasty	f. normal sinus rhythm
________	7. pericarditis	g. drug that reduces amount of fluid
________	8. dyspnea	h. pulse rate over 100 beats per minute
________	9. cardiotonic	i. drug that strengthens the heart
________	10. tachycardia	j. change or deviation of the heart rate
		k. inflammation of the outer layer of the heart
		l. may be related to stress

H. Mark the underlined word or words in the following statements either true or false. Correct any false statements.

________ 1. <u>Heart failure</u> occurs when the ventricles of the heart are unable to contract effectively and blood pools in the heart.

________ 2. If the left ventricle fails in heart failure, <u>edema</u> occurs.

________ 3. If the <u>right ventricle</u> fails in heart failure, an abnormal accumulation of serous fluid will occur in the abdominal cavity.

________ 4. In congestive heart failure, there is edema of the lower extremities and treatment is with <u>anticoagulants.</u>

________ 5. <u>Mitral valve prolapse is</u> due to the improper closing of the valve between the left atria and left ventricle.

________ 6. A heart block occurs when the conduction system between the <u>SA node</u> and the AV node is disrupted.

________ 7. <u>First-degree heart block</u> is characterized by a pattern of only every second, third, or fourth impulse being conducted to the ventricles.

________ 8. One form of <u>first-degree heart block</u> is characterized by a momentary delay at the SA node before the impulse is transmitted to the ventricles.

_________ 9. <u>Third-degree heart block</u> is characterized by no impulse carried over by the SA node.

_________ 10. The atria beat 72 times per minute, while the ventricles contract independently, beating 72 beats per minute; this occurs in <u>third-degree heart block.</u>

I. Fill in the blanks in the following statements.

1. When an area of the heart other than the pacemaker sparks and stimulates a contraction of the myocardium, it is known as a(n) ____________________ ____________________.
2. When abnormal impulses from the atria bombard the AV node, this condition is known as ____________________ ____________________.
3. Premature ventricular contractions (PVCs) originate in the ventricles and cause contractions ahead of the next anticipated beat; they may be ____________________ or ____________________.
4. When the heart rhythm breaks down and the muscle fibers contract at random without coordination, a life-threatening condition known as ____________________ exists.
5. The device used to discharge strong electric current through a patient's heart to shock the SA node to resume its normal rhythm is called a(n) ____________________.

J. Answer the following questions.

1. Describe the pain that occurs in angina pectoris and myocardial infarction. Are they the same?
____
____
____
2. Name the types of drugs used in the treatment of myocardial infarct.
____
____
3. Describe the two types of heart surgery.
____
____
____
____
4. What is the major problem in heart transplants?
____
____
5. What is the action of immunosuppressants?
____
____

6. What are the risks involved in taking immunosuppressants?

____

____

K. Complete the following word puzzle using the clues given. The numbers in parentheses tell how many letters are necessary to complete each statement. Some statements require two words.

1.	Abbreviated term for this condition		M	______	(2)
2.	Dilates blood vessels	______	y	______	(14)
3.	Count should be below 200	______	o	______	(11)
4.	Loss of elasticity of arterial walls	______	c	______	(16)
5.	Cardiotonic	______	a	______	(9)
6.	Another name for myocardial infarction	______	r	______	(11)
7.	Lack of this causes condition	______	d	______	(11)
8.	Tiredness	______	i	______	(7)
9.	Bed rest, oxygen, and medication	______	a	______	(9)
10.	Plaque buildup in arterial walls	______	l	______	(15)
11.	Therapy to dissolve clots	______	i	______	(13)
12.	Severe chest pain	______	n	______	(14)
13.	Change this to prevent heart attacks (per NIH)	______	f	______	(9)
14.	Blood vessel most involved in this condition	______	a	______	(14)
15.	Alleviates pain	______	r	______	(7)
16.	Heart muscle	______	c	______	(10)
17.	Classification of drugs to strengthen heart	______	t	______	(11)
18.	To reduce mortality, provide this type of care	______	i	______	(9)
19.	Surgical treatment	______	o	______	(11)
20.	Maintain blood pressure and weight	______	n	______	(10)

L. This cryptogram is a message in substitution code. Each letter is substituted for another letter. For example, the letter *k* is substituted for the letter *t*. Decipher the message.

Cryptogram for Cardiac Output

SJWMNJS LPKBPK NZ KIH KLKJO ALOPDH LY UOLLM HGHSKHM YWLD KIH IHJWK BHW DNVPKH. NY KIH IHJWK WJKH NZ 80, JOO KIH UOLLM NV KIH ULMR NZ BPDBHM KIWLPCI KIH IHJWK HAHWR DNVPKH.

APPLYING THEORY TO PRACTICE

1. a. How many quarts of blood are pumped through the heart in a 24-hour period with a heart rate of 72 bpm? If the heart rate was 60 bpm, how much blood would be pumped?

   ____

   ____

   ____

   b. Describe cardiac output.

   ____

   ____

   ____

2. Aliya is a cardiac nurse educator and is requested to prepare a brochure on "How to Reduce the Risk of Heart Disease" for the annual Health Fair. What information will Aliya include in this brochure?

   ____

   ____

   ____

   ____

   ____

3. Keith is 80 years old and uses a cardiac resynchronization therapy, a specialized type of pacemaker. What instructions can you give him regarding risks from external devices, such as smartphones?

   ____

   ____

4. A 70-year-old woman wants to know how nitroglycerine is going to help her heart. She had heard "nitro" was used as an explosive. Explain the difference to her.

   ____

   ____

5. Because you are employed at the Cardiac Care Center associated with your local hospital, you must be familiar with the diagnostic tests ordered for heart disease and circulatory problems.

   Describe the differences between the following pairs:

   a. Angiography and cardiac MRI

   ____

   ____

   b. Cardiac catheterization and IVUS

   ____

   ____

c. Arterial blood gases and C-reactive protein test

d. Lipid panel and BNP

e. Exercise stress test and use of Holter monitor

6. Fred Gander, age 75, complains of chest pain and dyspnea and has a fever. He goes to the ER and a diagnosis of pericarditis is made. Fred asks the doctor to explain pericarditis and how he got this illness. Describe pericarditis and its treatment.

7. Maureen Hague notices that her ankles are swollen. In addition, she is short of breath, has a cough, and seems tired most of the time. What heart condition may Maureen have? Describe the condition and its treatment.

8. Anthony is interested is a career as an EMT. He knows he must be certified in CPR. What is CPR, and how is it performed?

   What are the requirements to become an EMT?

SURF THE NET

For additional information and interactive exercises, use the following key words:

- structure and function of the heart
- conduction system of the heart
- electrocardiogram
- prevention of heart disease
- diagnostic tests for heart disease
- disorders of the heart—arrhythmias, inflammation of the heart, coronary artery disease, angina, myocardial infarction, heart attack, heart failure, conduction defects of the heart
- women and heart disease—atypical symptoms
- pacemakers and defibrillators
- heart surgery

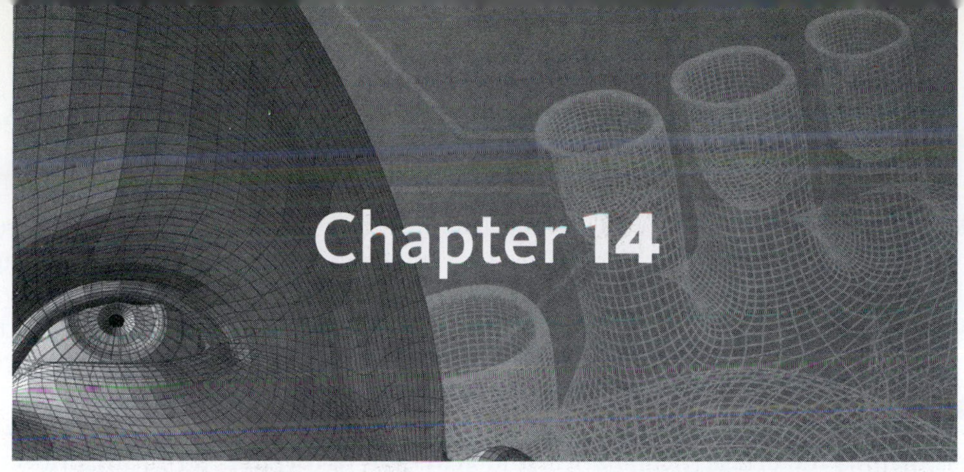

Circulation and Blood Vessels

OVERVIEW

The arteries, capillaries, and veins circulate the blood to all parts of the body through the cardiopulmonary and systemic circulation.

Circulation occurs through cardiopulmonary and systemic circulation. In *cardiopulmonary circulation*, blood travels from the heart to the lungs and back to the heart. In *systemic circulation*, blood travels from the heart to tissues and back to the heart. Specialized systemic routes are *coronary circulation, portal circulation,* and *fetal circulation.*

Cardiopulmonary Circulation

In **cardiopulmonary circulation**, deoxygenated blood returns to the heart through the superior and inferior vena cava to the right atrium, through the tricuspid valve to the right ventricle, through the pulmonary semilunar valve to the pulmonary artery, and finally to the lungs.

The gaseous exchange between carbon dioxide and oxygen takes place in the lungs. Oxygenated blood returns from the lungs through the pulmonary veins to the left atrium, through the bicuspid valve to the left ventricle, through the aortic semilunar valve to the aorta, and to all parts of the body.

Path of General Circulation. The *aorta,* the largest artery in the body, emerges from the heart and the first branch, the coronary artery, goes to the heart muscle. The aorta artery then forms an arch. Three arterial branches from the aortic arch are the brachiocephalic, the left common carotid, and the left subclavian arteries. The aortic arch descends and many arteries branch from it; for example, they go to the chest, organs of digestion, reproductive organs, and the rest of the body.

Systemic Circulation

Coronary Circulation. Two branches of the coronary artery, right and left, come from the aorta. Their branches feed the muscles of the heart. Blood returns to the right atrium through the *coronary sinus,* into which the coronary veins empty.

Portal Circulation. Portal circulation is a specialized circulation in which veins from the pancreas, stomach, small intestine, spleen, and colon empty into and form the *portal vein.* The portal vein carries blood to the liver, and glucose gets stored as glycogen. After going through the liver, the blood leaves through the *hepatic vein* to return to the heart via the inferior vena cava.

Fetal Circulation. In the fetus, the placenta acts like the lungs, and therefore cardiopulmonary circulation is not necessary. Specialized structures that enable the blood to bypass the lungs are the *foramen ovale,* an opening between the right atrium and the left atrium, and the *ductus arteriosus,* a structure between the pulmonary artery and the aorta. The structures usually close after birth.

Blood Vessels

Blood vessels include the arteries, capillaries, and veins. An **artery** has an elastic, muscular, thick wall that carries oxygenated blood (except for the pulmonary artery). It has three layers:

Tunica adventitia: outer layer; fibrous connective tissue with smooth muscle that gives it elasticity.

Tunica media: middle layer; muscle cells arranged in a circular fashion enable the vessels to dilate and constrict.

Tunica interna: inner lining; smooth and shiny.

Capillaries are the thinnest vessels; they connect the arteries and the veins. The exchange of gases and nutrients takes place in the capillaries.

Veins carry deoxygenated blood to the heart (except for the pulmonary veins). The structure of veins is similar to that of arteries, but the three layers are thinner. Within the veins are valves that prevent the backflow of blood.

The valves help push blood back to the heart. In addition, the contraction of skeletal muscles and the action of the diaphragm during respiration assist in *venous return.*

The Effects of Aging on the Circulation and Blood Vessels

As the body ages, the arteries become less elastic and the heart has to work harder to push the blood through them. Researchers believe that normal blood pressure for older persons may be 140/90.

Blood Pressure

Blood pressure is the pressure of the blood against the arterial walls when the heart contracts (*systolic*) and relaxes (*diastolic*). Blood pressure is recorded with the systolic number on top and the diastolic number on bottom. A normal blood pressure is 120/80. The difference between the systole and the diastole is the *pulse pressure.*

Pulse

Pulse is the alternating expansion and contraction of an artery as the blood flows through it. The pulse rate is usually the same as the heart rate. The pulse points are the temporal, carotid, brachial, radial, femoral, popliteal, and dorsalis pedis.

Disorders of Circulation and Blood Vessels

Congenital Heart Defects. Congenital heart defects occur when there is a malformation of the heart. *Cyanosis* is usually the first sign of a problem.

Disorders of the Blood Vessels. The following are disorders of the blood vessels:

Aneurysm—ballooning of the arterial wall.

Arteriosclerosis—the arterial walls thicken because of a loss of elasticity.

Atherosclerosis—deposits of fatty substances form along the arterial walls.

Gangrene—death of body tissue due to an insufficient blood supply.

Phlebitis—inflammation of the lining of a vein.

Embolism—a traveling blood clot.

Varicose veins—swollen veins.

Hemorrhoids—varicose veins of the rectum.

Cerebral hemorrhage—bleeding from blood vessels within the brain.

Peripheral vascular disease (PVD)—caused by a blockage in the arteries, usually in the legs.

Claudication—a cramping pain in the legs or buttocks that occurs when walking.

Hypertension—high blood pressure. It is called the "silent killer" because it has no symptoms. It leads to strokes, heart attacks, and kidney failure.

Transient ischemic attacks (TIAs)—temporary interruptions of the blood flow to the brain. Of people with TIAs, 50% have a major stroke within the following year.

Cerebrovascular accident (CVA)—a stroke; the sudden interruption of blood supply to the brain. Symptoms depend on which side of the brain has its blood supply interrupted.

Hypoperfusion/shock—inadequate blood flow to the organs and body systems, which leads to shock.

ACTIVITIES

A. Answer the following questions relating to circulation.

1. Name the two major circulatory systems.

___

2. Describe the three specialized systemic routes.

___

___

___

3. Describe coronary circulation.

___

___

4. What special structure is on the posterior wall of the right atrium?

___

5. In portal circulation, which veins form the portal vein?

___

6. Is arterial circulation related to portal circulation? If so, how?

___

7. The blood in the portal vein goes to the liver. What is the effect of the liver on glucose and blood glucose concentration?

___

___

B. 1. Label the diagram of fetal circulation from the mother to the heart of the fetus and back to the mother. Trace the flow of blood from the placenta to the umbilical arteries.

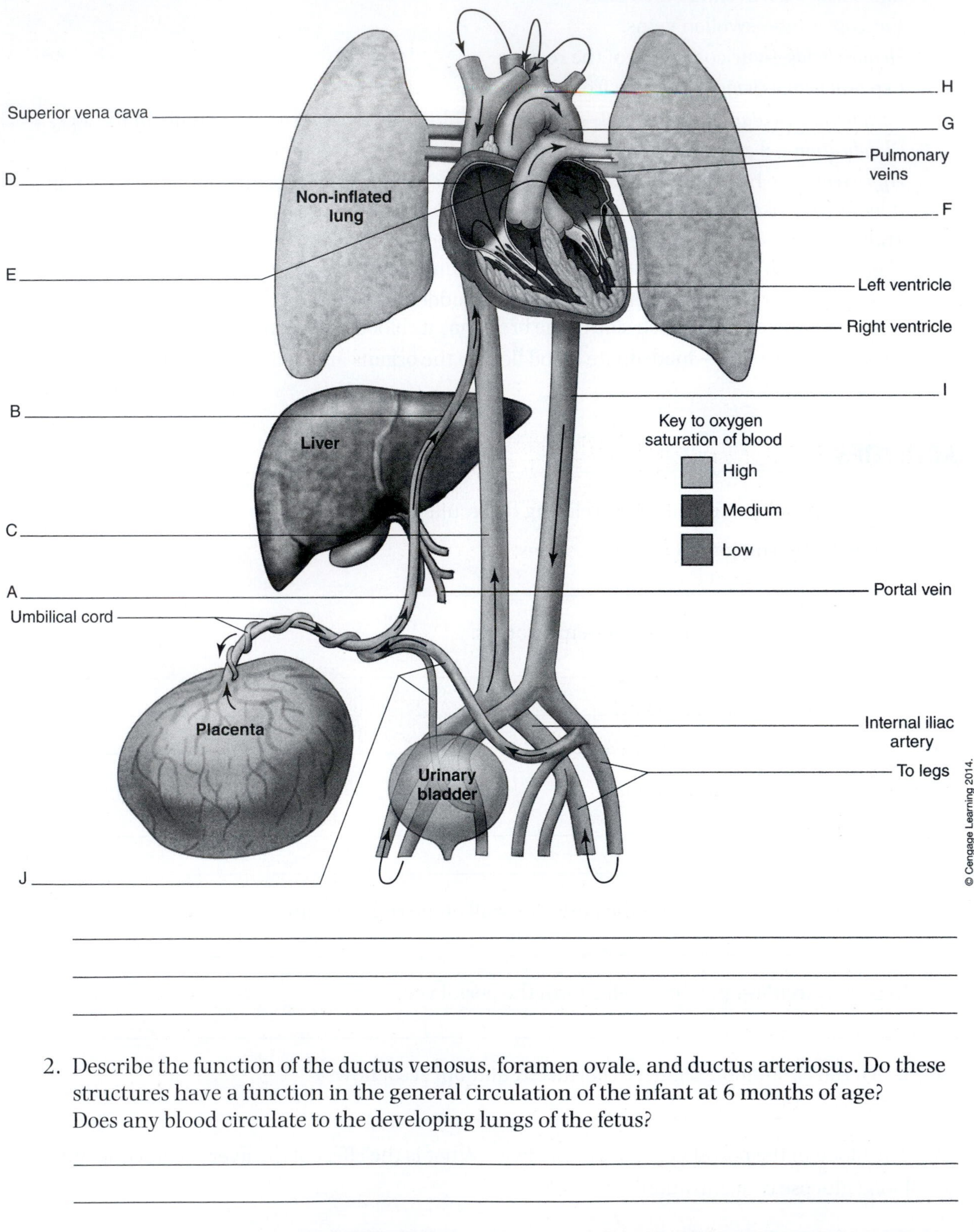

____

____

____

2. Describe the function of the ductus venosus, foramen ovale, and ductus arteriosus. Do these structures have a function in the general circulation of the infant at 6 months of age? Does any blood circulate to the developing lungs of the fetus?

____

____

____

____

C. Fill in the blanks to complete the following statements.

1. After the blood goes through the cardiopulmonary circulation, the blood then goes to the major artery, the ____________________.

2. The first branch is the ____________________ artery, which takes blood to the ____________________. The aorta now forms an arch.

3. The right branch off of the aortic arch is the ____________________ artery, which subdivides into the ____________________ artery to the shoulder and the ____________________ ____________________ artery to the ____________________ and ____________________.

4. The left branch off of the aortic arch has two arteries, the left ____________________ ____________________ artery to the ____________________ and ____________________ and the subclavian artery to the ____________________.

5. The arch turns downward and is called the descending aorta with the following arteries coming off as branches: the ____________________ artery to the chest cavity and the celiac artery to the ____________________, ____________________, ____________________, and ____________________.

D. Select the letter of the choice that best completes the statement.

1. The pulmonary artery carries deoxygenated blood from the
   a. right atrium to the lungs.
   b. right ventricle to the lungs.
   c. lungs to the left atrium.
   d. left ventricle to all parts of the body.

2. The outer layer of the arteries is the tunica
   a. adventitia.
   b. media.
   c. interna.
   d. intima.

3. The ability of the arteries to withstand a sudden large increase in pressure is accomplished by the
   a. elasticity of the smooth muscles.
   b. muscle cells being arranged in a circular pattern.
   c. smooth lining of the tunica interna.
   d. tunica media.

4. The ability of the arteries to dilate and constrict is accomplished by the
   a. elasticity of the smooth muscles.
   b. muscle cells being arranged in a circular pattern.
   c. smooth lining of tunica interna.
   d. tunica externa.

5. The capillaries are branches of the
   a. metarterioles.
   b. metavenuoles.
   c. arterioles.
   d. venules.
6. The thinnest of the capillary walls allows only ______________________ out of the capillary.
   a. oxygen
   b. metabolic wastes
   c. nitrogenous material
   d. oxygen, metabolic wastes, nitrogenous material, and carbon dioxide
7. Blood flow through the capillaries is controlled by the
   a. smooth muscles of the adventitia.
   b. precapillary sphincters.
   c. circular muscles in the media.
   d. skeletal muscles.
8. Which of the following is a true statement about arteries and veins?
   a. The walls are thicker in veins than in arteries.
   b. Valves are present only in veins.
   c. The walls are the same in arteries and veins, but valves are present only in veins.
   d. The walls are thinner in veins than in arteries, and valves are present only in veins.
9. The contractions of skeletal muscle
   a. help capillaries circulate blood.
   b. assist in venous return.
   c. assist in arterial distribution.
   d. have no role in circulation.
10. Blood flow through the capillaries is influenced by
   a. osmotic pressure.
   b. hydrostatic pressure.
   c. filtration.
   d. active transport.

E. Answer the following riddles, using the arteries from the list.

brachial
celiac
common iliac
dorsal pedalis
external carotid
femoral
internal carotid
popliteal
radial
vertebral

WHO AM I?

1. I run up and down the back,
   bringing blood to the central nervous system track. ________________
2. You feel me often at your wrist;
   running or jumping gives my numbers a lift. ________________
3. I struggle to get to all the parts of the brain,
   where intelligence and coordination reign. ________________
4. I run down and through the upper bone,
   get cuffed around, please leave me alone! ________________
5. They call me common, I go from place to place;
   I branch down the legs and into the pelvic space. ________________
6. I am really at the end of the line.
   My companion vein has an upward climb. ________________
7. If you reach down behind your knee,
   check around and you are sure to feel me. ________________
8. When you get embarrassed and your face turns red,
   my vessels have dilated, up to the hair roots on your head. ________________
9. I am hungry for nutrients from your food intake;
   I am now undecided, which of the four roads should I take? ________________
10. I sometimes get plugged and blood does not get through;
    the legs and the feet do not know what to do. ________________

F. Label the arteries in the following diagram.

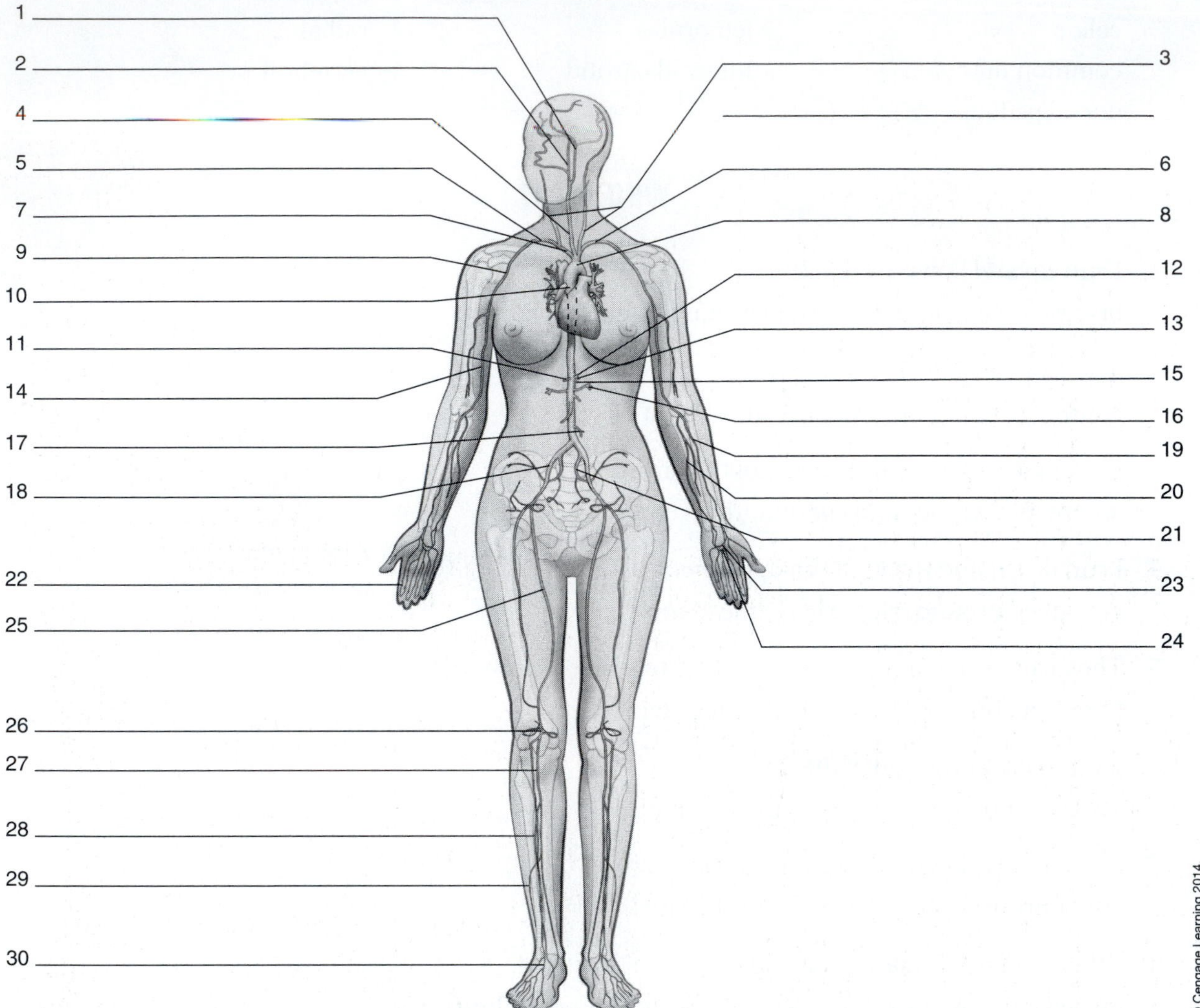

G. 1. Label the diagram of the layers of the walls of the arteries and veins and describe their structure.

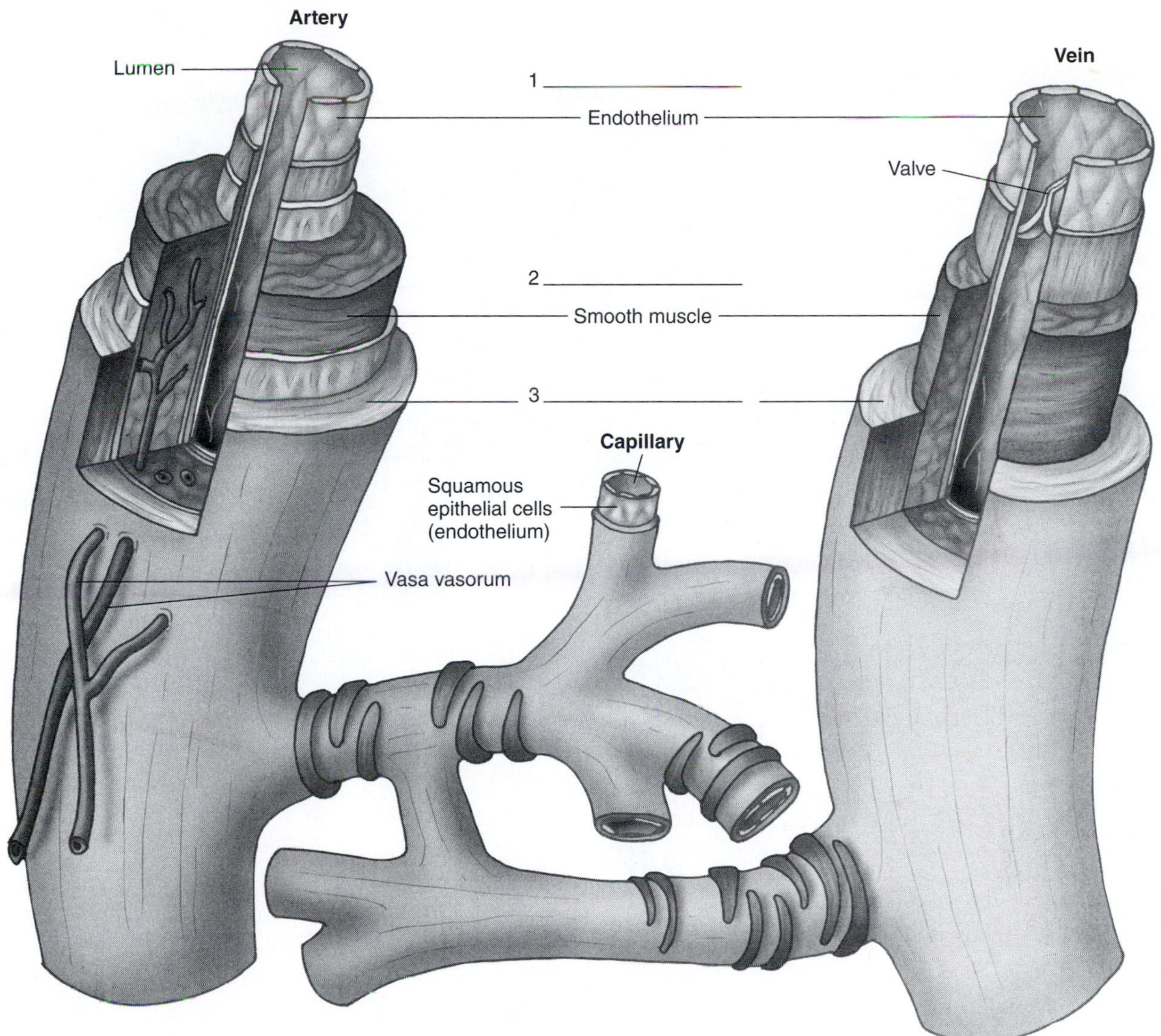

2. Explain the difference between the layers of the arteries and the layers of the veins.

____

____

____

H. Label the veins in the following diagram.

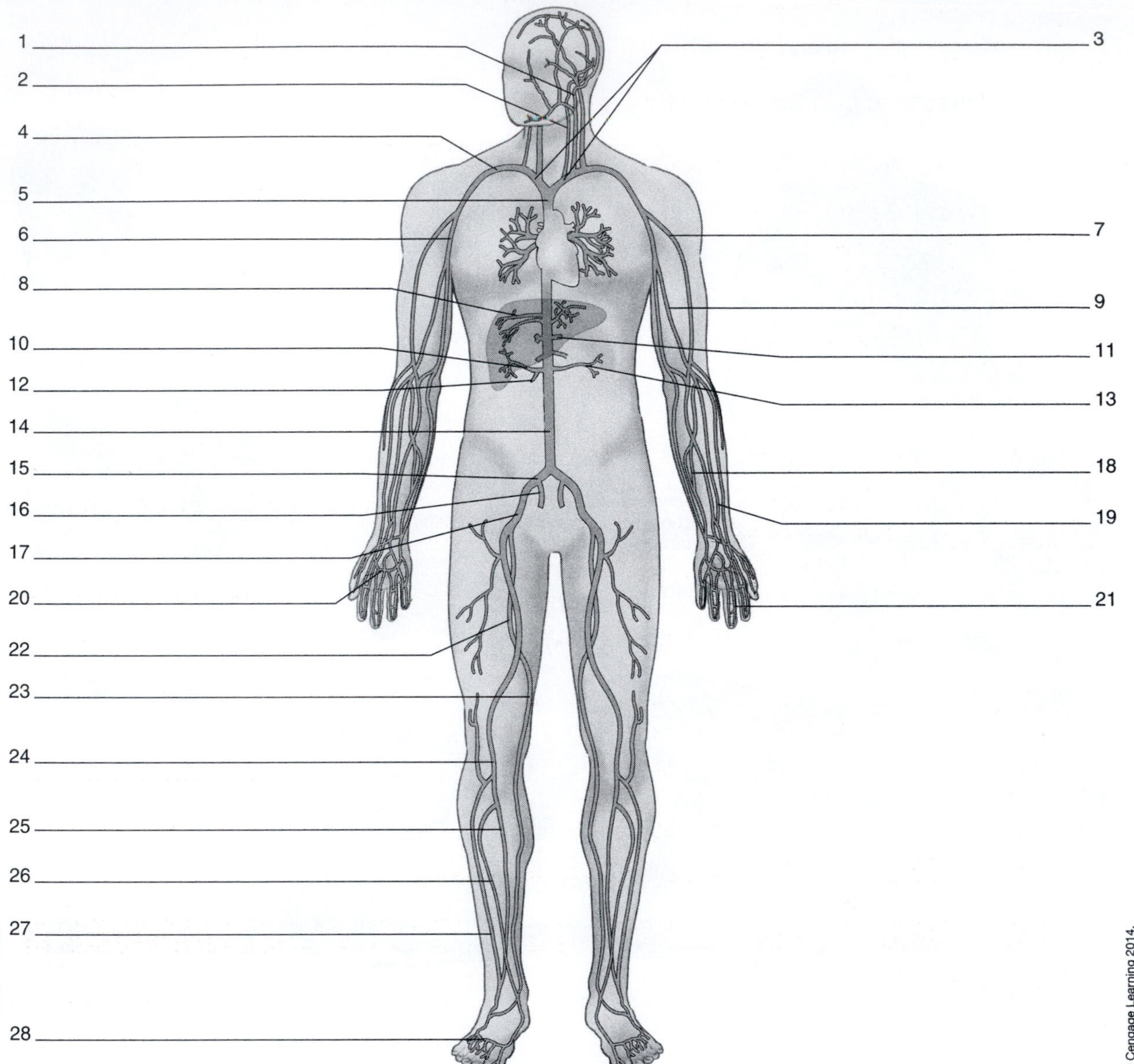

I. Using the previous diagrams as a guide, fill in the name of the vein that matches each description.

_________ 1. Affected in varicose veins

_________ 2. Furthest branch in feet

_________ 3. Largest vein in body

_________ 4. From the kidney

_________ 5. Returns blood to the right atrium

_________ 6. Branches into the shoulder and axilla

________ 7. Involved in portal circulation

________ 8. Branches into external and internal jugular

________ 9. Blood from small intestine and colon

________ 10. Blood from brain to superior vena cava

J. Fill in the blanks to complete the statements on blood pressure and pulse.

1. The pressure measured as the heart contracts is the systolic pressure; the pressure measured as the heart relaxes is the ____________________ pressure.
2. Pulse measures the alternating ____________________ and ____________________ of an artery as blood flows through it.
3. The pulse rate is usually the same as the ____________________ rate.

K. Answer the following questions.

1. Take the blood pressures of two of your classmates. Record the data. Are they within normal range?

____

____

2. What is pulse pressure?

____

____

L. The following questions relate to pulse points.

1. Take your pulse at the following pulse sites and describe their locations.

Pulse Point	Rate	Location
Temporal	____________	____________________
Carotid	____________	____________________
Brachial	____________	____________________
Radial	____________	____________________
Popliteal	____________	____________________
Dorsalis pedis	____________	____________________

2. Is there a difference in any of your readings?

____

M. Match the disorder in Column A with the explanation in Column B.

Column A	Column B
________ 1. aneurysm	a. cramping in buttocks while walking
________ 2. phlebitis	b. bleeding in blood vessels in brain
________ 3. hemorrhoids	c. fatty buildup in artery
________ 4. cerebral hemorrhage	d. ballooning of an artery
________ 5. varicose veins	e. inflammation of veins
________ 6. embolism	f. bluish discoloration of skin
________ 7. peripheral vascular disease (PVD)	g. death of body tissue
________ 8. claudication	h. traveling blood clot
________ 9. cyanosis	i. varicose veins in the walls of the rectum
________ 10. gangrene	j. swollen veins
	k. loss of elasticity
	l. blockage of artery in legs

N. Compare the following pairs.

1. Arteriole/venule

____

____

2. Phlebitis/thrombosis

____

____

3. Ischemia/gangrene

____

____

4. Embolism/thrombus

____

____

5. Transient ischemic attack/stroke

____

____

O. Label the diagram of affected sites and resulting complications of atherosclerosis.

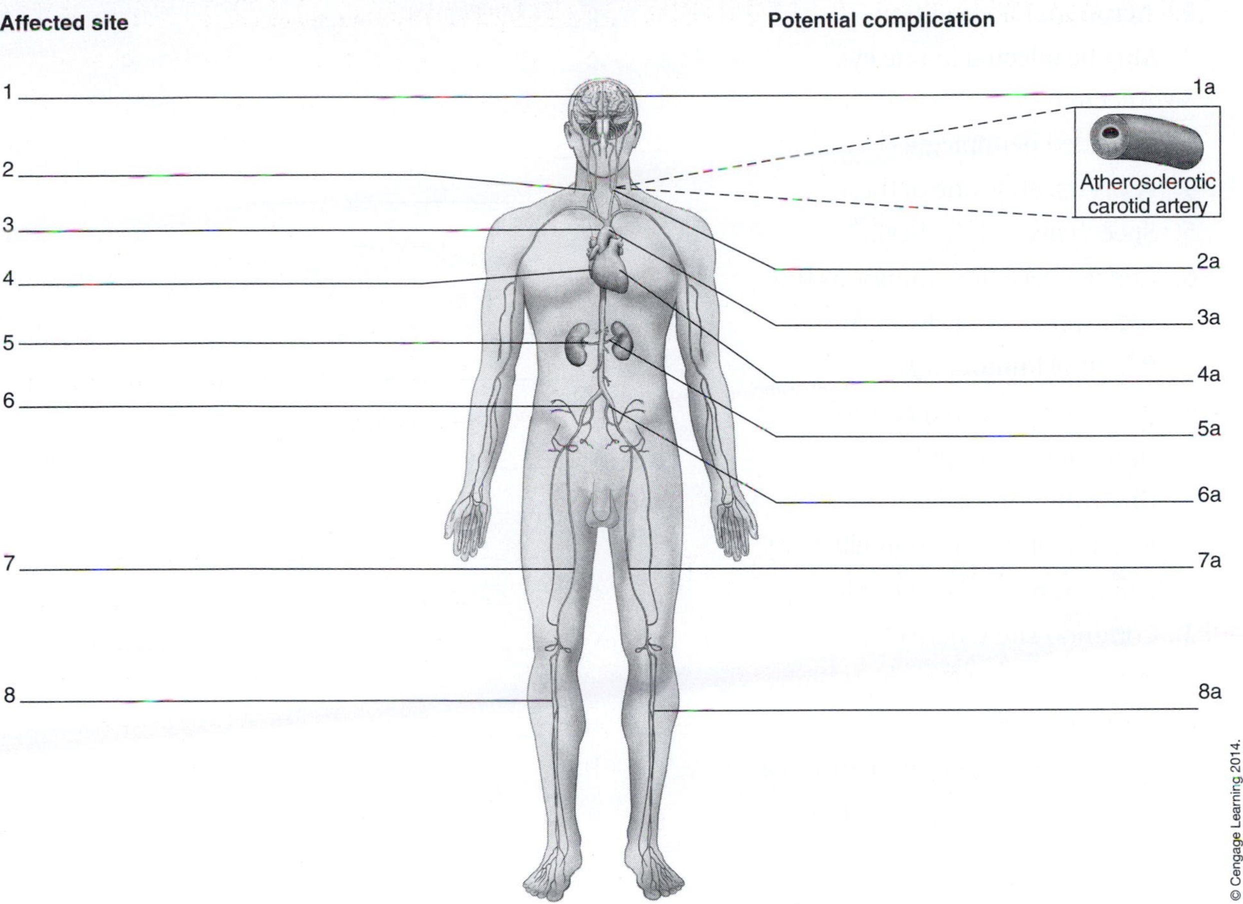

P. Match each disease in the following list with the correct description.

aphasia	hemiplegia
cyanosis	hypoperfusion
dysphasia	phlebitis
gangrene	orthostatic hypotension

1. Death of body tissue due to an insufficient blood supply ____________
2. Inadequate blood supply to organs and body systems ____________
3. Paralysis on one side of the body ____________
4. The inability to say what one wishes to say ____________
5. A bluish discoloration of the skin due to lack of oxygen ____________
6. Loss of speech or memory ____________
7. A drop in blood pressure that occurs when rising from a prone position to a standing position ____________
8. An inflammation of the lining of a vein ____________

Q. Complete the word puzzle relating to cerebral vascular accidents.

1. Acronym for condition C__ __
2. May be affected in one eye e__ __ __ __ __ __ __ __ __
3. Affected brain area causing left-sided hemiplegia r__ __ __ __ __ __ __ __ __ __ __ __ __ __
4. A CAT scan is one of these e__ __ __ __ __ __ __ __ __ __ __ __ __ __
5. Speech area of the brain B__ __ __ __ __'__ __ __ __ __ __
6. General term for conditions that predispose people to CVA r__ __ __ __ __ __ __ __ __ __ __
7. Result of immobility a__ __ __ __ __ __ __
8. Affected brain area causing right-sided hemiplegia l__ __ __ __ __ __ __ __ __ __ __ __ __
9. Dizziness v__ __ __ __ __ __ __
10. Risk factor; vessel loses elasticity a__ __ __ __ __ __ __ __ __ __ __ __ __ __ __ __ __ __ __ __
11. Another name for condition s__ __ __ __ __
12. Common site where clots form c__ __ __ __ __ __ __ __ __ __ __ __ __ __ __ __
13. Patient's complaint about limbs being affected u__ __ __ __ __ __ __
14. Changes necessary to reduce risk of CVA l__ __ __ __ __ __ __ __ __ __ __
15. Risk factor due to plaque buildup a__ __ __ __ __ __ __ __ __ __ __ __ __ __ __ __ __ __
16. Treatments necessary to return to activities of daily living after CVA r__ __
17. Loss of speech a__ __ __ __ __ __ __
18. Diagnostic test used to assess cause of stroke c__ __
19. Of CVAs, 90% result from this c__ __ __
20. When the brain is deprived of oxygen, this is the result i__ __ __ __ __ __ __ __ __ __ __
21. Inability to say what one wants to d__ __ __ __ __ __ __ __ __ __ __ __ in communicating
22. For treatment to be this, it must begin within 4 hours after stroke e__ __ __ __ __ __ __ __ __ __
23. Test to determine reflexes after CVA n__ __ __ __ __-__ __ __ __ __ __ __
24. Where CVA places as a leading cause of death t__ __ __ __

R. Explain the importance of the cardiovascular system to all other body systems in maintaining homeostasis.

____

____

____

APPLYING THEORY TO PRACTICE

1. Prepare a presentation for junior high school students regarding nursing careers, including registered nurses, nurse clinicians, licensed practical nurses, and nurse aides. Describe the educational requirements, the roles, and the future employment possibilities.

2. a. Why is hypertension called the "silent killer"?

   b. What risk factors predispose people to hypertension?

   c. What are the complications of hypertension?

   d. How can hypertension be prevented?

3. You are taking the blood pressure of a patient in the HMO where you are employed. The reading is 150/90. After she has rested for 5 minutes, you retake her pressure. It is the same. The patient asks what her blood pressure is. When you tell her the number, she states that it has never been that high. You suspect she may have "white coat" hypertension.

   a. Describe "white coat" hypertension.

b. Does medication help this situation?

c. How would you differentiate between true hypertension and "white coat" hypertension?

4. Tony has had a series of minor transient ischemic attacks (TIAs). His family has done some research and is concerned that a TIA may lead to a stroke.

   a. What acronym is helpful to use to assess whether someone is having a stroke?

   b. The family also wants to know whether there will be a chance of a complete recovery if Tony does have a stroke. How would you respond?

5. As a paramedic, you must be able to recognize the symptoms of shock. Define *shock*. What are the causes of and treatments for shock?

SURF THE NET

For additional information and interactive exercises, use the following key words:

- cardiopulmonary circulation
- specialized circulation—coronary, portal, fetal
- blood vessels—structure and function
- blood pressure—hypertension
- pulse rates and sites for measuring pulse
- disorders of the circulatory system—aneurysm, arteriosclerosis, atherosclerosis, blood clots, cerebral vascular accident (stroke), peripheral vascular disease
- aging effects on blood vessels
- Career profile: EMT and paramedic

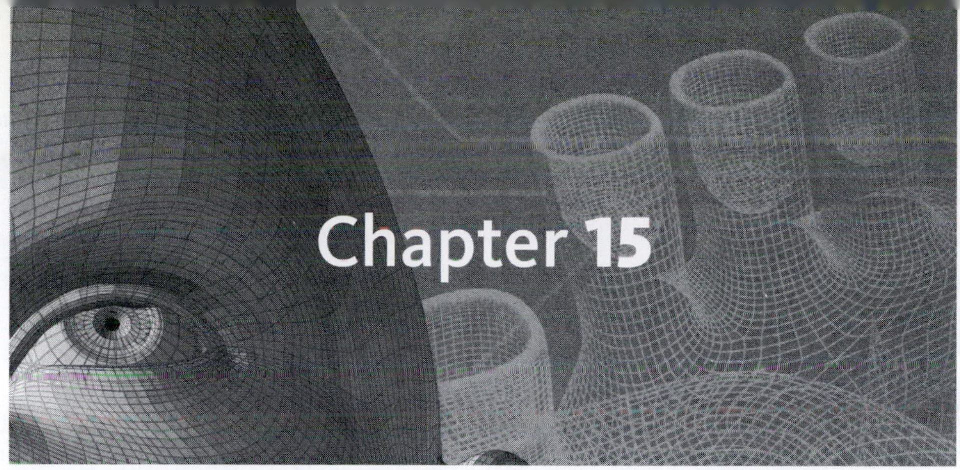

The Lymphatic and Immune Systems

OVERVIEW

The **lymphatic system** consists of the lymph, lymph nodes, vessels, spleen, thymus gland, tonsils, and lymphoid tissue in the intestinal tract.

Functions of the Lymphatic System

Functions of the lymphatic system include the following:

Lymph fluid serves as the intermediary between blood in the capillaries and tissue.

Lymph vessels transport excess tissue fluid back into the circulatory system.

Lymph nodes produce lymphocytes and filter out harmful bacteria.

The *spleen* produces lymphocytes and monocytes, acts as a reservoir for blood, and recycles red blood cells.

The *thymus gland* produces T lymphocytes.

Interstitial Fluid and Lymph

Lymph is a straw-colored fluid similar to blood plasma. **Intercellular** or **interstitial fluid** is lymph that bathes the spaces surrounding the tissue cells.

Lymph Vessels

Lymph vessels accompany and closely parallel the venous system; they are located in almost all the tissues and organs that have blood vessels. They form two main ducts, the thoracic and right lymphatic.

Lacteals are specialized lymph vessels in the villi of the small intestines that absorb digested fats.

The *thoracic duct* receives lymph from the left side of the chest, head, neck, abdominal area, and lower limbs and empties into the left subclavian vein.

The *right lymphatic duct* receives lymph from the right arm, right side of the head, and upper trunk and empties into the right subclavian vein.

Lymph Nodes

Lymph nodes are oval structures located alone or grouped in places along the lymph vessels. They provide a site for lymphocyte production and serve as a filter for screening out harmful substances.

Tonsils

Tonsils are masses of lymph tissue capable of producing lymphocytes and filtering out harmful bacteria. There are three pairs: the palatine, adenoids, and lingual.

Spleen

The **spleen** is a saclike mass of lymphatic tissue located in the upper-left area of the abdominal cavity. It forms lymphocytes and monocytes and stores and recycles large amounts of red blood cells.

Thymus Gland

The **thymus gland** is located in the thoracic area and produces T lymphocytes and thymosin.

Disorders of the Lymph System

Lymphadenitis is the enlargement of the lymph nodes.

Hodgkin's disease is a form of cancer of the lymph nodes.

Infectious mononucleosis is caused by the Epstein-Barr virus spread by oral contact; it is also known as the kissing disease.

The Effects of Aging on the Lymphatic and Immune Systems

As the body ages, the immune system cells are no longer able to undergo rapid cell division, which leaves every organ and tissue in the body more vulnerable to disease.

Immunity

Immunity is the ability of the body to resist disease.

Normal Defense Mechanisms

The individual's immune system is a normal defense mechanism. A unique feature of the immune system is its ability to recognize antigens that are not consistent with the genetic makeup of the host.

Nonspecific Immune Defense

The nonspecific immune defense is not dependent on prior exposure to the antigen. Examples include the skin and normal flora; mucous membranes; sneezing, coughing, and tearing reflexes; elimination and an acidic environment; and inflammation.

Specific Immune Defense

The specific immune defense is a response that is specific to the invading antigen and the production of T lymphocyte cells (T cells) and B cells.

T cells release substances called lymphokines that attract other lymphocytes to the area to assist in antigen destruction and stimulate production of B cells.

B cells cause formation of memory B cells that remember the antigen and prepare the host for future antigen invasion.

Natural and Acquired Immunities

There are two general types of immunity:

Natural is born-with immunity.

Acquired is immunity that results from exposure. Acquired immunity can be active or passive.

There are two types of *active acquired immunity:*

1. Natural—having the disease and recovering
2. Artificial—from a vaccination

There are also two types of *passive acquired immunity:*

1. Natural—may pass from the mother's milk to the baby
2. Artificial—receiving serum from another (i.e., gamma globulin)

Immunization is the process of increasing an individual's resistance to a particular infection by artificial means. See Tables 15-2 through 15-4 in the text for recommended immunization schedules.

Immunoglobulin is a protein that functions specifically as an antibody.

Autoimmunity

In **autoimmunity,** an individual's immune system forms antibodies against its own tissues, causing autoimmune disorders such as lupus and scleroderma.

Hypersensitivity

Hypersensitivity occurs when the body's immune system fails to protect itself against foreign material; instead, the formed antibodies irritate certain body cells.

Anaphylaxis or **anaphylactic shock** is a severe and sometimes fatal allergic reaction.

AIDS/HIV

AIDS is caused by the human immunodeficiency virus (HIV), which suppresses the body's own immune system. The patient becomes susceptible to opportunistic infections that can normally be fought off by a healthy individual with a normally functioning immune system. The most common infections are Kaposi's sarcoma (blood vessel malignancy) and pneumocystic pneumonia.

Diagnostic Tests for AIDS. Diagnostic tests include HIV antibody test, ELISA test, Western blot test, and Rapid test. Home-based test kits are available.

Symptoms of AIDS. Symptoms of AIDS are nonspecific and are very similar to those of other illnesses, such as influenza.

The *incubation period* (the time between becoming infected and when the actual symptoms appear) is quite long, ranging from 1 month to 10 years.

AIDS-related complex (ARC) develops when an individual contracts HIV and symptoms occur; some individuals may develop AIDS.

Some people infected with HIV do not develop symptoms; this is called **asymptomatic infection.**

Treatment for AIDS. Treatment for AIDS uses three classes of antiretroviral drugs.

High-Risk Groups for AIDS. High-risk groups for AIDS include:

Homosexual and bisexual men with multiple sexual partners
Male and female intravenous drug users who share needles
Infants born to parents with AIDS
Persons who received blood or blood products before all blood banks were required to test for HIV

Transmission is by sexual intercourse, sharing of hypodermic needles, and infants born to parents who are HIV positive.

Measures to *prevent* transmission include limiting sexual partners, using latex condoms, and avoiding practices that would place people at risk of acquiring this disease.

The lymphatic system affects other body systems to maintain homeostasis.

ACTIVITIES

A. Fill in the missing word or words in the following statements.

1. The lymph system differs from the circulatory system because it lacks a ______________.
2. Lymph fluid is the intermediary between the blood in the capillaries and the ______________.
3. The spleen produces ____________________ and ____________________.
4. If lymph is not reabsorbed, the tissue may swell; this condition is known as ______________.
5. The transportation of excess fluid back into the circulatory system is accomplished by the ____________________ ____________________ ____________________.
6. Lymph follicles in the walls of the small intestine that produce macrophages are known as ____________________ ____________________.
7. Lymph nodes help in the defense of the body by filtering out ____________________ ____________________.
8. The spleen helps the body in hemorrhagic conditions because it acts as a blood ____________________.
9. The organ of the lymph system located in the pharynx is the ____________________.
10. The type of white blood cell produced by the thymus gland is the ____________________.

B. Select the letter of the choice that best completes the statement.

1. Lymph is a straw-colored fluid that is also called
   a. plasma.
   b. serum.
   c. interstitial fluid.
   d. intracellular fluid.

2. The ________________ of the lymph node is (are) responsible for the production of lymph.
   a. germinal center
   b. trabeculae
   c. macrophage cells
   d. plasma membrane

3. The method by which lymph is pushed through the lymph vessels is via
   a. a muscular pump.
   b. contraction of the lymph vessels.
   c. contraction of skeletal muscles against the lymph vessels.
   d. contraction of smooth muscles against the lymph vessels.

4. Lymph vessels closely resemble veins and may be found in the
   a. central nervous system.
   b. epidermis.
   c. muscles.
   d. spleen.

5. Lymph in the thoracic duct area is carried to the ________________ vein.
   a. subclavian
   b. jugular
   c. brachial
   d. radial

6. Lymph travels in one direction: from the
   a. heart to the body organs.
   b. body organs to the pulmonary circulation.
   c. body organs to the heart.
   d. body organs to the liver.

7. Lacteals are specialized lymph vessels in the small intestines that
   a. produce lymphocytes.
   b. absorb fat and fat-soluble vitamins.
   c. carry away metabolic waste products.
   d. produce lymphokines.

8. Tonsils are masses of lymph tissue; the adenoid tonsils are located
   a. under the tongue.
   b. on the sides of the soft palate.
   c. on the sides of the hard palate.
   d. in the upper part of the throat.

9. Enlargement of the tonsils causes all of the following, *except*
   a. difficulty in swallowing.
   b. hoarseness.
   c. sore throat.
   d. pyrexia.

10. The thymus gland produces a special type of leukocyte called a(n)
    a. monocyte.
    b. eosinophil.
    c. B lymphocyte.
    d. T lymphocyte.

C. Label the diagram of the vessels and organs of the lymphatic system.

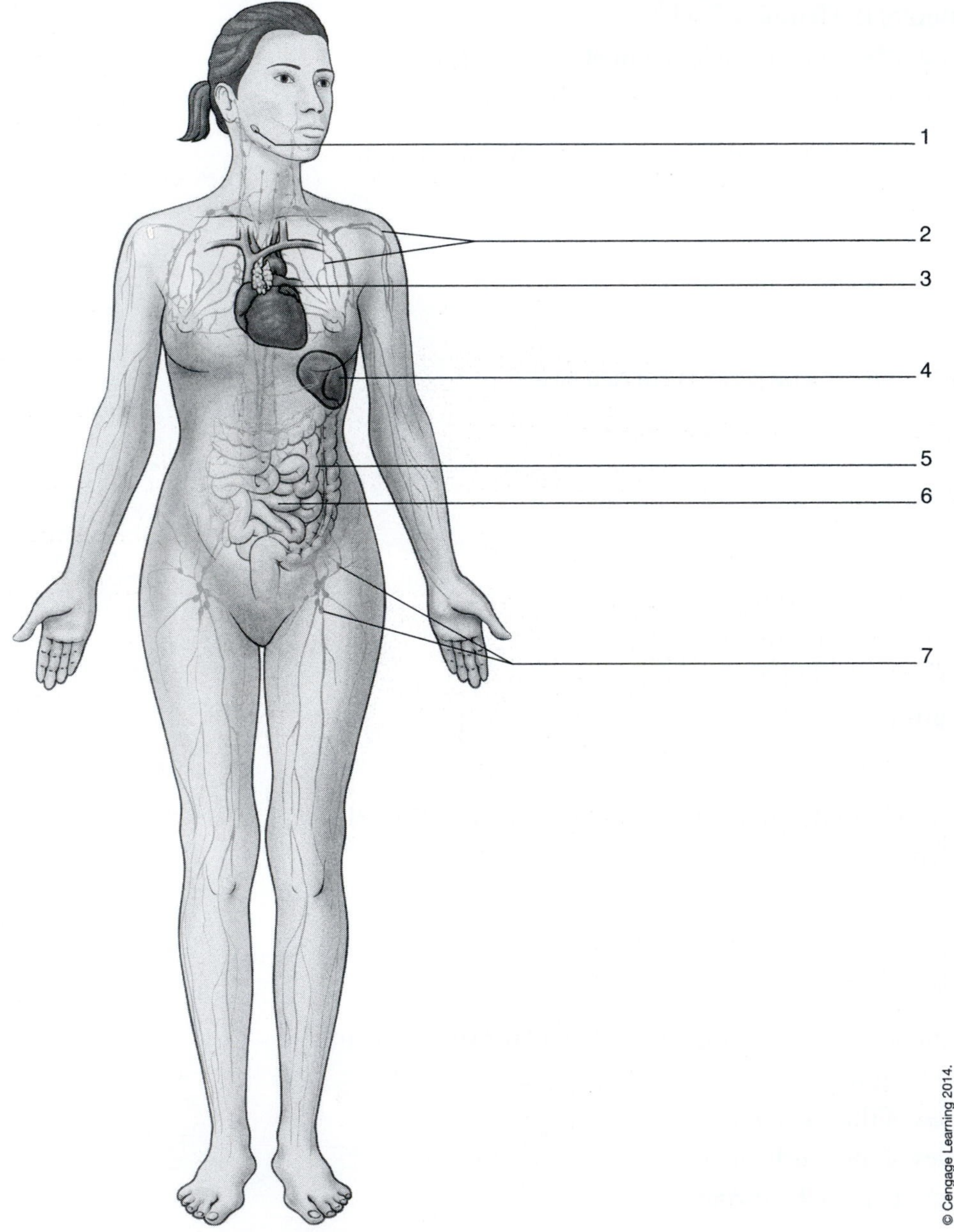

D. Compare the following items in terms of structure and function.

1. Blood capillary/lymph capillary

____

____

2. Antigen/antibody

____

____

3. Immunoglobulin/lymphokines

____

____

4. Immunity/autoimmunity

____

____

E. Label and color the diagram of lymph drainage. Color the thoracic duct yellow, the right lymph duct blue, and the lymph nodes orange.

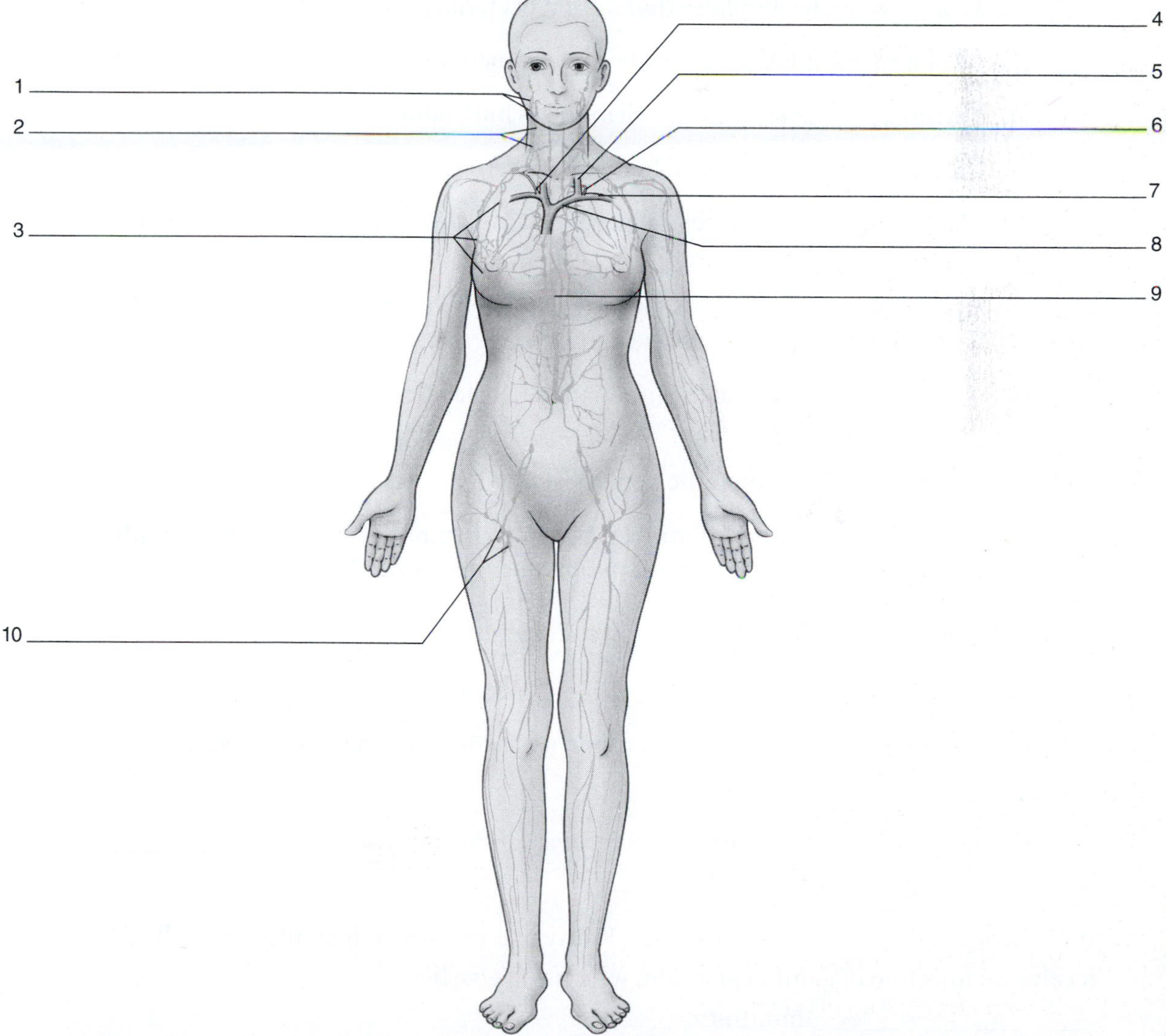

F. State the location and function of each of the following structures.

Structure	Location	Function
Spleen	______	______
Thymus	______	______
Axillary lymph node	______	______
Thoracic duct	______	______
Palatine tonsils	______	______
Right lymph duct	______	______
Lymph capillaries	______	______

G. Mark the statements either true or false. Correct any false statements.

______ 1. The skin and normal flora serve as physical barriers against infectious agents.

______ 2. Tears contain bactericides that inhibit bacterial growth.

______ 3. The large intestine has an acidic environment to prevent the growth of pathogens.

______ 4. The nonspecific response to cell injury is inflammation.

______ 5. Immunoglobulin E is found in the blood serum and lymph.

______ 6. Plasma cells are formed by helper T cells and produce large quantities of the same antibody.

______ 7. Macrophages exist in the body for years, enabling the body to respond quickly to any future infection from the same pathogen.

______ 8. Helper T cells stimulate the production of killer T cells and more B cells to fight invading pathogens.

______ 9. Killer T cells slow down the activity of B cells once the infection is controlled.

______ 10. B cells are lymphocytes found in the spleen, lymph nodes, and other lymphatic tissue. These clones form plasma cells and memory cells.

H. Fill in the blanks to complete the following statements.

1. Immunity is the ability to ______ disease.
2. Baby Anthony was born with anatomical barriers to disease; this is considered ______ immunity.
3. Rebecca, age 6, has had chickenpox and recovered; she now has ______ ______ immunity.
4. While working in the adult home center, Kathy was exposed to hepatitis; she will receive an injection of gamma globulin, which will give her ______ ______ immunity.

5. Bryan is going to camp. The physical form asks whether he has received immunizations for measles and mumps. This type of immunization is considered ____________________ ____________________ immunity.

6. Baby Megan's mother, Eileen, has had mumps, which will give Megan ____________________ ____________________ immunity; it will last only about 1 year.

I. The length of time immunity lasts varies; state the amount of time each type lasts.

1. Natural immunity ____________________
2. Natural passive immunity ____________________
3. Artificial acquired immunity ____________________
4. Natural acquired immunity ____________________

J. Circle the correctly spelled word in each of the following statements.

1. (Swollen, Swollan) glands is another term for lymph (adenitis, adanitis).
2. Treatments for Hodgkin's disease include chemotherapy and (radiation, rediation).
3. The lymph disease that often occurs in young adults and children is infectious (mononucleosis, mononuclosis).
4. Mono, or the "kissing disease," is treated (symptomatically, symptomaticaly).
5. In autoimmunity, an (individual's, indivedual's) immune system forms antibodies that attack healthy tissue.
6. In hypersensitivity reactions, the antibodies formed irritate certain body cells, causing an (alergic, allergic) reaction.
7. In asthma, antibodies bind to (bronchioles, broncholes); in hay fever they cause runny nose and (itcy, itchy) eyes.
8. A severe allergic reaction is called (anophylactic, anaphylactic) shock.
9. Patients should always be questioned regarding (sensativity, sensitivity) to allergens or drugs.
10. Medical-alert tags have saved the lives of people who are (unconsious, unconscious) or unable to communicate.

K. Unscramble the letters to form the word that matches the description.

Lymphatic System

1. Chronic inflammatory autoimmune disease — ULSAU
2. Disease with thickening of skin and blood vessels — ERCRASMDLOE
3. Occurs when the body's immune system fails to protect itself against foreign material — IPNSIERVTSEYYHI

4. A severe and sometimes fatal allergic reaction — LHYXSAPANAI
5. An antigen that causes an immune response — EAENLLRG
6. When a person's own immune system mistakenly targets normal cells — MIOUTHAUITMN
7. Specialized lymph vessels in the villi of the small intestines — TLAECLSA
8. The ability of the body to fight disease — YMITUIMN

L. The following symptoms occur in AIDS patients. For each, name another condition in which the symptom may also appear.

Symptom	Disorder
1. Prolonged fatigue	______________
2. Persistent cough	______________
3. Shortness of breath	______________
4. Chronic diarrhea	______________
5. Easy bruising or bleeding	______________
6. Discolored skin lesions	______________
7. Swollen glands	______________
8. Unexplained weight loss	______________

M. Complete the following related to AIDS and HIV.

1. AIDS and HIV are acronyms for: ______________________________________

____

____

2. How is AIDS transmitted? ______________________________________

____

____

3. Explain opportunistic infections and list the opportunistic infections an AIDS patient may develop. ______________________________________

____

____

N. Place the following words in the crossword puzzle.

3 Letters
ARC
cut

4 Letters
AIDS
gown
mask
mono

5 Letters
cough
lymph
ulcer

6 Letters
gloves
plasma
spleen
thymus
valves

7 Letters
caution
dyspnea
goggles
lingual
natural
needles
passive
tonsils
vaccine

8 Letters
acquired
adenitis
adenoids
allergen
axillary
bleeding
Hodgkins
immunity
palatine

9 Letters
isolation
lymphatic

10 Letters
autoimmune
incubation
leukopenia
lymph nodes

11 Letters
anaphylaxis

12 Letters
immunization
interstitial
thoracic duct
transmission

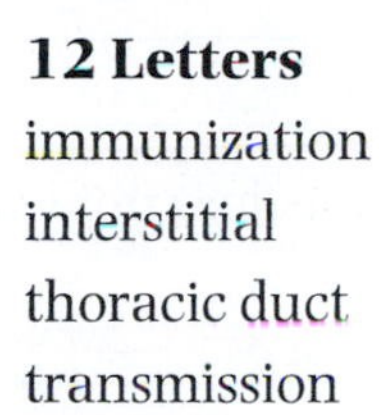

13 Letters
opportunistic

14 Letters
Kaposi's sarcoma

15 Letters
lymphatic system
natural acquired

16 Letters
acquired immunity
hypersensitivity

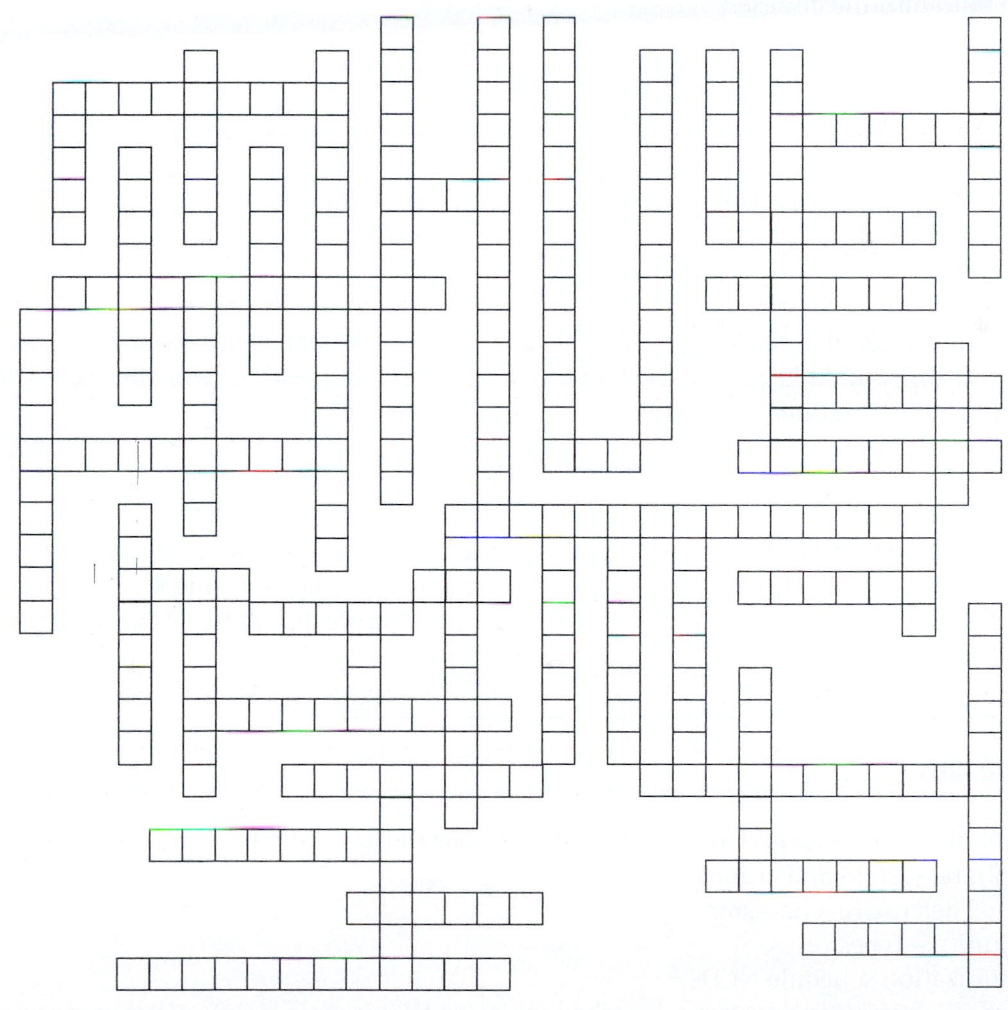

O. List one way in which the lymph system affects the other body systems.

____

____

____

APPLYING THEORY TO PRACTICE

1. The patient's mother says that, years ago, if you had many sore throats the doctors would remove your tonsils. This procedure is not done for sore throats today. Why has the standard changed?

   ____

   ____

2. A father states that he does not want his baby vaccinated. How would you respond regarding immunization?

   ____

   ____

   ____

3. Christopher has been diagnosed with Sjorgen's syndrome, and Dr. Bryan explains to him this is an autoimmune disease.
   a. Christopher wants to know what this means. He also want to know what other conditions are considered to be autoimmune diseases. How would you respond?

      ____

      ____

   b. Describe Sjorgen's syndrome, its symptoms, and its treatment.

      ____

      ____

4. Mike is a worker at an auto repair shop. While at work, he stepped on a board with several nails sticking out. Mike goes to the ER for treatment. What questions will Mike be asked regarding immunization?

   ____

   ____

5. Survey the adult members of your family and friends to find out whether they know what immunizations they should have. As a class, compare survey results and make up a list of the recommended immunizations for adults; the list can then be distributed as necessary.

   ____

   ____

SURF THE NET

For additional information and interactive exercises, use the following key words:

- lymphatic system and organs
- normal defense mechanisms
- immunity—types
- immunization schedule—CDC
- disorders of the lymph system—lymphadenitis, Hodgkin's disease, infectious mononucleosis
- autoimmune diseases—lupus, scleroderma, arthritis, Sjorgen's syndrome, and others
- AIDS

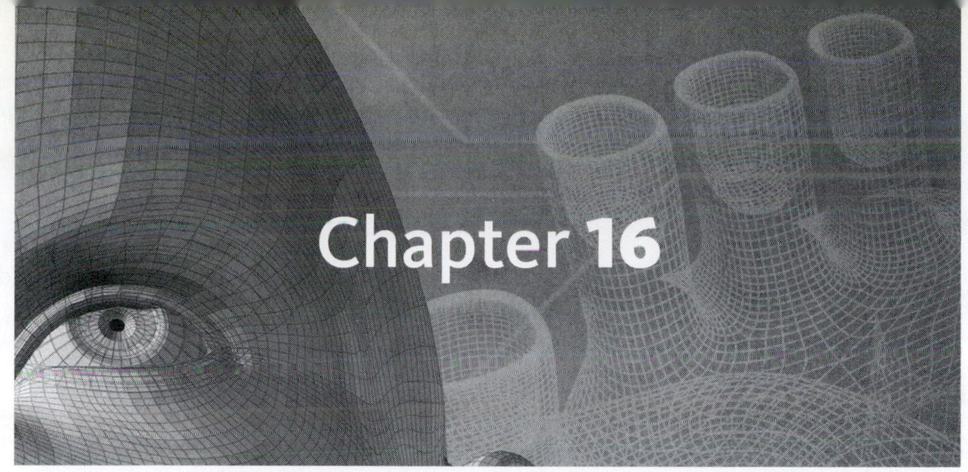

Infection Control and Standard Precautions

OVERVIEW

Infection control principles that relate to pathogenic microorganisms include chain of infection, normal defense mechanisms, the infectious process, nosocomial infections, and standard precautions.

Flora

Flora are microorganisms that occur in a specific environment. There are two types of flora:

Resident flora, or normal flora, are always present.
Transient flora occur in periods of limited duration.

Pathogenicity and Virulence

Pathogenicity is the ability of microorganisms to produce disease. **Virulence** is the frequency with which a pathogen may cause disease.

Types of Microorganisms. The six types of pathogenic microorganisms are bacteria, virus, fungi, protozoa, rickettsia, and helminths.

Bacteria are one-celled microorganisms that lack a true nucleus or mechanism to provide metabolism; some types produce spores.
A *virus* is a microorganism that can only live inside a cell; some viruses produce a protective coat called an envelope.
Fungi may grow in single cells or colonies and are found mainly in people who are immunologically impaired.
Protozoa are single-celled organisms with the ability to move.
Rickettsia are intercellular parasites that need to be in living cells to reproduce. Infection is spread through the bite of fleas, ticks, and lice.
Helminths, or parasitic worms, are microorganisms acquired by eating inadequately prepared meats.

Chain of Infection

The **chain of infection** describes the elements of an infectious process. This process includes several essential elements for transmission of microorganisms to occur.

Agent. An **agent** is an entity that is capable of causing disease, for example:

Biological agents are living organisms that invade the host, such as bacteria, viruses, fungi, protozoa, and rickettsia.

Chemical agents are substances that can interact with the body, such as pesticides.

Physical agents are factors in the environment, such as heat, light, noise, and radiation.

Reservoir. The **reservoir** is a place where the agent can survive and reproduce. The most common reservoirs are humans, animals, environment, and **fomites** (objects contaminated with an infectious agent). **Carriers** are humans and animals that have the infectious agent but are symptom free.

Portal of Exit. The **portal of exit** is the route by which an infectious agent leaves the reservoir through body secretions.

Mode of Transmission. The **mode of transmission** is the process that bridges the gap between the portal of exit of the agent and the portal of entry of the susceptible new host. Types include the following:

Contact—physical transfer from an infected person to an uninfected person.

Airborne—occurs when a susceptible person contacts contaminated droplets or dust particles suspended in the air.

Vehicle—occurs when the agent is transferred to a susceptible host by contaminated inanimate objects, such as water.

Vectorborne—occurs when an agent is transferred to a susceptible person by mosquitoes, fleas, and ticks.

Portal of Entry. The **portal of entry** is the route by which an infectious agent enters the new host.

Host. The **host** is an individual who is at risk of contracting an infection. A *susceptible host* is a person who lacks resistance and is vulnerable to disease. A *compromised host* is a person whose normal defense mechanisms are impaired and is more susceptible to infection.

Breaking the Chain of Infection

Health care workers focus on breaking the chain of infection by applying proper infection control practices to interfere with the spread of microorganisms.

Between Agent and Reservoir. The key to eliminating infection is through cleansing, disinfection, and sterilization.

Between Reservoir and Portal of Exit. Promoting proper hygiene, maintaining clean dressings and linen, and ensuring the use of clean equipment can break the chain.

Between Portal of Exit and Mode of Transmission. Maintaining clean dressings on all wounds, covering the mouth and nose when sneezing and coughing, using gloves with infectious secretions, and properly disposing of contaminated articles can break the chain.

Between Mode of Transmission and Portal of Entry. Break the chain by washing hands before and between patients and using barrier protection such as masks, gowns, gloves, and goggles.

Between Portal of Entry and Host. Maintain skin integrity and use sterile technique to prevent transmission from an infected person to an uninfected person.

Between Host and Agent. Proper nutrition, exercise, and immunization can maintain an intact immune system.

Stages of the Infectious Process

The two types of infectious responses are *localized* (confined to one area) and *systemic* (affects the entire body). The stages are as follows:

Incubation—time interval between entry of an infection and the onset of symptoms.

Prodromal—time interval from the onset of nonspecific symptoms until specific symptoms appear.

Illness—time when the person is showing specific signs and symptoms.

Convalescent—time from the beginning of disappearance of acute symptoms until the person returns to the previous state of health.

Nosocomial or Hospital-Acquired Infections (HAIs)

A **nosocomial** or **hospital-acquired infection** is acquired in a health care setting. Personnel who fail to follow proper handwashing techniques transmit most infections.

Bioterrorism

Bioterrorism is the use of bacteria, viruses, or germs to cause illness and spread fear. Terrorists use these methods because they can be spread through the air.

Standard Precautions

Standard precautions are the guidelines to be used during routine patient care and cleaning duties. They are required when there is possible contact with blood, any body fluid except sweat, mucous membranes, and nonintact skin. Standard precautions establish guidelines for handwashing, the use of protective barriers, care of patient equipment, occupational health, and blood-borne pathogens, as well as for patient placement.

ACTIVITIES

A. Complete the statement by filling in the correct answer.

1. Health care professionals are responsible for care that utilizes ______________________ ______________________ principles to provide a safe environment.
2. Organisms that live in a specific environment for a period of limited duration are known as ______________________ ______________________.
3. The ability of microorganisms to produce disease is known as ______________________.
4. ______________________ refers to the frequency with which a pathogen can cause disease.
5. An example of a resident flora is found on the ______________________.

B. 1. Name the factors that affect the virulence of a pathogen.

____

____

____

2. List the six types of pathogenic microorganisms.

____

____

____

____

____

____

C. State the classification of microorganisms that cause the following illnesses:

a. rubella
b. thrush
c. salmonella
d. *E. coli*
e. HIV
f. athlete's foot
g. Lyme disease
h. staphylococcus
i. mononucleosis
j. tapeworm
k. malaria
l. common cold

D. Select the letter of the choice that best completes the statement.

1. One-celled organisms that lack a true nucleus are
   a. protozoa.
   b. bacteria.
   c. viruses.
   d. fungi.

2. Organisms that can live only inside cells are
   a. helminths.
   b. protozoa.
   c. viruses.
   d. bacteria.
3. Which of the following pathogenic organisms are acquired by eating inadequately prepared meat?
   a. Helminths
   b. Protozoa
   c. Viruses
   d. Bacteria
4. Rocky Mountain spotted fever is caused by
   a. a virus.
   b. bacteria.
   c. protozoa.
   d. rickettsia.
5. A resistant state of bacterial production that can withstand unfavorable environments is known as
   a. mold.
   b. envelope.
   c. spore.
   d. parasite.
6. Urinary tract infections are mostly caused by
   a. rickettsia.
   b. fungi.
   c. viruses.
   d. bacteria.
7. Single-celled organisms that obtain food from dead or decaying organic matter are
   a. protozoa.
   b. viruses.
   c. fungi.
   d. rickettsia.
8. The disease caused by fungi may also be referred to as
   a. helminth.
   b. protozoa.
   c. rickettsia.
   d. mycoses.

9. An infection that is spread by the bites of fleas, ticks, and mites is a ____________ infection.
   a. fungal
   b. bacterial
   c. rickettsia
   d. protozoal
10. Individuals who are immunologically impaired may be more susceptible to disease caused by
   a. viruses.
   b. fungi.
   c. rickettsia.
   d. bacteria.

E. Label the following diagram of the chain of infection.

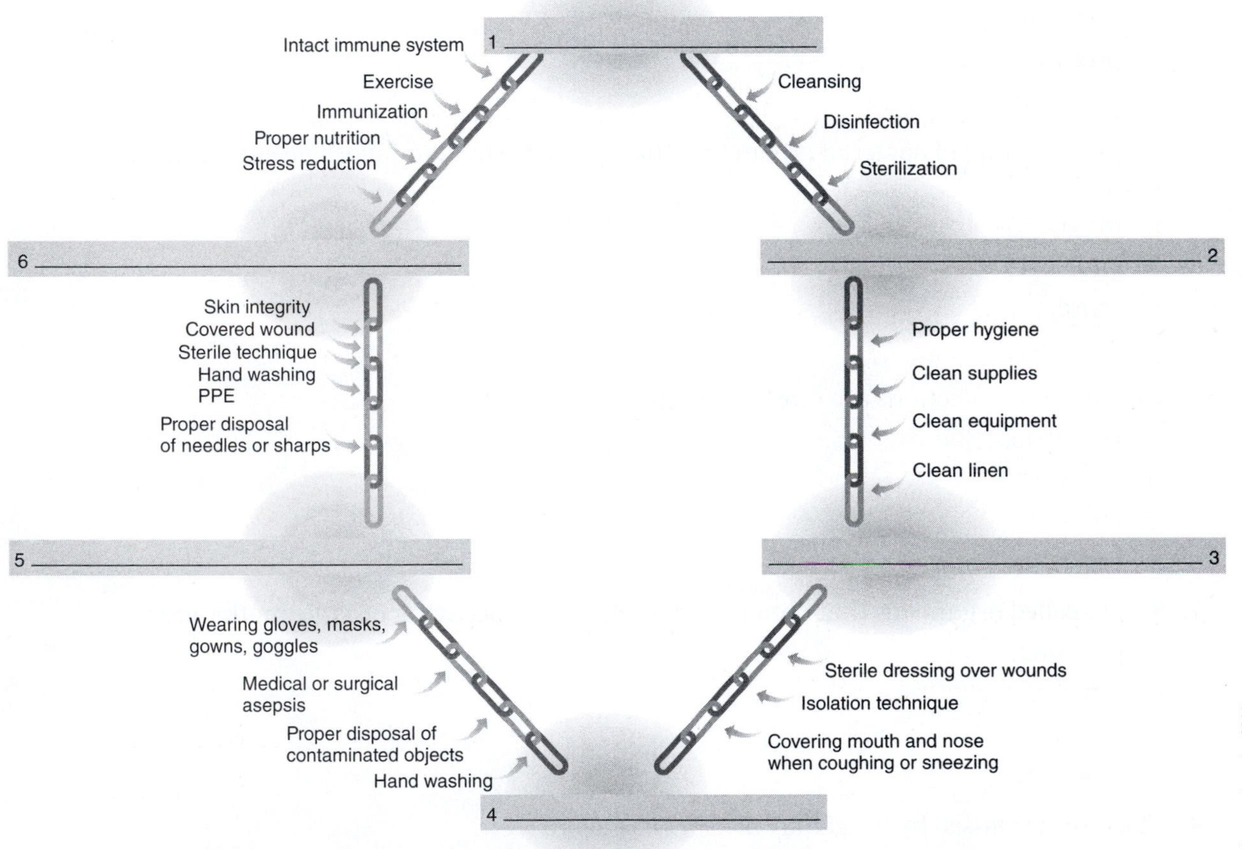

F. Place the numbers from the previous diagram beside the best description.
   a. ________ Place where the agent can survive
   b. ________ A simple or complex organism that can be affected by an agent
   c. ________ Process that bridges the gap between portal of exit and portal of entry
   d. ________ An entity that is capable of causing disease
   e. ________ Route by which an infectious agent enters the host
   f. ________ Route by which an infectious agent leaves the host

G. Use information on practices that will break the chain of infection to complete the following. Place your answer under the line for the rhyme.

Example: A clean dressing goes over the wound
Will help a person get well real soon
Between portal of entry and transmission
Make these as couplets the same as the preceding couplet

1. Immunization, exercise, and good nutrition
To keep healthy this is good ammunition

____

2. Disinfecting, sterilizing, and cleansing
Will keep this pathogen from growing

____

3. Covering mouths when sneezing or coughing
Will keep microbes from migrating

____

4. The pathogens cannot leave the scene
If you use clean dressings and practice good hygiene

____

5. Wearing masks and gowns and washing hands
Will keep germs from finding a new place to land

____

6. Skin integrity and sterile technique will help defeat
These little microbes from finding a new place to eat

____

H. Complete the following word puzzle using the clues given in the statement

a. single most effective way to prevent infection _ _ _ _ _ _ _ _ I _ _
b. elimination of pathogens except spores from inanimate objects _ _ _ _ N _ _ _ _ _ _ _
c. An interactive process that involves an agent, host, and environment is called a chain of _ _ F _ _ _ _ _ _
d. any change from normal function _ _ _ E _ _ _
e. infection acquired in a health care setting not present at the time of admission _ _ _ _ C _ _ _ _ _
f. ability of an organism to produce disease _ _ T _ _ _ _ _ _ _ _ _ _
g. pathogenic organism that can only live inside the cell _ I _ _ _
h. item worn when caring for a person who may have infectious secretions _ _ O _ _ _
i. removal of organic matter from equipment used in providing care _ _ _ _ N _ _ _ _

j. time interval between entry of an infection and appearance of symptoms __C_______

k. object contaminated with an infectious agent _O____

l. plant-like organism that may cause disease __N__

m. single parasitic organism with the ability to move ___T____

n. place where infectious agent can survive ____R____

o. use of bacteria, viruses, or organisms to cause illness and spread fear __O______

p. total elimination of all microorganisms, including spores _____L_______

J. Compare the following terms.

1. Susceptible host/compromised host

____

2. MRSA/*C. diff*

____

3. Disinfectant/sterilization

____

4. Direct contact transmission/indirect contact transmission

____

5. Fomite/carrier

____

K. Underline the correctly spelled words in the following statements.

1. Localized and (systemic, systamic) infection progress through four stages.
2. An infection limited to a defined area is a (localized, localezed) infection.
3. The incubation stage is the time interval between entry of an infectious agent into the host and the onset of symptoms in the (infectous, infectious) process.
4. The time interval from the onset of nonspecific symptoms until specific symptoms appear occurs in the (prodomal, prodromal) stage of infection.
5. The period of time from the beginning of disappearance of acute symptoms until the patient returns to the previous state of health is the (convalescent, convalesent) stage.

6. A (nosocomial, nosocommial) infection is acquired in a hospital or other health care facility.
7. (Personnal, Personnel) who fail to follow proper handwashing techniques transmit most infections.
8. The hospital environment provides exposure to a (variety, variaty) of virulent organisms.
9. The most common endemic infection is a (urinery, urinary) tract infection.
10. Individuals in long-term care facilities often have multiple illnesses, which decrease their (resistence, resistance) to infection.

L. 1. Handwashing is the single most effective way to prevent infection. Describe four rules that must be followed when handwashing.

____

____

____

____

2. What procedure must be used when using an alcohol-based hand-sanitizer?

____

____

____

3. When should a health care professional wear gloves?

____

____

____

4. Describe how a health care professional can prevent injuries from needles.

____

____

____

M. Word search: Circle the key words related to infection control and standard precautions.

INFECTION CONTROL

n	n	f	h	f	t	n	e	c	s	e	l	a	v	n	o	c
f	o	o	l	o	n	o	i	t	c	e	f	n	i	s	i	d
w	p	s	i	o	s	a	g	n	i	s	n	a	e	l	c	f
y	o	s	o	t	r	t	e	n	r	o	b	r	i	a	u	b
y	r	t	t	c	c	a	w	q	p	t	o	u	b	n	t	m
t	t	e	i	r	o	e	e	k	r	y	c	k	g	n	s	v
i	a	r	x	i	r	m	f	x	s	h	i	i	e	i	a	i
c	l	i	e	o	h	w	i	n	d	i	b	g	n	x	h	r
i	o	l	f	v	o	l	p	a	i	w	a	a	f	u	n	u
n	f	i	o	r	b	v	f	j	i	f	g	v	j	q	u	l
e	e	z	l	e	s	g	t	v	c	r	o	s	v	v	m	e
g	n	a	a	s	a	r	i	a	o	e	f	n	p	h	n	n
o	t	t	t	e	u	r	r	o	x	e	k	o	i	o	z	c
h	r	i	r	r	u	r	r	b	g	h	f	i	m	a	r	e
t	y	o	o	s	i	c	k	w	w	z	l	i	s	i	h	e
a	x	n	p	e	i	p	r	o	d	r	o	m	a	l	t	c
p	m	v	r	m	r	i	c	k	e	t	t	s	i	a	e	e

agent
airborne
carrier
chain of infection
cleansing
convalescent
disinfection
flora
fomite
fungi
host
microorganism
nosocomial
pathogenicity
portal of entry
portal of exit
prodromal
reservoir
rickettsia
spore
sterilization
virulence
virus

APPLYING THEORY TO PRACTICE

1. Nichole is in charge of a unit at the local hospital.

   She must be certain that her staff members know about standard precautions and infection control.

   Nichole has prepared a chart for staff members regarding standard precautions and posted it on the unit for reference.

   Complete Nichole's chart for standard precautions. [Use Table 16-5]

Recommendations for Application of Standard Precautions for the Care of All Patients in All Health Care Settings

COMPONENT	RECOMMENDATION
Hand hygiene (washing)	
Personal protective equipment (PPE)	
	For touching blood, body fluids, secretions, excretions, contaminated items; for touching mucous membranes and nonintact skin
Gown	
Mask, eye protection, face shield	
	Handle in a manner that prevents transfer of microorganisms to others and to the environment; wear gloves if visibly contaminated; perform handwashing
Environmental control	
	Handle in a manner that prevents the transfer of microorganisms to others and the environment
Needles and other sharps	
	Use mouthpiece, resuscitation bag, other ventilation devices to prevent contact with mouth and oral secretions
Patient placement	
Respiratory hygiene/cough etiquette (source containment of infectious respiratory secretions in symptomatic patients beginning at the initial point of contact)	

2. Vincent is the father of four children. He explains that colds in his household go from one person to another. Describe some of the methods of preventing colds from spreading in the household.

___

___

___

___

3. There is much fear in the public about bioterrorist attacks. Kreg works for a lumber supply company and asks Alyia, the nurse in the personnel department, what he should do in case of such a bioterrorist attack. What should Alyia tell Kreg?

___

___

___

___

4. We frequently hear about the emergence of a new disease. In reality, the incidence of infectious disease has been drastically reduced over the past few years.
   a. List the reasons why infectious diseases have declined in number.

   ___

   ___

   ___

   b. What are some emerging infectious disease threats?

   ___

   ___

   ___

SURF THE NET

For additional information and interactive exercises, use the following key words:

- normal flora
- pathogenic microorganisms—bacteria, viruses, fungi, protozoa, rickettsia helminths
- chain of infection
- nonspecific immune response
- specific immune response
- stages of the infectious process
- emerging infectious diseases
- bioterrorism agents of infection
- CDC—standard precautions

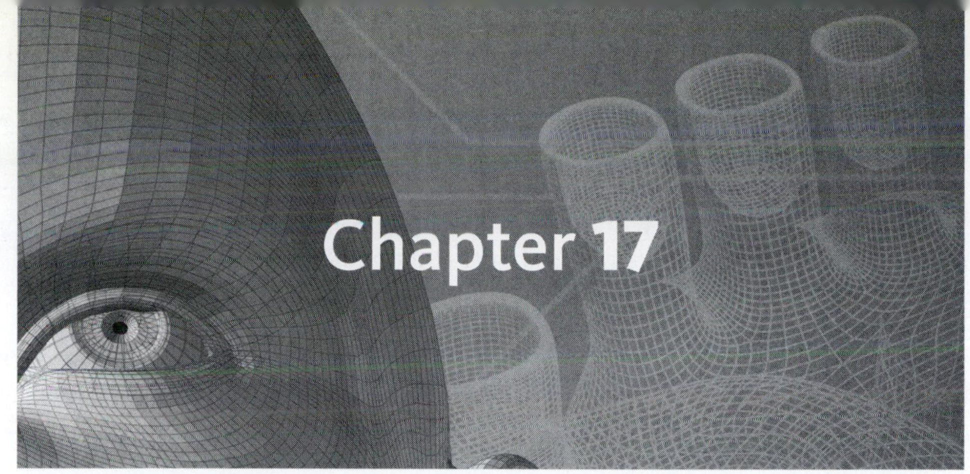

Respiratory System

OVERVIEW

The structures of the respiratory system allow for the exchange of oxygen and carbon dioxide for use by the cells of the body. This process is essential for the body to survive.

Functions of the Respiratory System

Functions of the respiratory system include the following:

To provide structures for the exchange of oxygen and carbon dioxide in the body and cells
To be responsible for the production of sound

Respiration

Human respiration is divided into three stages:

External respiration is breathing or ventilation; exchange of CO_2 and O_2 occurs between the lungs and the outside environment.

Internal respiration is the exchange of O_2 and CO_2 between the cells and the lymph surrounding them.

Cellular respiration or *oxidation* is the use of oxygen to release energy stored in nutrient molecules. When food is oxidized, it gives off carbon dioxide and water as waste.

Respiratory Organs and Structures

Organs of respiration include the nasal cavity, sinuses, pharynx, larynx, trachea, bronchi, bronchioles, alveolar ducts, alveoli, lungs, pleura, diaphragm, and mediastinum.

Nasal Cavity. Air enters through the nasal cavity, which filters, moistens, and warms the air.

The anterior nares are the two oval openings in the nose; also called the *nostrils.*

The nasal septum divides the nasal cavity into a right and left chamber.

The nasal concha or *turbinates* are three scroll-like bones that increase the surface area of the nasal cavity, causing turbulence.

The olfactory nerve is the upper part of the nasal cavity; it provides the sense of smell.

Sinuses. Sinuses are cavities lined with mucous membranes. They are located in the bones of the skull, around the nasal region, and are referred to as the *frontal, ethmoidal, maxillary,* and *sphenoidal* sinuses. They give tone to the voice.

Pharynx. The pharynx, or throat, is the common passageway for food and air. Air goes from the nasal cavity to the pharynx, which is divided into three parts: the *nasopharynx, oropharynx,* and *laryngopharynx.*

Larnyx. The larnyx, or voice box, is inferior to the pharynx. A cartilage lid, the *epiglottis,* is pushed by the tongue when you swallow to close the larynx, preventing food from entering the trachea. The larynx contains the *vocal cords;* air passes over the vocal cords to create sound.

Trachea. The trachea, or windpipe, is a ciliated passageway that extends from the larynx to the bronchi. It is composed of 15 to 20 C-shaped cartilage rings.

Bronchi and Bronchioles. The lower end of the trachea divides into the right and left bronchi. These bronchi further subdivide into smaller structures, the bronchioles. At the end of each bronchiole is an alveolar duct.

Alveolar Duct and Sacs. At the end of each alveolar duct is the alveolar sac, which resembles a cluster of grapes and consists of many alveoli.

Alveoli. The alveoli are a single layer of epithelial cells. The exchange of oxygen and carbon dioxide occurs between the capillaries around the alveoli by the process of diffusion. *Surfactant* is a lipid material that lines the inner surface of the alveoli.

Lungs. The lungs are right and left cone-shaped organs in the thoracic cavity. Lung tissue is porous and spongy because of the tremendous amount of air it contains. The right lung is divided into three lobes, the left into two lobes.

Pleura. The pleura is a double-layered membrane covering the lungs. The parietal pleura lines the thoracic cavity, and the visceral pleura covers the lung. Pleural fluid in this space prevents friction as the lungs expand and contract.

> *Pleurisy* is inflammation of the lining of the pleura.
>
> *Pneumothorax* is buildup of excess air in the pleural cavity on one side of the chest. The excess air increases pressure on the lung, causing it to collapse.

Diaphragm. The *diaphragm* is a dome shaped sheet of muscle separating the thoracic cavity from the abdomen; it is the contraction and relaxation of the diaphragm that makes breathing possible.

Mediastinum. The mediastinum, or interpleural space, is located between the lungs and extends from the sternum to the vertebrae.

The Breathing Process

Pulmonary ventilation allows the exchange of oxygen between the alveoli and the red blood cells.

> *Inhalation,* or *inspiration,* occurs when muscles in the thoracic cavity contract, increasing the space within the chest cavity. This results in a decrease in pressure; atmospheric pressure is now greater and air rushes in, all the way down to the alveoli.
>
> *Exhalation* or *expiration* is the opposite of inhalation. The muscles relax, space in the thoracic cavity decreases, and the increased pressure forces air out of the lungs.

Respiratory Movements. An inspiration and an expiration are one respiratory movement; the average rate is 14 to 20 breaths per minute. Factors that affect the rate are exercise, temperature, age, body position, emotions, coughing, sneezing, and hiccoughing.

The Effects of Aging on the Respiratory System

As the body ages, the lung tissue loses elasticity and muscle strength decreases. These factors compromise oxygen and carbon dioxide exchange, which causes signs of activity intolerance. There is a change in lung capacity. The elderly are more prone to respiratory disease.

Control of Breathing

The rate of breathing is controlled by neural and chemical factors.

Neural factors are controlled by the medulla oblongata in the brain. There are two centers, inspiratory and expiratory. An increase of carbon dioxide and a decrease of oxygen will trigger the respiratory center.

Phrenic nerves stimulate the diaphragm and the intercostal muscles.

Vagus nerves are involved in the Hering-Breuer reflex: when the lungs are inflated, the nerve endings of the lungs are stimulated, which then stimulate the vagus nerve to inhibit the inspiratory center.

Chemical factors occur as the level of carbon dioxide in the blood passes through the brain, stimulating the inspiration center.

Chemoreceptors are chemical regulators in the carotid arteries and aorta sensitive to the oxygen level; as oxygen decreases, impulses are sent to the respiratory center to stimulate inspiration.

Lung Capacity and Volume

Terms used to determine the amount of air in the lungs include *tidal volume, inspiratory reserve volume (IRV), expiratory reserve volume (ERV), vital capacity, residual volume, functional residual capacity,* and *total lung capacity.* See Figure 17-11 in your textbook for further explanation of these terms.

Types of Respiration

The following terms relate to types of respiration.

Apnea: temporary stoppage of respiration.

Dyspnea: difficulty in respiration.

Eupnea: normal or easy breathing.

Hyperpnea: increase in the depth and rate of breathing.

Orthopnea: difficult or labored breathing in the horizontal position.

Tachypnea: abnormally rapid and shallow breathing.

Hyperventilation: condition caused by stress—rapid breathing causes a rapid loss of carbon dioxide, leading to alkalosis, which results in dizziness and fainting.

Disorders of the Respiratory System

The *common cold* is the most common respiratory infection caused by a virus; it is often the basis for more serious disorders.

Infectious Causes. Infectious causes include the following:

Pharyngitis: red, inflamed throat.

Laryngitis: inflammation of the larynx or voice box.

Sinusitis: infection of the mucous membrane lining the sinuses.

Bronchitis: inflammation of the mucous membrane lining of the bronchial tubes; may be acute or chronic.

Influenza or "*flu*": inflammation of the respiratory system.

Pneumonia: infection of the lungs caused by a virus or bacteria.

Tuberculosis: disease of the lungs caused by the tubercle bacillus.

Diphtheria: rarely seen today because children are immunized against this condition shortly after birth.

Pertussis or whooping cough: highly contagious; the vaccine DTaP limits the number of cases.

Severe Acute Respiratory Syndrome (SARS): a contagious disease caused by the corona virus.

Anthrax: caused by the inhalation of the bacterium bacillus and its spores; spores convert to active bacillus and infect the lungs, leading to death.

Noninfectious Causes. Noninfectious causes include the following:

Rhinitis: inflammation of the nasal mucous membrane caused by an allergen or cold virus.

Asthma: airway becomes obstructed due to an inflammatory response to a stimulus that may be an allergen or stress.

Atelectasis: failure of the lungs to expand normally due to bronchial occlusion.

Bronchiectasis: dilation of a bronchus caused by an inflammation.

Asbestosis: caused by inhaling asbestos fibers.

Silicosis: caused by breathing dust containing silicon dioxide; the lungs become fibrosed, which results in reduced lung capacity.

Pulmonary embolism: a blood clot that travels to the lung; may occur after a person has been immobile.

Chronic Obstructive Pulmonary Disease (COPD).

Emphysema is when the alveoli become overdilated, lose their elasticity, cannot rebound, and eventually rupture. In this process, air becomes trapped, making it difficult to exhale.

Chronic bronchitis is also classified as COPD.

Cancers of the Respiratory System.

Cancer of the lung is a malignant tumor that forms in the bronchial epithelium; the most common cause of lung cancer is smoking.

Cancer of the larynx is a malignant tumor of the voice box.

Sudden Infant Death Syndrome (SIDS). Sudden infant death syndrome, or *crib death*, usually occurs between the ages of 1 week and 1 year; the infant stops breathing during sleep. The exact cause is unknown.

ACTIVITIES

A. Select the word or words from the following list to complete the statements. A word or words may be used more than once.

alveoli	diffuses	internal respiration
bicarbonate	exhalation	oxidation
breathing	external respiration	oxygen
carbon dioxide	inhalation	water
cellular respiration	inspiration	

1. The exchange of oxygen and carbon dioxide between the lungs and the environment is called ____________ ____________ or ____________.
2. The ventilation process consists of taking air in, or ____________ (____________), and breathing air out, or ____________.
3. In ventilation, oxygen ____________ from an area of higher concentration in the alveoli to an area of lower concentration in the bloodstream.
4. In the process of exhalation, ____________ ____________ and ____________ are exhaled.
5. The exchange of carbon dioxide and oxygen between the cells and the surrounding lymph is called ____________ ____________.
6. Deoxygenated blood produced during internal respiration carries carbon dioxide in the form of ____________ ions.
7. The use of ____________ to release energy stored in nutrient molecules is called ____________ ____________ or ____________.
8. The waste products of oxidation are carried away through the process of ____________ ____________.

B. Describe the functions of the respiratory system.

____

____

____

____

C. Label the diagram of the respiratory system. Trace air from the external environment to the alveoli. Color the diagram.

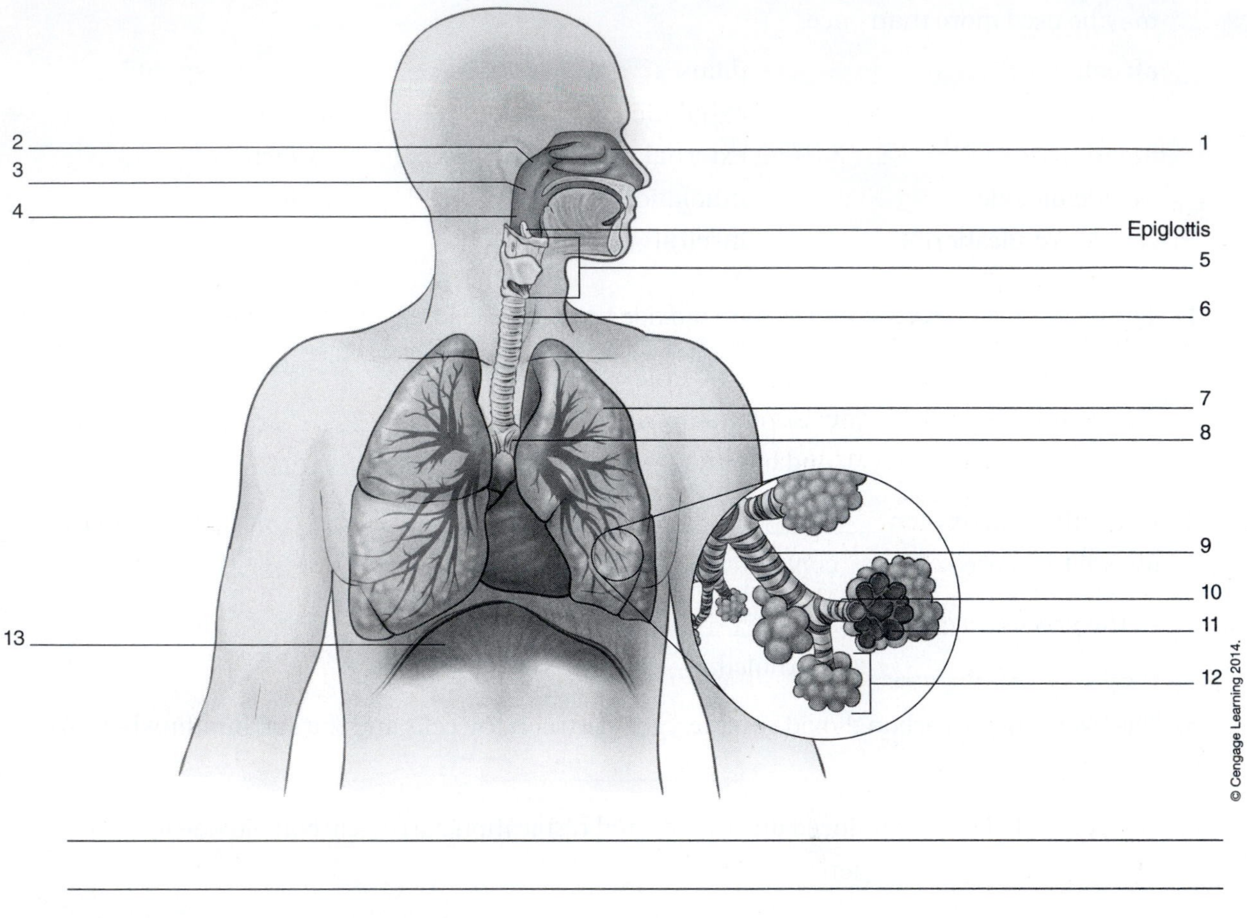

____

____

____

D. Select the letter of the choice that best completes the statement.

1. The nasal cavities are lined with mucous membrane, and the air is ____________ as it passes through.
   a. warmed and moistened
   b. cooled and moistened
   c. warmed and dried
   d. cooled and dried
2. The turbinates, or nasal concha, are responsible for
   a. cooling the air in the nares.
   b. filtering the air in the nasal cavity.
   c. decreasing the surface area of the nasal cavity, causing turbulence.
   d. increasing the surface area of the nasal cavity, causing turbulence.
3. The structure that filters the air in the nasal cavity is the
   a. concha.
   b. cilia.
   c. septum.
   d. mucous membrane.

4. Located in the upper part of the nasal cavity are the endings of the ____________ nerve.
   a. optic
   b. olfactory
   c. oculomotor
   d. auditory
5. The diaphragm contracts because it is stimulated by the ________________ nerve.
   a. sciatic
   b. phrenic
   c. glossopharyngeal
   d. humoral
6. The four nasal sinuses are the
   a. frontal, ethmoidal, sphenoidal, and maxillary.
   b. frontal, ethmoidal, sphenoidal, and mandible.
   c. frontal, parietal, sphenoidal, and maxillary.
   d. frontal, ethmoidal, sphenoidal, and temporal.
7. The pharynx is also known as the
   a. voice box.
   b. windpipe.
   c. throat.
   d. nares.
8. The eustachian tube connects the middle ear and the
   a. laryngopharynx.
   b. larynx.
   c. nasopharynx.
   d. propharynx.
9. The structure also known as the interpleural space is the
   a. parietal pleura.
   b. mediastinum.
   c. visceral pleura.
   d. diaphragm.
10. Sound is produced when the air is
    a. inhaled into the lungs.
    b. exhaled from the lungs.
    c. vibrated by the glottis.
    d. acted on by the lips and tongue.

E. The various sinuses are shown in the following diagram.

1. Label the sinuses.

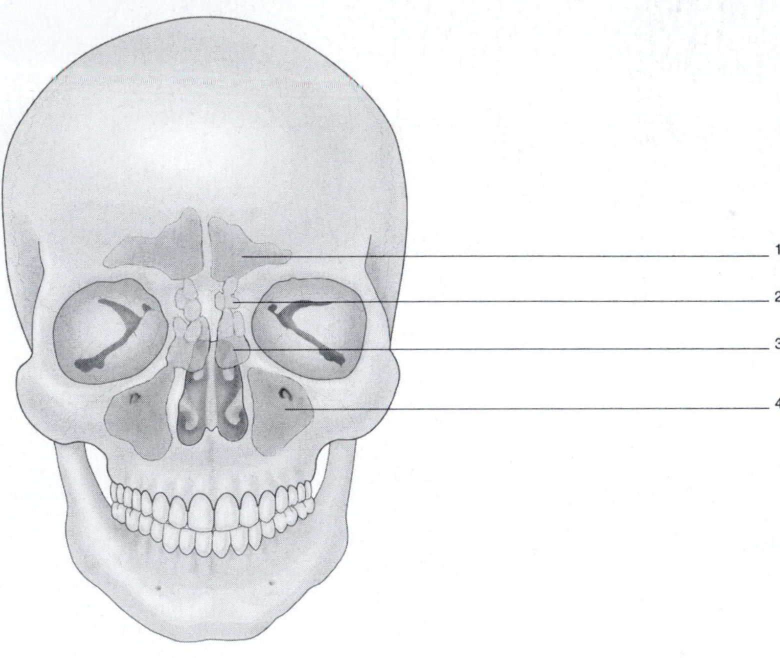

2. Describe the functions of the sinuses.

____

____

____

____

F. Fill in the blanks to complete the statements on the respiratory system.

1. The trachea conducts air from the larynx to the ____________
2. The walls of the trachea are composed of 15 to 20 C-shaped rings of ____________, which prevent the trachea from collapsing.
3. The process by which dust-laden mucus is expelled is ____________.
4. The lower end of the trachea divides into the ____________ ____________ and the ____________ ____________.
5. The terminal ends of the bronchi are the ____________.
6. The bronchiole walls are made from ____________ ____________ and elastic tissue lined with ____________ epithelium.
7. At the end of the bronchiole there is an alveolar duct, which ends in a ____________ ____________.
8. There are about ____________ times the number of alveoli necessary to sustain life.

9. The inner surfaces of the alveoli are covered with ____________________.

10. It is through the moist walls of the ____________________ and the ____________________ that rapid exchange of carbon dioxide and oxygen occurs.

G. Label the diagram of the bronchial tree.

1 ____________________

Cartilage ring

2 ____________________

3 ____________________

4 ____________________

6 ____________________

5 ____________________

8 ____________________

7 ____________________

9 ____________________

A

H. Compare the following according to structure and function.

1. Right bronchus/left bronchus

____

____

2. Sound/speech

____

____

3. Alveolar duct/alveoli

____

____

4. Parietal pleura/visceral pleura

____

____

5. Right lung/left lung

____

____

6. Lung tissue/heart tissue

____

____

7. Pleurisy/pneumothorax

____

____

I. Use the words from the following list to complete the statements.

atmospheric pressure	elasticity	inspiration
compliance	expanded	internal intercostals
decrease	external intercostals	negative pressure
diaphragm	flattened	surface tension
downward	increases	upward

1. The normal pressure within the pleural space is always ____________ ____________, which is less than ____________ ____________; this helps keep the lungs expanded.
2. There are two groups of intercostal muscles; during ____________, the ____________ ____________ lift the ribs ____________ and outward.
3. During inspiration, the ____________ contracts and becomes ____________.
4. The action of the muscles and the diaphragm results in a ____________ in pressure in the pleural space; the atmospheric pressure is greater and air rushes in.
5. In expiration, the ____________ ____________ of the fluid lining the alveoli reduces the elasticity of the lung tissue, causing the alveoli to collapse.
6. The ability of the lungs to change capacity as the size of the thoracic cavity is altered is known as ____________.

J. Answer the following questions on respiration.

1. What actions are considered as one respiratory movement?

____

2. What is the normal respiratory rate?

____

3. How is the respiratory rate affected by the following?
   a. Age ______
   b. Body position ______
   c. Increased body temperature ______
   d. Gender ______
   e. Emotions ______
4. Explain how coughing, sneezing, and hiccoughing affect respirations.

______

______

______

K. Breathing is controlled by neural factors and chemical factors. Explain the role of the following in respiratory control.

1. Medulla oblongata

______

______

2. Phrenic nerve

______

______

3. Vagus nerve

______

______

4. Hering-Breuer reflex

______

______

5. Increase in carbon dioxide

______

______

6. Chemoreceptor

______

______

7. Depressant drugs

______

______

L. Label the diagram of lung capacity and include the amount of air involved.

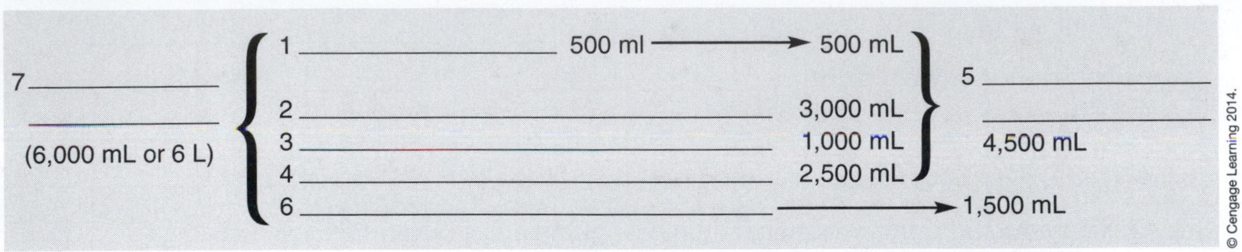

M. Match the terms in Column A with the statements in Column B

Column A	Column B
_______ 1. spirometer	a. Tidal volume + IRV + ERV + functional capacity + residual air
_______ 2. tidal volume	b. the total amount of air involved with tidal volume, IRV, and ERV
_______ 3. inspiratory reserve volume	c. air that cannot be voluntarily expelled from the lungs
_______ 4. expiratory reserve volume	d. amount of air that moves in and out of the lungs with one breath
_______ 5. total lung capacity	e. amount of air you can force a person to take in
_______ 6. residual volume	f. instrument that measures lung capacity
_______ 7. functional residual volume	g. amount of air you can force a person to exhale
	h. sum of the ERV plus the residual volume

N. Fill in the blanks with the correct terms describing types of breathing.

1. _________ temporary stoppage of breathing
2. _________ normal breathing
3. ___________ difficult or labored breathing
4. _____________ an abnormally rapid and shallow rate of breathing
5. ________________ difficult or labored breathing when the body is in a horizontal position
6. _______________ an increase in the rate and depth of breathing
7. ________________ rapid breathing that causes the body to lose carbon dioxide too quickly, lowering the blood level of CO_2, which leads to alkalosis and possibly fainting

O. How do you correct hyperventilation?

____

____

____

____

P. Use the words from the following list to complete the rhymes.

alveolar duct	bronchus	larynx	trachea
alveoli	capillary	mucus	vein
artery	cilia	nasal cavity	voice box
bronchi	inhaled	pharynx	

I was floating by in the evening breeze
when I got inhaled by a great big sneeze.

Next thing I knew I was inhaled inside
to the ____________ ____________ on the right side.

The place was warm, moist, and had ____________ so thick
with little hairs called ____________; they make you want to itch.

I did not have much chance to look around;
I went over the cliff and down, down, down.

I landed in a place called the ____________ or throat;
it was so full of watery juice, I thought I needed a boat.

I was quickly pulled through a place with a high pitch,
the ____________, or voice box, where air rushes by real quick.

Off to another tube, lined with those little hairs, the
windpipe or ____________; I spent little time there.

I landed then on what looked like a tree,
the ____________, I believe; what side should it be?

The ____________ branches keep getting narrower and end in the
____________ ____________, into the air sacs or ____________
I quickly get sucked.

I pass through the wall onto the ____________ train;
off to a new adventure as I board an ____________ and not a
____________.

Q. Circle the correctly spelled word in each of the following statements.

1. The common cold, a (resperatory, respiratory) infection, results in the greatest loss in production hours each year.
2. To treat a common cold you should stay in bed, drink plenty of fluid, and eat (wholesome, holesome), nourishing food.
3. (Pharyngitis, pharynxitis) is an inflammation of the throat that may occur as the result of an (irritant, irritent), such as too much smoking or speaking.

4. The most common form of laryngitis is (catarrhal, catarhal).
5. Symptoms of laryngitis include dryness, hoarseness, coughing, and (disphagia, dysphagia).
6. Sinusitis is an infection of the mucous membrane lining the sinus cavity or (cavities, cavites).
7. Acute bronchitis is characterized by fever, cough, substernal pain, and (rails, rales).
8. Chronic bronchitis differs from acute bronchitis in that the cough must be (persistent, persistence) for 3 months and have occurred for 2 consecutive years.
9. In (neumonia, pneumonia), an infection of the lung, the alveoli become filled with thick fluid called exudate.
10. An inflammation of the mucous membrane of the respiratory system is called the flu or (influenza, influinza).

R. Mark the underlined word or words in the statements true or false. Correct any false statements.

1. ________ <u>TB</u> is an infectious disease diagnosed by a Mantoux test.
2. ________ In the treatment of <u>emphysema</u>, a humidifier is recommended to relieve congestion.
3. ________ <u>Anthrax</u> is considered to be a disease that might be spread by terrorists.
4. ________ Respiratory illnesses account for approximately <u>20%</u> of all acute illnesses.
5. ________ SARS is a respiratory disease caused by corona virus.
6. ________ <u>Bronchitis</u> is characterized by a cough, substernal pain, and rales.
7. ________ A yearly vaccine for <u>pertussis</u> is recommended for the elderly and people who work or live with high-risk individuals.
8. ________ The CDC states that pertussis currently is seen at the highest level in <u>25</u> years.
9. ________ In <u>emphysema</u>, the lungs become over-dilated and lose their elasticity.
10. ________ In <u>pneumonia</u>, the alveoli become filled with a thick fluid called exudate.

S. Match the following respiratory disorders in Column A with the correct descriptions in Column B.

Column A	Column B
________ 1. nasal polyps	a. lungs fail to expand normally
________ 2. rhinitis	b. alveoli of lungs lose their elasticity
________ 3. asthma	c. lungs become fibrosed, leading to reduced capacity
________ 4. atelectasis	d. inflammation of the nasal mucous membrane
________ 5. emphysema	e. growth that occurs in the nasal cavity
________ 6. silicosis	f. airway obstructed due to an inflammatory response to a stimulus

T. Fill in the blanks to complete the following statements about lung cancer.

1. Cancer of the lungs is found mainly in people who ____________________.
2. Diagnosis of cancer of the lung usually is made by a ____________________. During this procedure, the throat is anesthetized; therefore it is important to be certain that the ____________________ ____________________ has returned before the person takes fluid or food.

U. Explain the role that the respiratory system has in the function of the other body systems.

____

____

____

APPLYING THEORY TO PRACTICE

1. Kathy has been a smoker for over 35 years. She goes to her physician because of her chronic cough. The physician orders a CAT scan of the lungs and pulmonary function studies. The diagnosis is chronic obstructive pulmonary disease (COPD) due to emphysema.
   a. Name and describe the two conditions that are considered to be COPD.

   ____

   ____

   ____

   b. Explain pulmonary function studies.

   ____

   ____

   ____

   c. Explain the treatment for emphysema.

   ____

   ____

   ____

2. Smoking is the leading cause of lung cancer and COPD. Many establishments both public and private are now "smoke free," no smoking allowed. How does smoking affect the respiratory system?

   ____

   ____

   ____

   ____

3. A patient who has been in bed recovering from hip surgery complains of sudden severe chest pain and is having dyspnea. What could be occurring?

____

____

4. The Jones family is very upset. They feel responsible for their infant's death from sudden infant death syndrome. Explain to the Jones family what you know about this condition.

____

____

____

____

5. Emary's parents say she is having a great deal of difficulty in breathing. Emary, age 7, has been previously treated in the ER for asthma. What are the causes of asthma? Describe the physiological changes that occur in an asthmatic attack. Describe the usual treatment and a possible adjunct treatment for asthma. How can the nurse help Emary understand her illness?

____

____

____

6. Maria is 78 years old; she has been very active at the senior center and loves to dance. Lately, Maria is having some difficulty in breathing after her dancing. As the LPN who is assigned to the senior center, explain to Maria what is occurring as she ages.

____

____

____

7. Mr. Gonzales is 65 years old. He has come to the HMO because he is falling asleep during the daytime. His wife is complaining that his snoring is so loud that it keeps her awake. The doctor orders a sleep apnea test. Mr. Gonzales asks you, the health educator, to explain sleep apnea and asks if it can be treated.

____

____

____

____

8. Daniel is in middle school and comes home with a note stating that there has been an outbreak of pertussis in the school. His mother Victoria calls the school nurse and asks her to explain pertussis. Victoria says "I thought that Daniel was vaccinated against that disease." Explain to Victoria what changes are occurring regarding vaccination.

____

____

____

____

9. Kieran attends a Career Day function featuring the career of respiratory therapist. What information will Kieran find out about this career?

____

____

____

SURF THE NET

For additional information and interactive exercises, use the following key words:

- respiratory system—structure and function
- external and internal respiration
- breathing process
- control of breathing—neural and chemical factors
- lung capacity and volume
- types of respiration
- effects of aging on the respiratory system
- disorders of the respiratory system—common cold, infections of the passageway, bronchitis, influenza, pneumonia, tuberculosis, diphtheria, pertussis, anthrax, chronic obstructive pulmonary disease (COPD), asthma
- lung cancer and smoking

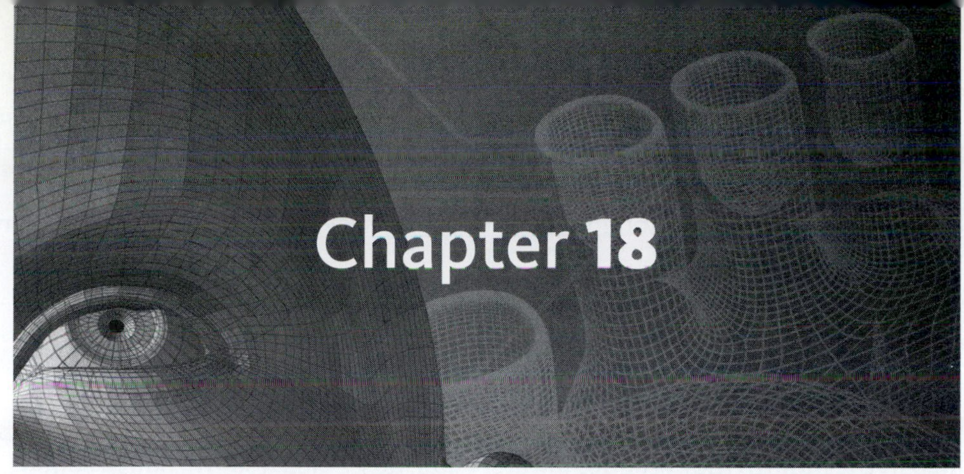

Digestive System

OVERVIEW

The organs of digestion change food into a simple form that can be used by the cells of the body and eliminate the waste products of the digestive process.

Digestion. Digestion is the process of changing complex solid foods into simple soluble forms that can be absorbed by the body cells.

The **digestive system** consists of the main organs of digestion: mouth, pharynx, esophagus, stomach, small intestine, large intestine, and anus. The accessory organs of digestion are the tongue, teeth, salivary glands, pancreas, liver, and gallbladder.

Layers of the Digestive System

The digestive system is composed of four layers:

Mucosa: the innermost lining; made of epithelial cells.

Submucosa: connective tissue.

Circular muscle: third layer; made of skeletal and smooth muscle.

Longitudinal muscle: fourth layer; also called visceral peritoneum.

Lining of the Digestive System

The **peritoneum** is a serous double membrane lining the abdominal cavity. Specialized layers are as follows:

Mesentery: intestines attached to the lining, which is attached to the posterior wall of the abdominal cavity.

Greater omentum: double fold of peritoneum that hangs down over the abdominal organs like an apron.

Organs of Digestion

Mouth or Buccal Cavity. The mouth is the oral cavity. It is composed of several parts:

Hard palate: roof of the mouth, formed from maxillary and palatine bones.

Soft palate: made from a movable mucous fold; separates the mouth from the nasopharynx.

Uvula: conical flap that hangs from the soft palate.

Tongue (Accessory Organ). The tongue is a bundle of skeletal muscles lying in many different planes.

Papillae are projections of the tongue containing the nerve endings for taste buds.

Taste buds are organs that sense salty, bitter, sour, sweet, and savory flavors.

Salivary Glands (Accessory Organ). The three salivary glands, parotid, sublingual, and submandible, are located in the mouth; they produce a watery substance called saliva. Saliva softens, lubricates food, and dissolves it. Saliva contains salivary amylase, which digests starch to simpler substances.

Teeth (Accessory Organ). Teeth cut and shred food, a process called mastication.

Gingivae, or **gums,** are fleshy tissue, covered with mucous membrane, that support and protect the teeth. **Deciduous teeth** or **baby teeth** begin to erupt at 6 months and continue to erupt through 2 years of age. **Permanent teeth** begin to replace deciduous teeth at about 5 years; the adult mouth has 32 permanent teeth. Types of teeth are as follows:

Incisors: sharp edges for biting.

Canines: pointed for tearing.

Molars: ridges or cusps designed for crushing and grinding.

Bicuspids: premolars that are broad and have two cusps.

Esophagus. The esophagus is a muscular tube about 10 inches long. It begins at the pharynx or throat and runs to the cardiac sphincter of the stomach.

Stomach. The stomach lies in the upper quadrant of the abdominal cavity and is divided into the *fundus, body,* and *pylorus.* When the stomach is empty, it hangs in folds called *rugae.* The opening between the esophagus and the stomach is controlled by the *cardiac sphincter*; the opening between the pylorus and the duodenum is controlled by the *pyloric sphincter.*

Gastric Glands. The gastric glands are located in the mucosal lining; they secrete pepsinogen, mucus, hydrochloric acid, and the intrinsic factor.

Pepsinogen converts to pepsin by the action of hydrochloric acid.

Mucus neutralizes the effects of hydrochloric acid.

Hydrochloric acid destroys bacteria in food.

Intrinsic factor is necessary for vitamin B_{12} absorption.

Small Intestine. The small intestine is a coiled portion of the digestive system about 20 feet long and 1 inch in diameter. It is divided into the duodenum (first 12 inches), the jejunum (8 feet), and the ileum (10 to 12 feet). A few inches into the duodenum is the hepatopancreatic ampulla, the site where the pancreatic duct and the common bile duct empty their contents into the small intestine. The digestive juices in the small intestine are the following:

Secretin and cholecystokinin are enzymes that stimulate the digestive juices of the pancreas, liver, and gallbladder.

Pancreatic juices break down protein, starch, and fats; they also contain sodium bicarbonate, which neutralizes the food content of the stomach.

Bile emulsifies fat.

Intestinal juices work on protein, starches, and fats.

Absorption in the Small Intestine. Absorption in the small intestine is possible because of the *villi*, which contain blood capillaries and lymph capillaries that absorb the end products of digestion, including the following:

Starch: absorbed as glucose.

Protein: absorbed as amino acids.

Fat: absorbed as fatty acids and glycerol.

See Table 18-1 of your textbook for additional information.

Accessory Organs of Digestion. The accessory organs of digestion are the tongue, teeth, salivary glands, pancreas, liver, and gallbladder.

Pancreas. The pancreas, a feather-shaped organ behind the stomach, produces digestive juices, insulin, and glucagon.

Liver. The liver is located in the upper-right quadrant and is the largest organ in the body. Its functions include:

Manufacturing bile
Manufacturing plasma proteins
Detoxifying drugs and alcohol
Storing glucose in the form of glycogen and storing vitamins A, D, and B complex
Preparing urea
Breaking down hormones
Removing worn-out red blood cells (RBCs) and recycling the iron content

Gallbladder. The gallbladder is a small organ on the inferior surface of the liver. It stores and concentrates bile.

Large Intestine. The large intestine, or *colon*, is about 5 feet long and 2 inches in diameter and includes the following:

Ileocecal valve: connects the ileum to the colon.

Cecum: blind pouch below the ileocecal valve; projecting from it is the vermiform appendix.

The **colon** is divided into *ascending, transverse,* and *descending* parts. The large intestine absorbs water and contains normal flora that synthesize B-complex vitamins and vitamin K.

The **sigmoid** portion is the end portion of the colon; it enters the iliac region and continues as the rectum.

The **rectum** opens exteriorly to the anus, which contains the internal (involuntary) and the external (voluntary) muscle sphincters.

Defecation is the reflex triggered when the rectum becomes distended, resulting in emptying of the bowels.

General Overview of Digestion

Food enters the mouth and is mechanically broken up by the teeth and chemically digested by saliva, at which point the food is called a *bolus*. The bolus moves into the pharynx and slides down to the esophagus, stomach, and small intestine, where the food becomes totally fluid and is transported across the small intestine villi to the bloodstream. Undigested food goes to the large intestine and leaves through the anus as feces. Food is pushed through the system by peristalsis and segmented movement.

Action in the Organs. The following organs are involved in digestion:

Mouth: the teeth and tongue begin mechanical digestion by breaking food apart.

Salivary glands: in the mouth, the glands begin chemical digestion as salivary amylase begins to change starch to maltose or glucose.

Pharynx: swallowing.

Esophagus: peristalsis and gravity move food into the stomach.

Stomach: hydrochloric acid prepares the area for action. Pepsin breaks up protein, and lipase acts on emulsified fats. Food leaves as chyme.

Liver: produces bile.

Gallbladder: stores and releases bile as needed.

Pancreas: enzymes are released into the small intestine; amylase breaks down starch, protease breaks down protein, and lipase breaks down fat.

Small intestine: produces enzymes and prepares food for absorption, breaking it into glucose, amino acids, fatty acids, and glycerol; site for absorption.

Large intestine: absorbs water and collects food residue for excretion.

The Effects of Aging on the Digestive System

As the body ages, there is a decrease in the sensory ability of the taste buds and in the production of saliva. There may be a loss of teeth, which leads to poor nutrition. A slowdown in peristalsis may make it more difficult to swallow, digest food, and eliminate waste products.

Metabolism

Nutrients from the digestive system are changed into energy.

Common Disorders of the Digestive System

The following are the common disorders of the digestive system:

Stomatitis is inflammation of the soft tissue of the mouth.

Gingivitis, or gum disease, begins with plaque that hardens into tartar on the teeth.

Periodontal disease is a chronic bacterial infection of the gums and surrounding tissue that causes oral bacteria by-products to enter the bloodstream.

Gastroesophageal reflux (GERD) occurs when the cardiac sphincter muscle relaxes, and food flows back into the esophagus.

A hiatal hernia occurs when stomach tissue protrudes above the diaphragm through the esophageal opening.

Heartburn is backflow of acidic gastric juice into the lower end of the esophagus.

Pyloric stenosis is the narrowing of the pyloric sphincter.

Gastritis is inflammation of the lining of the stomach.

Gastroenteritis is inflammation of the lining of the stomach and intestines.

Enteritis is inflammation of the lining of the small intestine.

Peptic ulcers are lesions that occur in the stomach or duodenum; a common cause is bacteria, *H. pylori.*

Irritable bowel syndrome (IBD) is an inflammation of the intestinal tract; the most frustrating symptom is chronic diarrhea. The two types are: (1) Crohn's disease, in which inflammation occurs anywhere in the digestive tract; and (2) ulcerative colitis, in which inflammation typically occurs in the colon and rectum.

Appendicitis is inflammation of the vermiform appendix.

Hepatitis is inflammation of the liver. Types are as follows:

Hepatitis A, viral hepatitis: spread through contaminated food and water.

Hepatitis B, serum hepatitis: caused by a virus found only in the blood.

Hepatitis C: caused by hepatitis virus; steadily growing disease.

Hepatitis D: requires coinfection with hepatitis B.

Hepatitis E: transmitted through intestinal secretions.

Standard precautions are required for all types of hepatitis.

Cirrhosis is a chronic progressive disease of the liver; normal tissue is replaced by fibrous connective tissue.

Cholecystitis is inflammation of the gallbladder.

Gallstones are a collection of crystallized cholesterol that may block the bile duct.

Pancreatitis is inflammation of the pancreas.

Diverticulosis occurs when little sacs form in the intestine; if they become inflamed, diverticulitis develops.

Hemorrhoids are a condition in which the veins around the anus and lower rectum are swollen and inflamed.

Diarrhea is loose, watery, frequent bowel movements.

Constipation is when defecation is delayed; the colon absorbs excessive water from the feces, rendering them dry and hard; defecation thus becomes difficult.

Cancer may occur in any part of the digestive system. Surgery, chemotherapy, and radiation are available treatments.

ACTIVITIES

A. Use the words in the following list to complete the statements.

colon	30 feet	peritoneal
muscle circularis	greater omentum	small intestine
digestion	mesentery	submucosa
enzyme	insoluble complex	visceral peritoneum
15 feet	mucosa	

1. To change food into simpler soluble molecules, physical and chemical changes occur; this process is known as ____________________.

2. Substances that promote chemical reactions in living things but are not affected by the reactions are ____________________.

3. The serosa lining that covers the outside of each organ in the abdominal cavity is the ____________________.

4. The layer of the digestive system that consists of connective tissue, blood vessels, and nerve endings is the ____________________.

5. The length of the alimentary canal is________feet.

6. The innermost layer of the digestive tract insulates it from powerful enzymes and secretes digestive juices. It is known as the ____________________.

7. The third layer of the digestive system that consists of both skeletal and smooth muscle is the ____________________ ____________________.

8. Lining the abdominal cavity is the ____________________ membrane.

9. A specialized layer of the membrane to which the small intestine is attached, and that is attached to the posterior wall of the abdominal cavity, is the ____________________.

10. This layer of the membrane hangs over the organs like a protective apron; it is known as the ____________________ ____________________.

B. Complete the following regarding the digestive system.

1. Label the organs of the digestive system.

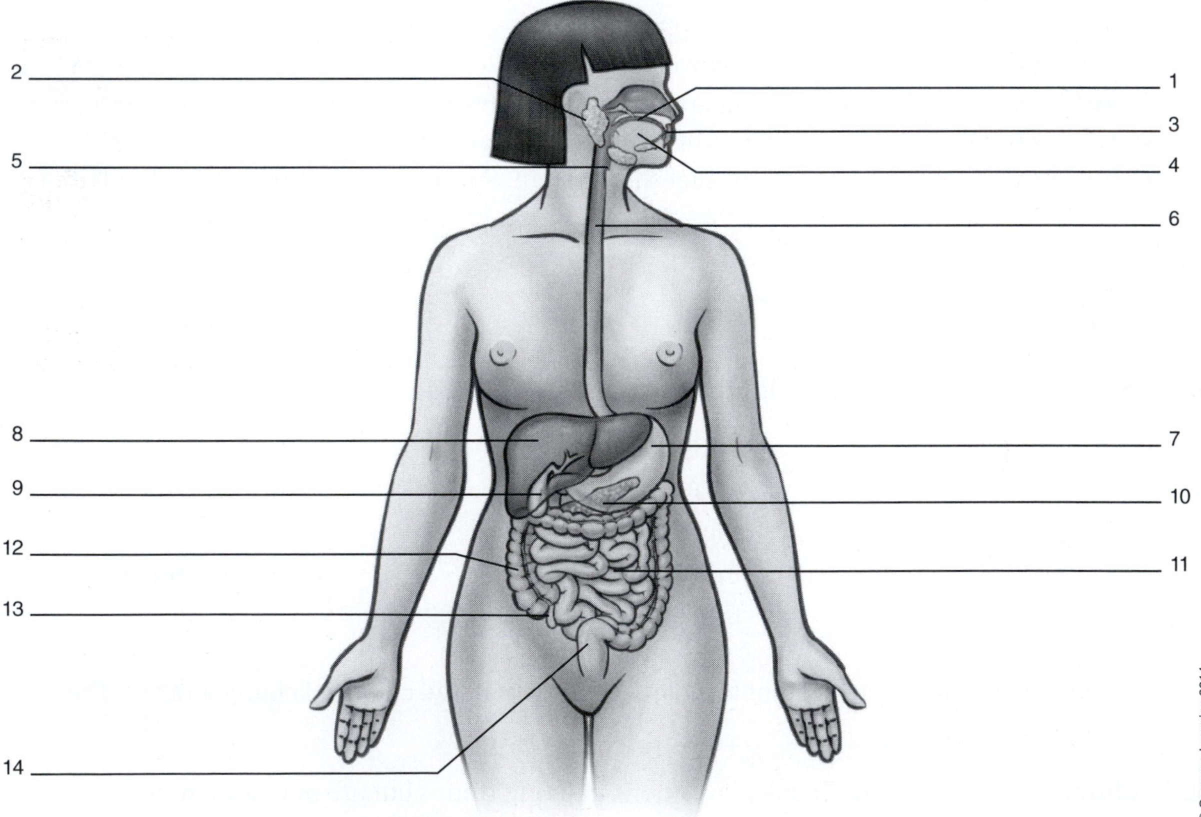

2. Name the functions of the digestive system.

____

____

____

____

3. Name the main organs of digestion.

____

____

4. Name the accessory organs of digestion.

____

C. Circle the correctly spelled word in each of the following statements.

1. Food enters the digestive tract through the (bugle, buccal) cavity.
2. The hard palate is formed by the (maxilary, maxillary) and palatine bones.
3. The tongue and its muscles are attached to the floor of the mouth and assist in both chewing and (swallowing, swalowing).
4. The tongue is attached to four bones, the (hyod, hyoid), mandible, and two (tempral, temporal) bones.
5. The taste buds respond to the bitterness, (saltiness, saltyness), sweetness, savoriness, and (soreness, sourness) in food.

D. Label the diagram of the tongue and oral cavity.

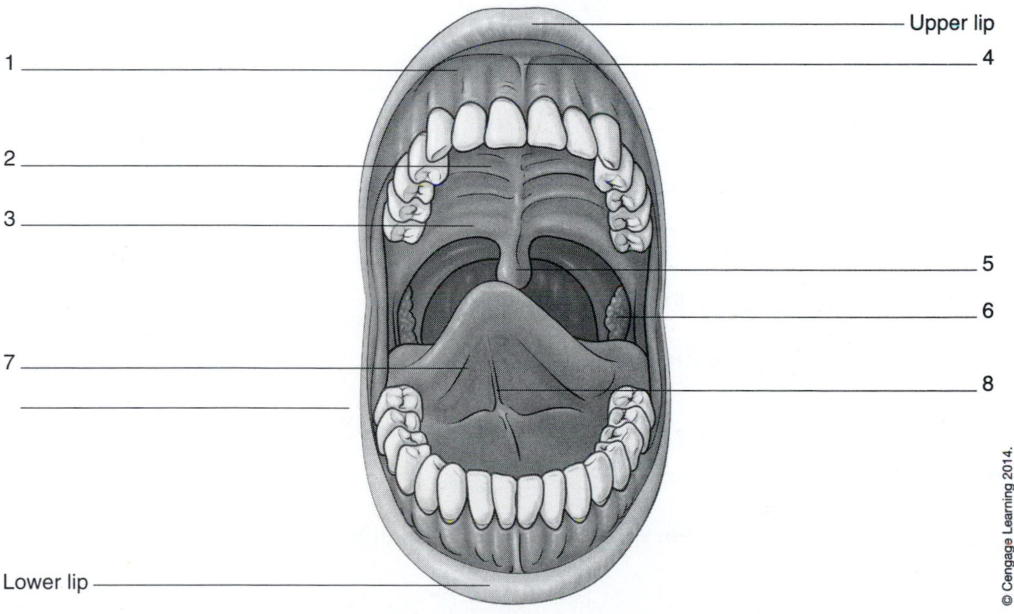

E. Using the labels from the previous diagram, match the numbers with the following descriptions. Letters may be used more than once.

_________ a. This structure is formed from the maxillary and palatine bones.

_________ b. This prevents food from entering the nasal cavity when swallowing.

_________ c. This structure supports and protects the teeth.

_________ d. Attaches the tongue to the floor of the mouth.

F. Label the salivary glands, and state where they are located and their function.

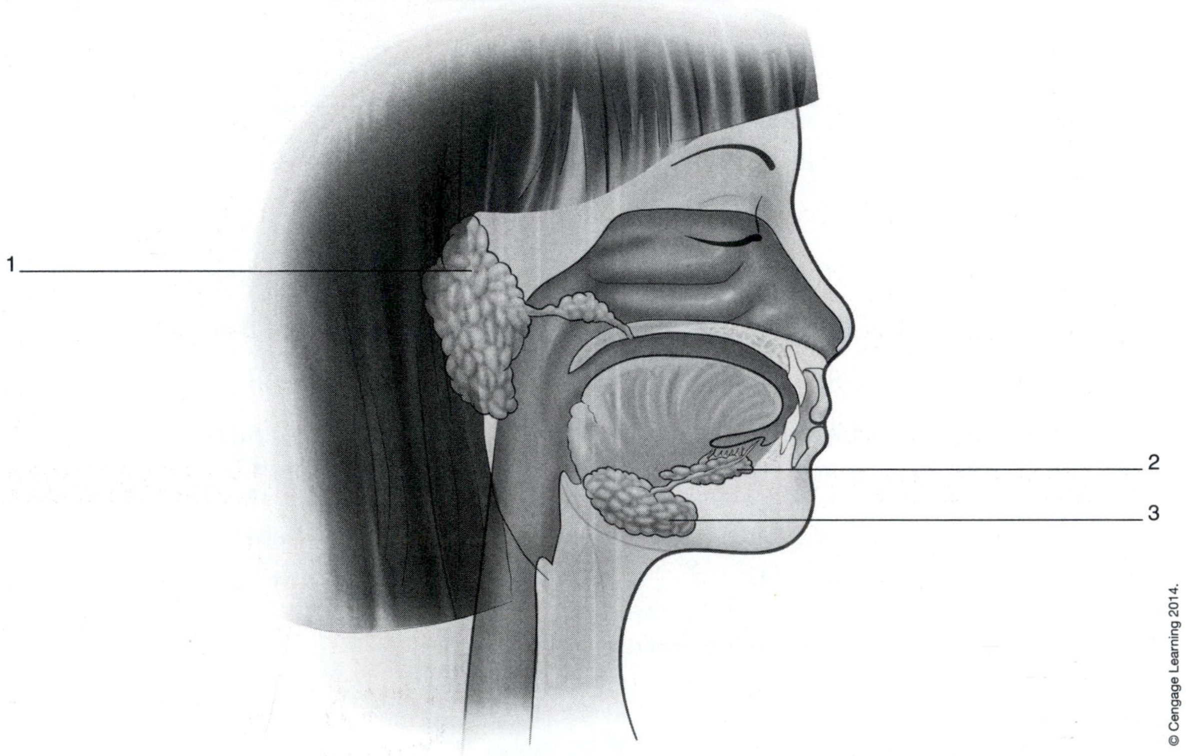

1 ____________________

2 ____________________

3 ____________________

© Cengage Learning 2014.

____

____

G. Fill in the blanks to complete the following statements.

1. The gland infected in mumps is the ____________________.
2. The other name for saliva is ____________________.
3. The salivary glands secrete the enzyme_______________, which destroys bacteria.
4. The ____________________ salivary gland contains no salivary amylase.

H. Label the tooth.

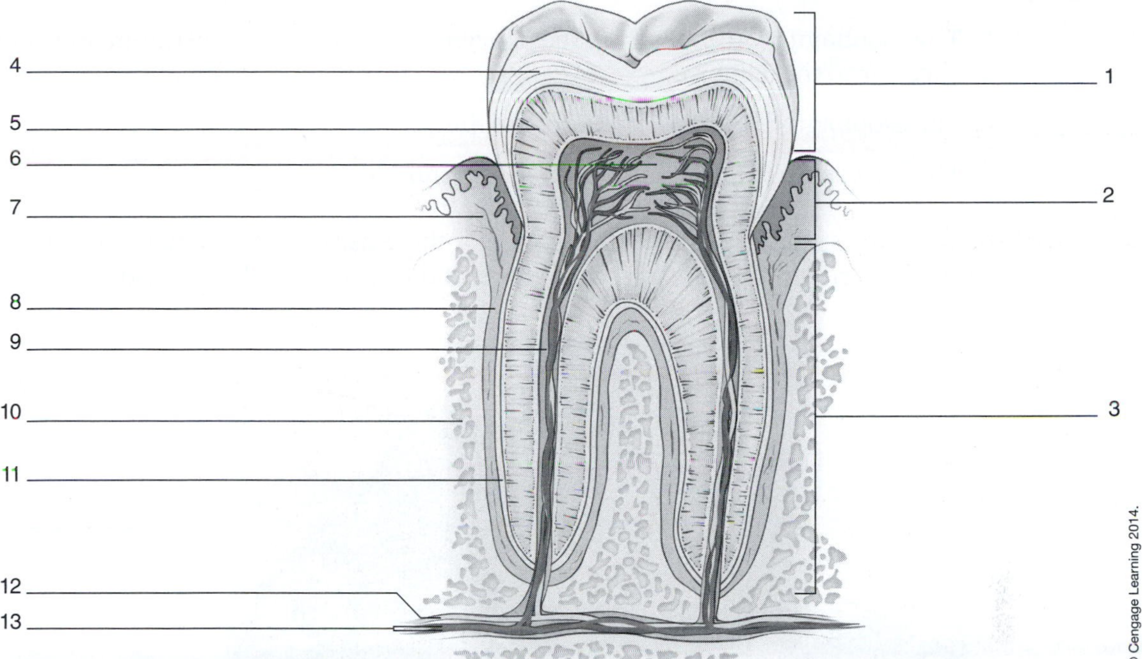

I. Match the terms in Column A with the correct descriptions in Column B.

	Column A	Column B
________	1. deciduous	a. mastication
________	2. gingivae (gums)	b. sharp edges for biting
________	3. chewing	c. support the teeth
________	4. canines	d. eight
________	5. number of permanent bicuspids	e. crushing and grinding
________	6. incisor teeth	f. milk teeth
________	7. number of deciduous canine teeth	g. four
________	8. molars	h. tearing and shredding food

J. Fill in the blanks to complete the following statements.

1. The structure that anchors the teeth in place is the ____________________ membrane.
2. The ____________________ ____________________ contains the nerve and blood supply.
3. The hardest substance in the body is ____________________.
4. The calcified tissue surrounding the pulp cavity is ____________________.
5. The root of the tooth is embedded in the ____________________ ____________________ of the jaw.

K. Mark the following statements either true or false. Correct any false statements.

________ 1. The esophagus is a muscular tube about <u>20</u> inches long, posterior to the trachea.

________ 2. The esophagus continues from the pharynx through the mediastinum and ends <u>superior</u> to the diaphragm.

________ 3. The esophagus joins with the cardiac sphincter of the stomach.

________ 4. The muscles in the esophagus are <u>smooth</u> muscles.

L. Label and color the structures of the stomach. Color the muscle layers using three different colors. Outline the rugae in black. Write the name of the part on the line provided.

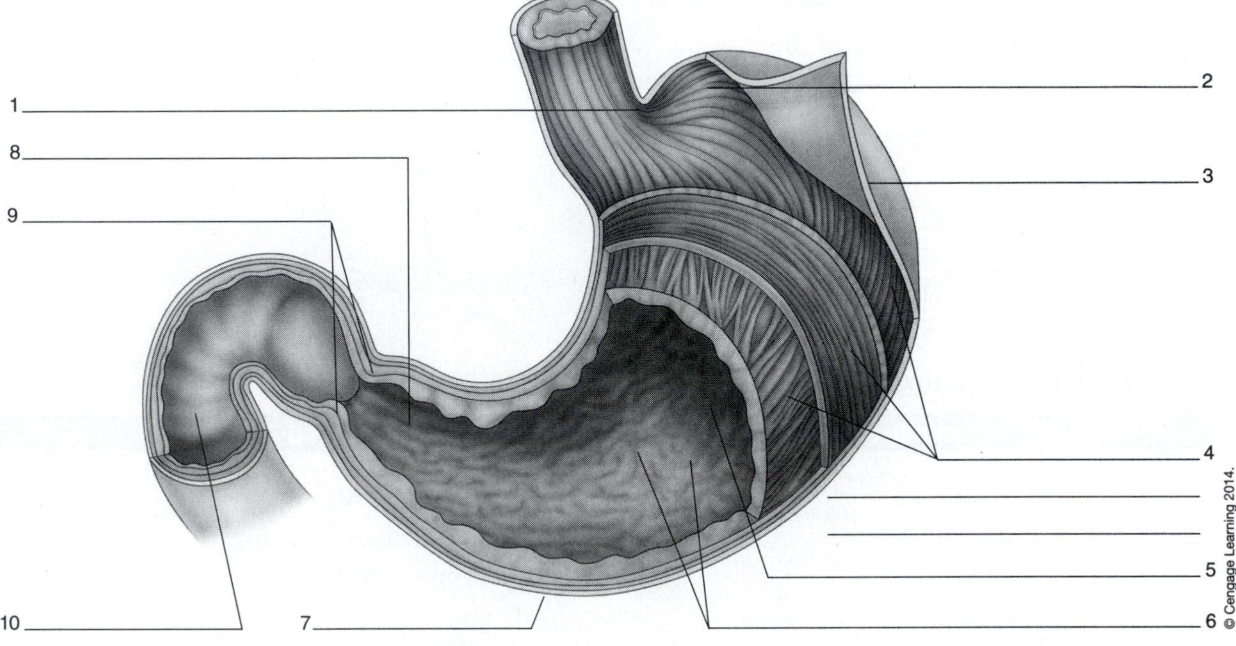

M. Compare the following structures.

1. Esophageal sphincter/pyloric sphincter

____

____

2. Mesentery/greater omentum

____

____

3. Chief-type cells of stomach/parietal cells of stomach

____

____

4. Mucosa layer/muscularis layer

____

____

N. Complete the following word puzzle, using the clues provided to fill in the missing words regarding the gastric glands.

1. G astrin ________ Stimulates the production of hydrochloric acid and pepsinogen
2. A lkaline ________ Mucus from the mucous cells help neutralize hydrochloric acid.
3. S terilizer ________ Hydrochloric acid is the body's natural one

GASTRIC

4. R ennin ________ Found in infants; prepares milk protein
5. I ntrinsic ________ Factor necessary for absorption of vitamin B_{12}
6. C hief ________ type ________ Cells that produce pepsinogen that converts to pepsin

O. Select the letter of the choice that best completes the statement.

1. Pancreatic digestive juices are carried by
   a. the bloodstream into the duodenum.
   b. a duct into the duodenum.
   c. the bloodstream into the ileum.
   d. a duct into the ileum.
2. If the common bile duct is blocked, the skin will become
   a. cyanotic.
   b. jaundiced.
   c. ischemic.
   d. icteric.
3. The liver manufactures all of the following plasma proteins, *except*
   a. albumin.
   b. fibrinogen.
   c. prothrombin.
   d. hemoglobin.
4. The liver prepares urea, the chief waste product of
   a. protein metabolism.
   b. glucose metabolism.
   c. fatty acids.
   d. glycerol.
5. The gallbladder stores bile, which is released when foods
   a. high in fat enter the stomach.
   b. with protein content enter the stomach.
   c. high in fat enter the duodenum.
   d. low in fat content enter the stomach.
6. The large intestine connects with the small intestine at the
   a. ileocecal valve.
   b. pyloric sphincter.
   c. cecum.
   d. cardiac sphincter.

7. The large intestine is
   a. longer in length and larger in diameter than the small intestine.
   b. the same size as the small intestine.
   c. shorter in length and larger in diameter than the small intestine.
   d. shorter in length but with the same diameter as the small intestine.

8. The pancreatic juice that neutralizes the acid content of the stomach is
   a. sodium bicarbonate.
   b. amylase.
   c. protease.
   d. lipase.

9. The pancreatic juice that breaks down fat to fatty acid and glycerol is
   a. sodium bicarbonate.
   b. amylase.
   c. protease.
   d. lipase.

10. Below the ileocecal valve is a blind pouch called the
    a. appendix.
    b. cecum.
    c. sigmoid.
    d. rectum.

P. Complete the story about the gastrointestinal (GI) tract using the words from the following list.

amino acid	duodenum	protease	rectum
bile	esophagus	peptones	rugae
buccal	fatty acid	peristalsis	stomach
canines	glucose	pepsin	tongue
cardiac sphincter	hydrochloric acid	salivary amylase	uvula
chyme	jejunem	pyloric sphincter	villi
colon			

THE TRIP THROUGH THE GI TRACT

My friends and I decided to try a new ride on the GI tract. I am Taco Corn Chip, and they are Meat and Cheese. We paid admission to Ms. Lips, who looked good enough to kiss, and then entered the GI tract. Standing in the big ____________________ cavity, all around us were strange white things. They really looked like mad scientists in long white coats, and we were the juicy specimens.

Just then the thick-muscled ____________________ platform started to move, pushing us up and down toward the white things, which bit and tore at us like angry ____________________. Next, I was squirted with ______________ ______________, which came at me through a thin tube, and I began to get gooey. I grabbed my friends, who also looked gooey, and we started moving further back in this cavity. "Wait!" someone shouted, "grab your rain gear off the ____________________ rack, which hangs down from the roof at the rear of the buccal."

Now we are going down the roller coaster called ____________________ and find ourselves at this strange door marked ____________________ ____________________. It slowly opens and we go inside. This ________________ room is even stranger; the walls are all draped in ____________________ folds. Upon our arrival we take a bath using ____________________ ____________________; we can now proceed since we are all cleaned up. My friend Meat is hit with ____________________, which has him singing "I am a peppy little ____________________," and Cheese is getting softened up. A big voice announces, "You are no longer who you once were. Your name is now ____________________." "Who cares," I think, "just get me out of here." A big tidal wave called ____________________ hits just then, pushing us through the exit marked ____________________ ____________________.

Now I am really scared, because this tube goes on forever. We are in the first part of it, the ____________________. I look around and see a slitlike opening. Look! Cheese is standing right behind me and gets a big squirt of ____________________ all over him. He is starting to come apart. At this point, we are being hit with all sorts of stuff that breaks us up into strange parts. I transform into ____________________. Meat is a(n) ____________________ ____________________ and Cheese is ____________________ ____________________ and glycerol. What will become of us? We get pushed again into the next part of the tunnel, the ____________________, and our fate is sealed. Awaiting us like a welcome mat are many little fingers called ____________________. They are now walking right through us, picking us apart. "Goodbye my friends," I shout, as we get sucked up.

There were some pieces of us left over. They were shoved into a bigger tunnel, the ________________, where they were dried out and then dumped out through the ________________.

RING!! RING!! That is my alarm clock. Oh what a nightmare. I should not have stayed up so late studying for my GI test and stuffing myself with tacos and pizza.

Q. In the following exercise, state what process of digestion takes place in the labeled organs in figure 18-13

1. Mouth: ____
____
____

2. Salivary glands: ________________________________
____
____

3. Esophagus: ______________________________
____
____

4. Stomach: ______________________________
____
____

5. Liver: ______________________________
____
____

6. Gallbladder: ______________________________
____
____

7. Pancreas: ______________________________
____
____

8. Small intestine: ______________________________
____
____

9. Large intestine: ______________________________
____
____

R. Write the word for inflammation of the following organs:

1. mouth ______________________________
2. stomach ______________________________
3. liver ______________________________
4. gallbladder ______________________________
5. pancreas ______________________________
6. appendix ______________________________
7. small intestine ______________________________
8. colon ______________________________

S. Fill in the blanks to complete the following statements on digestion.

1. The passage of food through the digestive tract is pushed through by ____________________ and ____________________ movement.
2. The purpose of the ____________________ is to cover the ____________________ to prevent food from entering the trachea.
3. The complex process of changing nutrients into energy is called __________.
4. The large intestine absorbs ____________________, ____________________, and potassium, which helps in the regulation of ____________________ balance.
5. The bacterial population of the colon is also referred to as the normal ____________________.
6. The action of the bacteria on undigested food turns the food into ____________________, ____________________, ____________________, and other waste products.
7. Bacteria in the colon help to ____________________ moderate amounts of vitamins ____________________ and ____________________.
8. Gas passed through the rectum is called ____________________.
9. Cellulose contributes ____________________ to feces, which ____________________ the muscular activity of the colon, resulting in ____________________.
10. When the rectum becomes distended with the accumulation of feces, it triggers the ____________________ ____________________. This action results in the relaxation of the ____________________ ____________________. For defecation to occur, the ____________________ ____________________ must also be relaxed.

T. Unscramble the letters to form the word that matches each statement.

1. Condition caused by a buildup of plaque on the teeth	IIISGTGIVN
2. Inflammation of the lining of the wall of the colon	TIVERITICULISDN
3. The liver disease that causes portal hypertension with ascites	RSOSIRCIH
4. Hidden blood in a stool specimen	LHOTCCMEU
5. Varicose veins of the lower rectum	MORRSOIHDEH

U. Using words from the following list, complete the statements on digestive disorders.

antacids	diverticula	histamine	pyloric stenosis
cirrhosis	heartburn	*H. pylori*	stomach cancer
constipation	hepatitis A	gallstones	stress
Crohn's disease	hepatitis B	gastroesophageal reflux	ulcer
diarrhea	hiatal hernia		

1. Many symptoms of digestive problems are caused by ____________________.
2. When the sphincter muscle is weak and the stomach contents flow up into the esophagus, the condition is ____________________ ____________________.
3. ____________________ ____________________ occurs in many people over age 50; the stomach protrudes above the diaphragm.
4. A backflow of the acidic gastric juices causes indigestion, or ____________________.
5. A narrowing of the sphincter at the lower end of the stomach causing projectile vomiting is ____________________ ____________________.
6. A lesion that occurs in the lining of the stomach or small intestine is a(n) ____________________.
7. Research shows that most ulcers are caused by the bacteria ____________________.
8. Drugs that reduce the amount of acid produced by the stomach are called ____________________ blockers.
9. Chronic dehydration, ulceration of the bowel, and personal embarrassment are symptoms of ____________________ ____________________.
10. ____________________ is a viral infection of the liver, spread through contaminated food and water; enteric precautions must be followed.
11. ____________________ is a viral infection of the liver, spread through contaminated blood; standard precautions must be taken at all times of exposure.
12. Liver disease, characterized by replacement of the normal tissue with fibrotic connective tissue, usually caused by excessive consumption of alcohol, is known as ____________________.
13. The majority of people over the age of 60 have little sacs, called ____________________, that develop in the wall of the colon.
14. Loose, watery bowel movements that can lead to dehydration are called ____________________.
15. A condition of hardened stool that can be caused by anxiety, fear, or fright is known as ____________________.
16. The treatment of ____________________ ____________________ may also lead to pernicious anemia.

V. Find the following words relating to the digestive system in the puzzle.

s d p e x m j s n b i l e d m u c e c l d y a r

p i e a s i u e i i a k d r e c l u e i o b e x

a a s f x o d n j g s f e c e s q m g u s d s d

o m n l e g p n e u m p c x h z a e r o d i i e

w z y c a c r h e d n o e o f n s e r a t a a s

l e r l r t a e a p o u i p e t t p l i r v i o

a v e e a e s t t g p u m d i c t b t r i t m c

n l c e s s a i i c u a d o n i l a h g i e a c

a a t r l a e s r o n s n i o l p e n l n n h h

c v u j i s p x r e n i h n a e a i o t i s v y

y l m x v o v i k f p p h g h d g c u n w w u m

r a a m e u i j l g s b c p h m e m e z o e a e

a c n u r r u m s c u z c o s e a c d t h e l v

t e u e q z o i a c c m i i n c a s i e q t u t

n c s l q l t i c o e n j p r s i r t d n g v l

e o t i a i d a s s t a r s q r t r t i u t u a

m e a r r r l d e r u o y p t s h i o b c o i s

i l s t a c i n i n t r h c a e r o p l u a u n

l i s c a p t n d e a c h p z p a o s a y r t s

a a b v s e s i a v a f D R E G i p s i t p n e

g o i u r i c s i m v i l l i d q l s i s i s i

m t c y c e e l o c o l o n q k f y l i c r o n

y i p w y p a t t e t s a t s u l o b a n n a n

b a r u h s s i n t r i n s i c f a c t o r i z

absorption
alimentary canal
amylase
anus
appendix
biscuspids
bile
bolus
buccal cavity
canine
cardiac sphincter
cecum
chyme
cirrhosis
colitis
colon
constipation
deciduous
defecation
dentin
diarrhea
digestion
duodenum
enamel
esophagus
feces
gallbladder
gastritis
GERD
gingivae
heartburn
hepatitis
illeocecal valve
ileum
incisors
intrinsic factor
jaundice
jejunum
lipase
liver
masticate
mesentery
molars
omentum
pancreas
papilla
pepsin
peristalsis
protease
pyloric sphincter
rectum
salivary
salt
sigmoid
sour
steapsin
stomach
sweet
taste
ulcer
uvula
villi

W. Match the system in Column B with the statement in Column A that shows how the digestive system interacts with other body systems.

Column A	Column B
1. __________ end products of amino acids converted to urea and excreted	A. Integumentary system
2. __________ provides oxygen necessary for metabolism to occur	B. Skeletal system
3. __________ manufacture of plasma proteins	C. Muscle system
4. __________ helps to form vitamin D	D. Nervous system
5. __________ protects the organs of digestion	E. Endocrine system
6. __________ provides nutrients for secondary sex characteristics	F. Circulatory system
7. __________ tissue in appendix helps to control bacteria	G. Lymphatic system
8. __________ nose receptors stimulate the salivary response	H. Respiratory system
9. __________ peristalsis and segmented movements	I. Urinary system
10. __________ insulin and glucagon maintain glucose metabolism	J. Reproductive system

APPLYING THEORY TO PRACTICE

1. Career opportunities exist in the field of dentistry. Prepare a career exploration seminar for junior high school students describing the jobs of dentists, dental hygienists, dental assistants, and dental laboratory technicians.

2. Riley is thinking of becoming a health care professional, but he is concerned about hepatitis. He wants to know his chances of contracting the disease. Explain hepatitis, the various types, and to which types health care professionals are susceptible. What is the current recommendation for workers in the health care field?

3. Margaret tells her son Jack not to talk while eating. Why is this good advice to follow? What happens when one swallows food?

4. The treatment for cancer of the colon frequently involves colostomy surgery. What are some of the difficulties patients have in accepting this procedure? How can you relieve some of this anxiety?

5. Keisha goes to the dentist because her gums bleed when she brushes her teeth. What is causing her gums to bleed? What can this problem lead to and how can it be prevented? What is the function of the teeth and periodontal membrane?

6. Linda has been losing weight and decides to visit her physician. After doing abdominal sonograms, the doctor suspects cancer of the stomach. Linda is distressed and questions the doctor regarding her lack of symptoms. What responses does the doctor give Linda? How is cancer of the stomach treated, and what is the prognosis?

7. Eileen is being treated for peptic ulcers. Where do peptic ulcers occur? What is the treatment for peptic ulcers?

8. Hector, age 75, has been complaining to Daniel, the health care worker at the senior center, that he has a problem with constipation. Hector tells Daniel that in the past, fruit was very effective in producing regular bowel movements. What information does Daniel need to give Hector regarding how aging affects the process of defecation?

____

____

____

____

SURF THE NET

For additional information and interactive exercises, use the following key words:

- digestive organs—structure and functions
- process of digestion
- chemical process of digestion
- digestive disorders—gingivitis, periodontal disease, hiatal hernia, heartburn, gastritis, enteritis, ulcer, inflammatory bowel disease, Crohn's disease, appendicitis, hepatitis (types), cirrhosis, cholecystitis, pancreatic, diverticulosis, diarrhea, constipation, hemorrhoids
- effects of aging on the digestive system

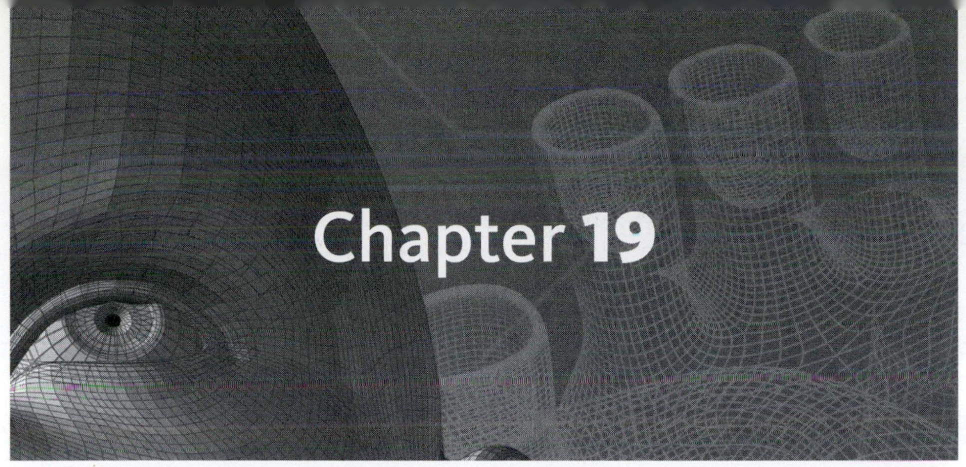

Nutrition

OVERVIEW

Nutrients. Nutrients are materials needed by the individual cells for optimal cell functioning. Nutrients include water, carbohydrates, lipids, proteins, vitamins, trace elements, and minerals.

Water makes up about 55% to 60% of the body. It is an essential component of body tissue. Its functions include:

Acting as a solvent for all biochemical reactions.

Serving as a transport medium for substances.

Lubricating joint movement and the digestive tract.

Controlling body temperature.

Serving as a cushion for the lungs and the brain.

Carbohydrates include the simple and complex sugars. They are the main source of energy for the body.

A **calorie** is a unit that measures the amount of energy contained within the chemical bonds.

Lipids, or **fats,** are a group of compounds of fatty acids combined with an alcohol. They are a storehouse of energy, cushion internal organs, insulate against cold, and contain the fat-soluble vitamins A, D, E, and K. Fats are classified as saturated, polysaturated, monosaturated, or trans fats.

Cholesterol is a fat found in animal products, including milk, meat, and cheese. It is a white, waxlike substance used to build cells and make hormones. If cholesterol builds up in the body, it causes atherosclerosis. High-density lipoprotein (HDL) helps to remove excess cholesterol.

Proteins are more complex than carbohydrates and fats and contain an amino group. They are synthesized in the cell cytoplasm from constituent molecules called amino acids. Proteins are important in the growth and repair of body tissue and make up the enzymes that regulate the rate of chemical reactions. They cannot be stored and are excreted as urea.

Minerals, trace elements, and **vitamins** are necessary for normal growth and maintenance of the body.

Mineral: chemical element that is obtained from inorganic compounds in food such as sodium, potassium, and so forth.

Trace element: present in the body in small amounts (e.g., zinc; see Table 19-2 in the textbook).

Vitamin: biologically active organic compound (see Table 19-3 in the textbook).

Fiber is found only in plant foods, such as whole-grain breads and fruit. It is important to include fiber in the diet for normal bowel functioning.

Recommended Daily Dietary Allowances

Recommended Dietary Allowances (RDAs) contain the daily recommendations for protein and fat-soluble and water-soluble vitamins and minerals.

The ***basal metabolic rate*** is the measure of the total energy utilized by the body to maintain body processes that are necessary for life.

Body mass index (BMI) is a better predictor of health than body weight.

The Effects of Aging on Nutrition

Chronic disease and social, economic, physical, and emotional factors affect the diet of the elderly.

Dietary Guidelines for Americans

The Dietary Guidelines for Americans are shown graphically in the MyPlate design, which has replaced the food guide pyramid. The plate is divided into five areas: fruits, vegetables, grains, protein, and dairy. These new dietary guidelines recommend the food necessary to provide essential nutrients.

Organic food is produced without using most conventional pesticides, fertilizers with synthetic ingredients, bioengineering, and ionizing radiation. Farms must be government certified to call themselves "organic."

Natural food is made with minimal processing and contains no additives or artificial coloring. It does not require government inspection.

Nutrition Labeling

Nutritional labeling must include information on total calories from a variety of foods.

Food Safety and Poisoning

Food poisoning occurs when microscopic organisms grow in food undetected and then cause illness after they are eaten.

Eating Disorders

Obesity: If a person's weight is 15% more than the optimum body weight for gender, height, and bone structure, then he or she is considered obese.

Anorexia nervosa is a disorder involving the refusal to eat because of a distorted body image and fear of weight gain.

Bulimia is episodic binge eating followed by behavior such as self-induced vomiting, which the bulimic believes will maintain body weight.

ACTIVITIES

A. Fill in the blanks to complete the following statements.

1. For our cells to function properly, they need ____________________.
2. These materials include ____________________, ____________________, ____________________, ____________________, ____________________, and ____________________.
3. Water is lost in the body through ____________________, ____________________, and ____________________.

B. Answer the following questions relating to nutrients.

1. Name five important functions of water.

____

____

____

____

____

2. Describe the functions of carbohydrates, fats, and proteins.

____

____

____

C. Water makes up between 55% and 65% of our total body weight. Calculate the water weight of the following:

1. A person weighing 200 pounds, with 62% water weight

____

2. A person weighing 140 pounds, with 57% water weight

____

3. A person weighing 90 pounds, with 60% water weight

____

D. Select the letter of the choice that best completes the statement.

1. The recommended dietary intake of carbohydrates is __________ of the daily intake of calories
   a. 40–50%
   b. 50–60%
   c. 60–70%
   d. 70–80%

2. Five grams of fat equal _____ calories.
   a. 45
   b. 36
   c. 25
   d. 24

3. A female is 24 years old, weighs 128 pounds, and is moderately active. Her daily requirement for calories is _______________ calories.
   a. 2,000–2,200
   b. 2,200–2,400
   c. 2,500–2,800
   d. 2,800–3,000

4. A 50-year-old male weighs 174 pounds and is very active. His daily requirement for calories is ______ calories.
   a. 1,800–2,000
   b. 2,000–2,500
   c. 2,400–2,600
   d. 2,800–3,000

5. Starch and cellulose provide all of the following, *except*
   a. roughage.
   b. minerals.
   c. empty calories.
   d. vitamins.

6. The measure of total energy utilized by the body is called
   a. blood pressure.
   b. basal metabolic rate.
   c. the Krebs cycle.
   d. anabolism.

7. Excess protein is
   a. eliminated by the body.
   b. stored in the body as an amino acid.
   c. stored in the body as fat.
   d. stored in the body as a complete protein.

8. The "good" lipoprotein that removes excess cholesterol is
   a. VLDL.
   b. LDL.
   c. HDL.
   d. LTH.

9. An example of a polyunsaturated fat is
   a. butter.
   b. olive oil.
   c. sunflower oil.
   d. peanut oil.

10. All of the following foods help lower cholesterol, *except*
    a. olive oil.
    b. peanut oil.
    c. safflower oil.
    d. cheese.

E. Answer the following questions regarding foods, minerals, and vitamins.

1. If your diet included all of the following foods listed in question E-2, would it meet your nutritional needs? Are all the essential amino acids present?

____

____

____

2. When your menu includes the following foods, which minerals and vitamins are being provided? Fill in the table.

Food	Mineral	Vitamin
A. milk	________	________
B. cheese	________	________
C. eggs	________	________
D. green leafy vegetables	________	________
E. table salt	________	________
F. liver	________	________
G. meat	________	________
H. poultry	________	________
I. fish	________	________
J. shellfish	________	________
K. shrimp	________	________
L. yellow vegetables	________	________
M. legumes	________	________
N. fruit	________	________
O. molasses	________	________
P. drinking water	________	________
Q. cherries	________	________
R. nuts	________	________

F. Match the mineral in Column A with the result of a deficiency in that mineral in Column B. Use each item in Column B only once.

Column A	Column B
______ 1. calcium	a. muscular weakness
______ 2. chlorine	b. deficiency in amino acid
______ 3. chromium	c. muscular cramps
______ 4. copper	d. weakness
______ 5. fluorine	e. demineralization of the bone
______ 6. iodine	f. lack of sexual maturity
______ 7. iron	g. poor appetite
______ 8. magnesium	h. impaired ability to metabolize glucose
______ 9. phosphorous	i. anemia
______ 10. potassium	j. deficiency is rare
______ 11. selenium	k. goiter
______ 12. sodium	l. convulsions
______ 13. sulfur	m. iron-deficiency anemia
______ 14. zinc	n. tooth decay

G. List vitamins necessary for each of the following:

1. Normal bone and teeth ______________________
2. Normal blood clotting ______________________
3. Nucleic acid synthesis ______________________
4. Cellular respiration ______________________
5. Night vision ______________________
6. Nervous system ______________________
7. Normal growth ______________________
8. Red blood cell synthesis ______________________

H. Complete the table on vitamins.

VITAMIN	FOOD SOURCE	FUNCTION	DEFICIENCY
______	Butter, fortified margarine, green and yellow vegetables, milk, eggs, liver	______	Night blindness, dry skin, slow growth, poor gums and teeth
B_1 (thiamine)	Chicken, fish, meat, eggs, enriched bread , whole-grain cereals	______	______
______	______	Needed in cellular respiration	______
B_3 (niacin)	Eggs, fish, liver, meat, milk, potatoes, enriched bread	______	Indigestion, diarrhea, headaches, mental disturbances, skin disorders
______	Milk, liver, brains, beef, egg yolk, clams, oysters, sardines, salmon	______	______
Folic acid	Liver, yeast, green vegetables, peanuts, mushrooms, beef, egg yolk, clams, oysters, sardines, salmon	______	
______	Citrus fruits, cabbage, green vegetables, tomatoes, potatoes	______	______
D	______	Needed for normal bone and teeth development, controls calcium and phosphorous metabolism	Poor bone and teeth structure, soft bones, rickets
E	Margarine, nuts, leafy vegetables, vegetable oils, whole wheat	______	______
K	Synthesized by colon bacteria, green leafy vegetables, cereal	______	______

I. Mark the underlined word or words in the following statements as either true or false. Correct any false statements.

_________ 1. The MyPlate idea recommended by the dietary guidelines is to help you visualize how food should appear on a plate.

_________ 2. The recommended serving of fruit is 1 cup every day when following a 2,000-calorie diet.

_________ 3. The recommended guideline for dairy is 3 cups daily when following a 2,000-calorie diet.

_________ 4. When we experience stress, we need a lesser amount of certain nutrients to maintain homeostasis.

_________ 5. Nutrition labels include information and total calories listed in a specific order.

_________ 6. The amount of each nutrient as a percentage of the recommended daily values is based on a 2,500-calorie diet.

_________ 7. The definition of overweight is a BMI of between 26 and 28.

_________ 8. In anorexia nervosa, there is a loss of appetite.

_________ 9. Bulimia is characterized by episodic binge eating followed by induced vomiting.

_________ 10. Barley may be an effective food to lower cholesterol.

J. Compare and contrast the following.

1. Trans fat/monounsaturated fat

____

____

2. Organic food/natural food

____

____

3. Cholesterol/triglycerides

____

____

4. BMR/BMI

____

____

5. Fiber/roughage

____

____

APPLYING THEORY TO PRACTICE

1. A person has an intake of 3,100 calories per day. If 25% is fat and 15% is protein, what percentage is carbohydrates? How many grams of fat, protein, and carbohydrate are in this diet?

2. Your friend is a vegetarian and has iron-deficiency anemia. Recommend a diet that will meet her needs.

3. Obesity + excessive weight has become a number one public health care problem.

   What are the statistics regarding this problem?

   What are some of the contributing factors?

   List some ways to eradicate this problem.

4. Much has been written about the healing power of foods. What foods are thought to be good in lowering cholesterol, fighting tooth decay, helping with arthritis, and preventing colds?

5. Dominick is 17 years old and has a family history of heart disease; he asks the school nutritionist, Kayla, what dietary guidelines he should follow to reduce his risk of heart disease. Explain the guidelines Kayla can give Dominick to reduce the risk.

6. Margaret had lunch with her 12-year-old son, Joseph, at a fast-food restaurant. After a few hours they both experienced flulike symptoms. Margaret thought they might have had a touch of food poisoning. What can Carolyn, the medical assistant, tell Margaret about safety factors regarding food?

____

____

____

7. Calculate the BMR for Mike, an active 40-year-old male who is 5′10″ and weighs 170 pounds. Calculate Mike's BMI; is it within normal limits?

____

____

____

SURF THE NET

For additional information and interactive exercises, use the following key words:

- nutrients—water, carbohydrates, proteins, fats, minerals, vitamins
- Recommended Dietary Allowances and dietary guidelines
- MyPlate
- organic food and natural food
- basal metabolic rate
- CDC—overweight epidemic

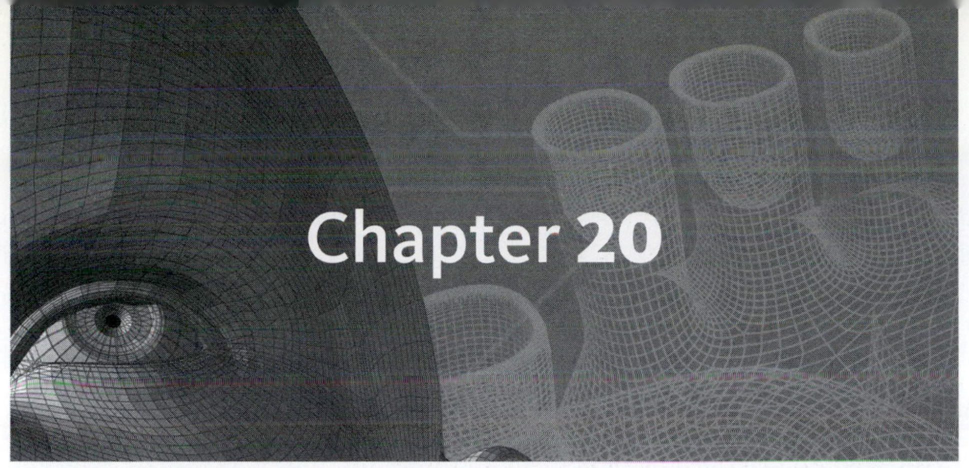

Urinary System

OVERVIEW

The **urinary and other excretory system** includes those organs that eliminate waste products. **Elimination of waste products** is through the following:

The *kidneys* excrete nitrogenous waste, salts, and water through urination; maintain the acid–base balance; and produce rennin and erythropoietin.

The *skin* excretes water and salt through perspiration.

The *intestines* excrete indigestible food, water, and bacteria through defecation.

The *lungs* excrete carbon dioxide and water vapor through exhalation.

Urinary System

The organs of the urinary system include two kidneys, two ureters, a bladder, and a urethra.

Kidneys. The kidneys are two bean-shaped organs located in the retroperitoneal area.

The *adipose capsule* is a mass of fat tissue that encloses the kidney and blood vessels.

The *renal fascia* is fibrous tissue that covers the adipose capsule.

The *hilum* is an indentation along the medial border; it serves as a passageway for lymph vessels, nerves, arteries, and veins.

The *renal pelvis* is a funnel-shaped structure at the upper end of each ureter.

The kidney is divided into two layers. The outer granular layer is called the cortex and the inner striated layer is called the medulla.

The **cortex** consists of millions of functional units called *nephrons.*

The **medulla** consists of renal pyramids, whose apexes empty into cuplike structures (calyces) which in turn empty into the renal pelvis.

Nephron. The nephron is the structural and functional unit of the kidney. It begins with the afferent arteriole, which carries blood from the renal artery to *Bowman's capsule,* a double-walled, hollow structure. Within the capsule, the arteriole divides, forming a ball of capillaries called the *glomerulus,* and then leaves the area as the *efferent arteriole* and forms the *capillary network* around the tubules.

The *proximal convoluted tubule* is a twisted tubular branch extending from the Bowman's capsule.

The *loop of Henle* is a proximal convoluted tubule that descends and forms a loop (the loop descends into the medulla part of the kidney).

The *distal convoluted tubule* is where the ascending loop of Henle returns to the cortex of the kidney.

The *collecting tubule* is a straight collection tubule that empties into the renal pelvis and then into the ureter.

The Path of the Formation of Urine

Blood enters the afferent arteriole, passing through the glomerulus to Bowman's capsule, as filtrate. It continues through the proximal convoluted tubule to the loop of Henle, on to the distal convoluted tubule, the collecting tubules, the renal pelvis, the ureter, the bladder, the urethra, and finally the urinary meatus.

Urine Formation in the Nephron

In urine formation in the nephron, the nephron uses three processes: filtration by the glomerulus, reabsorption within the renal tubules, and secretion by the tubular cells.

In *filtration,* blood enters the afferent arteriole and plasmalike fluid filters from the blood into the glomerulus, then through Bowman's capsule. The fluid, called filtrate, does not contain red blood cells or plasma proteins.

In *reabsorption,* substances are reabsorbed as they pass through the tubules. The proximal tubules reabsorb 80% of the water filtered out of the blood in the glomerulus, called obligatory reabsorption. Other substances are also reabsorbed.

In the loop of Henle and distal tubule, substances continue to be absorbed. In the distal tubules another 10% to 15% of water is reabsorbed, which is called optimal reabsorption. This process is controlled by ADH and aldosterone.

In *secretion,* the opposite of reabsorption, substances secreted are ammonia, hydrogen, and potassium ions. If a person is taking medication, the drugs may also be secreted.

Control of Urinary Secretion

Chemical Control. Chemical control includes hormones that promote reabsorption in the distal convoluted tubules, namely, aldosterone and ADH.

Aldosterone promotes the excretion of potassium and reabsorption of sodium, which causes reabsorption of water. As blood passes through Bowman's capsule, receptors can detect a drop in blood pressure. Renin is then released by the capsule into the bloodstream, which triggers the release of aldosterone (from the adrenal cortex).

ADH is released when the osmoreceptors in the hypothalamus detect an increase in the osmotic blood pressure due to salt retention. This causes an increase in the reabsorption of water in the tubules.

Nervous Control. Nervous control is accomplished directly through the action of nerve impulses on the blood vessels leading to the kidney and on those within the kidney leading to the urethra.

Urinary Output

Urinary output is, on average, approximately 1,500 to 2,400 ml/day. One milliliter of urine is formed per minute.

Ureters

The ureters are two narrow tubes running from the renal pelvis to the bladder.

Urinary Bladder

The urinary bladder acts like a reservoir, storing urine until approximately 500 ml is accumulated; the act of urination then occurs.

Urethra

The urethra is a narrow canal running from the bladder to the outside urinary meatus.

Disorders of the Urinary System

Acute kidney failure is caused by nephritis, shock, injury, bleeding, sudden heart failure, or poisoning; symptoms include oliguria and anuria. *Uremia* is a toxic condition in which the blood retains urinary waste products because the kidneys fail to excrete them.

Chronic renal failure is a gradual loss of function of the nephrons.

Glomerulonephritis is inflammation of the glomerulus of the nephron.

Acute glomerulonephritis usually occurs in children, 1 to 3 weeks after a bacterial infection.

Chronic glomerulonephritis may permanently affect the filtration membrane.

Hydronephrosis results in the renal pelvis and calyces becoming distended due to an accumulation of fluid.

Pyelonephritis is an inflammation of the kidney tissue along with its renal pelvis.

Kidney stones are also called renal calculi; stones form in the kidney. *Lithotripsy* is the use of ultrasound techniques to pulverize the stone, which then may be passed in the urine.

Cystitis is inflammation of the mucous membrane lining of the urinary bladder, leading to dysuria and polyuria.

Neurogenic bladder is caused by a damaged nerve that controls the urinary bladder.

Urethritis is inflammation of the urethra.

The Effects of Aging on the Urinary System

There is a decrease in nephrons and the glomerular filtration rate, which results in a decrease in renal blood flow. This compromises the ability of the kidney to eliminate waste. Loss of muscle tone leads to urinary incontinence and nocturia.

Dialysis

Dialysis is the passage of dissolved molecules through a semipermeable membrane. This treatment serves as a substitute kidney.

Hemodialysis: Blood is removed from an artery, passes through a dialyzer, and is returned to a vein.

Peritoneal dialysis: The peritoneal membrane acts as the semipermeable membrane.

Kidney Transplants

Kidney transplants require a donor organ from an individual who has a similar immune system to prevent rejection.

ACTIVITIES

A. Answer the following questions regarding the urinary system.

1. Name the excretory organs, the process of elimination, and the waste products excreted.

Organ of Excretion	Process of Elimination	Products Excreted

2. Describe the function of the urinary system.

____

____

____

____

____

B. Label the structures of the urinary system.

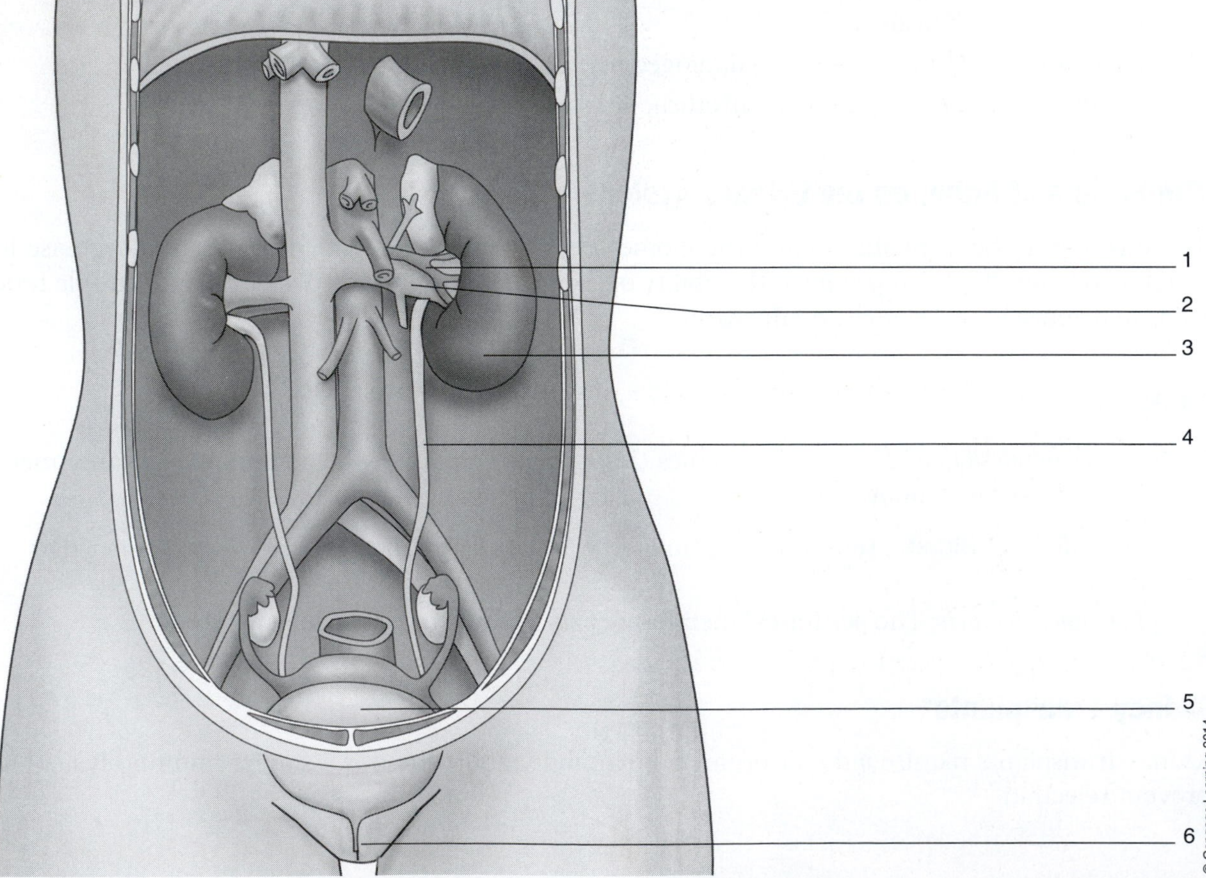

C. Using the previous figure, match the function to the letter of each structure.

_________ a. Takes urine to the outside of the body

_________ b. Organ that removes nitrogenous waste

_________ c. Stores urine

_________ d. Brings blood to the kidney

_________ e. Takes blood from the kidney

_________ f. Transports urine from the kidney to the bladder

D. Label the diagram of the kidney.

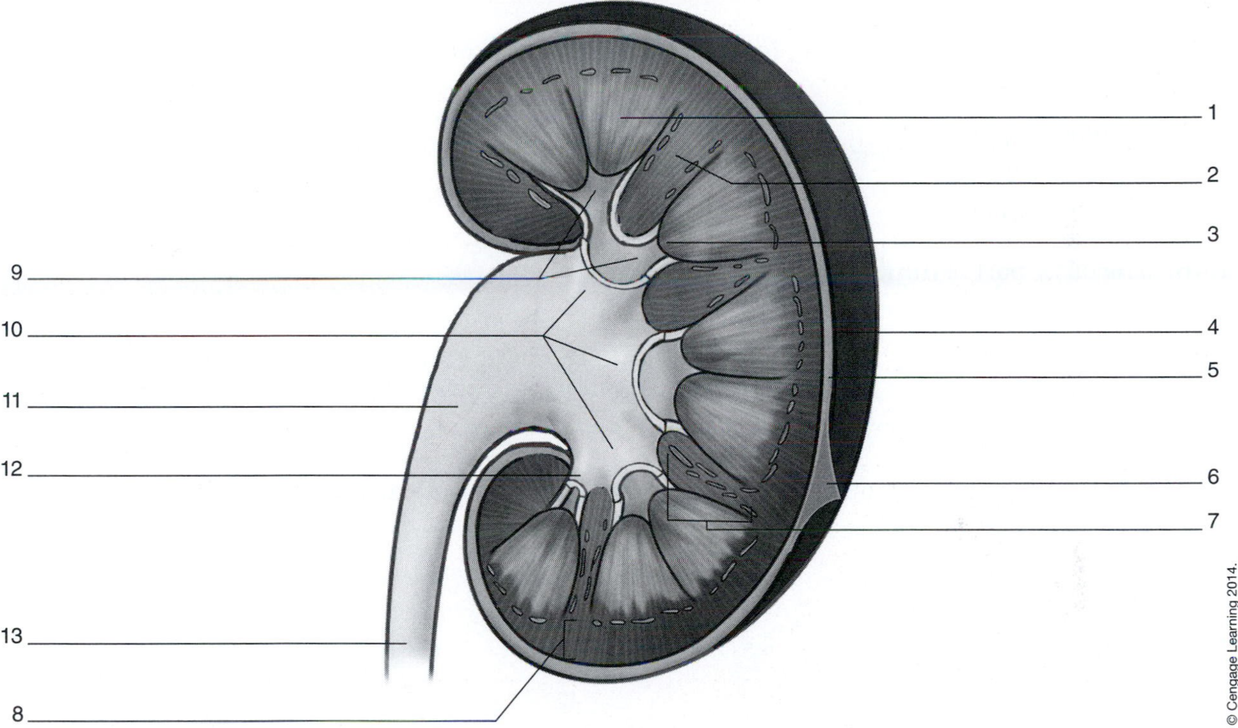

E. Select the letter of the choice that best completes the statement.

1. The kidneys are said to be retroperitoneal, which means they
   a. are located inside the peritoneal cavity.
   b. are located behind the peritoneal cavity.
   c. lie on either side of the vertebrae.
   d. rest high against the anterior wall of the abdominal cavity.

2. Each kidney is covered with a tough fibrous tissue called the
   a. adipose capsule.
   b. omentum.
   c. renal fasciae.
   d. mesentery.

3. The upper end of each ureter flares into a(n)
   a. funnel-shaped structure, the pelvis.
   b. outer granular layer, the cortex.
   c. long tube called the urethra.
   d. concave medial border, the hilum.

4. The kidney is divided internally into the medulla and cortex. The medulla consists of individually striated cones called the
   a. renal pyramids.
   b. pelvis.
   c. renal papillae.
   d. calyces.

5. Cuplike structures that empty into the renal pelvis are known as
   a. renal pyramids.
   b. renal papillae.
   c. renal calyces.
   d. renal fascia.

6. The outer part of the kidney, the cortex, consists of
   a. pyramids.
   b. papillae.
   c. calyces.
   d. nephrons.

7. The blood pressure in most of the capillaries in the body is 25 ml of mercury; in the glomerulus it is _________ ml.
   a. 30–60
   b. 60–90
   c. 90–120
   d. 120–150

8. Obligatory reabsorption of water by osmosis is when ________ is absorbed in the proximal convoluted tubule.
   a. 60%
   b. 70%
   c. 80%
   d. 90%

9. Optimal reabsorption takes place in the
   a. Bowman's capsule.
   b. glomerulus.
   c. proximal convoluted tubule.
   d. distal convoluted tubule.

10. The Bowman's capsule filters 125 ml of fluid per minute; 99% of the fluid is reabsorbed. How much filtrate is produced per minute?
    a. 1 ml
    b. 2 ml
    c. 12.5 ml
    d. 7.5 ml

F. Label and color the structure of the nephron. Color the glomerulus red; Bowman's capsule and the proximal convoluted tubule yellow; and the loop of Henle, distal convoluted tubule, and collecting tubules orange.

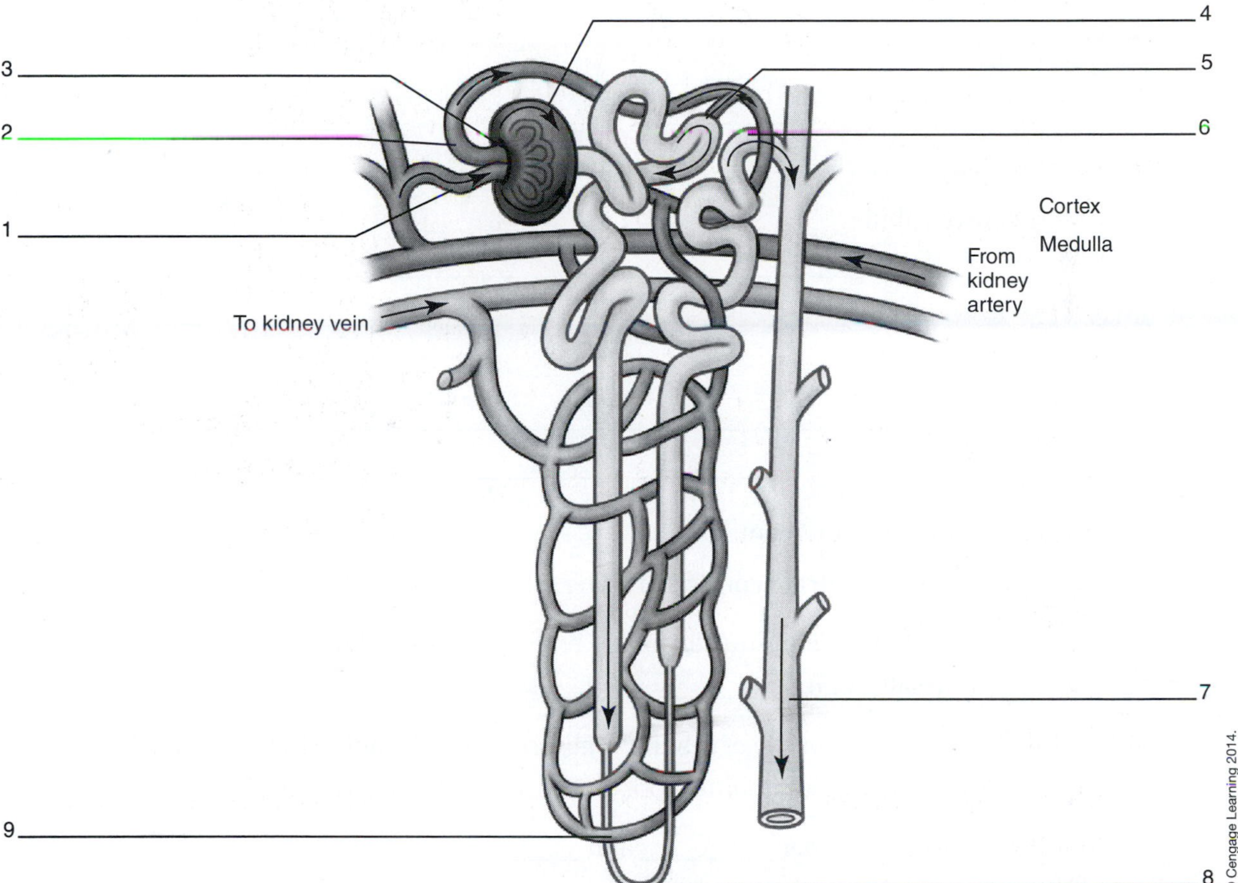

G. Describe the structures and functions of the following:

1. Afferent arteriole

____

____

2. Glomerulus

____

____

3. Efferent arteriole

____

____

4. Bowman's capsule

____

____

5. Proximal convoluted tubule

____

____

6. Loop of Henle

____

____

7. Distal convoluted tubule

____

____

8. Collecting tubule

____

____

H. Complete the following statements.

1. In tubular filtration, the filtrate consists of water, glucose, amino acids, salts, and ________.
2. In tubular reabsorption, useful substances are reabsorbed, including glucose, amino acids, vitamins, chloride salts, and ________________ ions.
3. Tubular secretion is the opposite of tubular reabsorption. Substances that are added to the filtrate include some drugs, ammonia, potassium ions, hydrogen ions, and ______.
4. The secretion of urine is under _________ and ___________ control.
5. The chemical control of the secretion of urine is influenced by the hormones ____ and _______.

I. List the steps in the process of urine formation.

1. _______________
2. _______________
3. _______________
4. _______________
5. _______________

6. ______________________________

7. ______________________________

8. ______________________________

9. ______________________________

10. ______________________________

11. ______________________________

12. ______________________________

13. ______________________________

14. ______________________________

J. Using the words from the following list, complete the statements regarding the formation of urine. Words may be used more than once.

ADH	filtrate	peritubular capillaries
afferent arteriole	glomerulus	proximal convoluted
blood	glycosuria	plasma protein
Bowman's capsule	increase	red blood cell
collecting tubule	loop of Henle	renal artery
decrease	obligatory	renal vein
distal convoluted tubule	optional	therapeutic
exceeds	osmosis	threshold
125 ml	100 ml	7,500 ml
80	10–15	60%

1. Blood from the ____________ ____________ goes to the ____________ ____________, which then becomes a ball of capillaries, the ____________.

2. The blood vessels become narrower leaving the renal artery, which results in a(n) ____________ in blood pressure in the capillaries.

3. This action forces blood from the ____________ into the ____________ ____________. The fluid is now called a(n) ____________.

4. The filtrate contains all the elements of the blood except ____________ ____________ and ____________ ____________ ____________.

5. Bowman's capsule filters about ____________ of fluid from the blood in 1 minute, or about ____________ of filtrate per hour.

6. Reabsorption begins in the ____________________ ____________________ tubule (a continuation of the Bowman's capsule) and continues through the ____________________ ____________________ ____________________, ____________________ ____________________ tubule, and the collecting tubule.

7. The proximal tubules reabsorb ____________________ % of the water filtered out of the ____________________.

8. This is considered ____________________ water absorption by ____________________, the fluid the body needs to survive.

9. The selective cells lining the tubules and the loop of Henle reabsorb other material until a certain level is reached. The term used to describe this level is ____________________. Passing the level is referred to as spilling over the level.

10. For example, glucose is absorbed until the ____________________ is reached, above which it will no longer be absorbed and ____________________ occurs. This may also explain why some medications must be taken several times daily to maintain a ____________________ dosage of the drug in the blood.

11. The ____________________ ____________________ tubule reabsorbs ____________________ ____________________ % of water, depending on the needs of the body. This is called ____________________ reabsorption, which is controlled by ____________________.

12. Secretion, the opposite of reabsorption, transports material from the blood in the ____________________ ____________________ into the distal convoluted tubule, which then is added to the filtrate, then passed on to the collecting tubules.

K. Circle the correctly spelled word in each of the following statements.

1. The smooth muscles of the (ureter, uretre) contract, (initialing, initiating) peristalsis, and urine is pushed from the pelvis of the kidney to the bladder.

2. The urinary bladder is a hollow muscular organ that acts like a (resevoir, reservoir) and stores urine.

3. When 500 ml of urine (accumulates, acumulates), the bladder must be emptied.

4. (Voiding, Voieding) is the act of urination.

5. The (reabsorbtion, reabsorption) of water in the distal convoluted tubule is (influenced, influinced) by ADH.

6. ADH increases the size of the cell membrane pores in the distal convoluted tubules, which increases the (permebility, permeability) to water.

7. The (osmoticreceptors, osmoreceptors) in the hypothalamus are sensitive to the osmotic blood pressure of the blood plasma. An increase in the osmotic blood pressure due to salt retention causes an increase in ADH, which inhibits normal water retention.

8. Aldosterone promotes the (excretion, escretion) of potassium and hydrogen ions and the reabsorption of sodium, chloride, and water ions.

9. The hormone renin is (released, relesed) by the kidneys and into the bloodstream when the cells in Bowman's capsule detect a drop in blood pressure. Renin stimulates the release of aldosterone from the adrenal gland.

10. Any (disfunction, dysfunction) of the adrenal cortex produces pronounced changes in the salt and water content of body fluids.

L. Mark the underlined word or words in the following statements as either true or false. Correct any false statements.

_________ 1. A major symptom of acute kidney failure is <u>oliguria</u>, which is the absence of urine formation.

_________ 2. <u>Uremia</u> is a toxic condition that occurs when the blood retains urinary waste products.

_________ 3. In <u>chronic renal failure</u>, there is a gradual loss of function of the nephron.

_________ 4. <u>Glomerulonephritis</u> may be acute or chronic; in both conditions, protein is found in the urine.

_________ 5. Hydronephrosis occurs when the renal pelvis and calyces become distended due to an accumulation of fluid; this condition may occur 1 to 3 weeks after a <u>bacterial infection</u>.

_________ 6. An inflammation of the kidney tissue in the renal pelvis is <u>pyelonephritis</u>.

_________ 7. Renal calculi are accumulations of crystals of calcium phosphate, which clump together and may fill the <u>renal papillae</u>.

_________ 8. Diagnostic tests for kidney stones include <u>KUB and IVP</u>.

_________ 9. Treatment for kidney stones includes <u>decreased</u> fluid intake, medication to dissolve the stones, and lithotripsy if necessary.

_________ 10. The most common cause of cystitis is <u>*E. coli*</u>. Symptoms include dysuria and polyuria.

_________ 11. <u>Cystitis</u> is an inflammation of the urinary bladder.

_________ 12. <u>Incontinence</u> is also known as involuntary urination, which occurs in stroke patients and babies.

M. Match the disorder in Column A with the treatment in Column B.

	Column A	Column B
_________	1. acute kidney failure	a. antibiotics
_________	2. hydronephrosis	b. increasing fluids
_________	3. pyelonephritis	c. proper hygienic techniques
_________	4. kidney stones	d. removal of obstruction
_________	5. cystitis	e. dialysis

N. Fill in the blanks to complete the following statements regarding dialysis.

1. Dialysis involves the passage of blood through a(n) ____________________ membrane to rid the body of harmful wastes.
2. In hemodialysis, substances in the blood pass through the membranes into the lesser concentrated ____________________ in response to the laws of ____________________.
3. The patient is connected to the dialysis unit by means of a(n) ____________________ or ____________________, which are surgical constructions to provide a site for inserting the needle.
4. Dialysis is usually done ____________________ to ____________________ times per week and lasts from ____________________ to ____________________ hours.
5. The patient on dialysis must take medications and follow a(n) ____________________ diet.
6. In peritoneal dialysis, the person's own ____________________ lining is used to filter the blood.
7. In peritoneal dialysis, a ____________________ solution fills the abdominal cavity. Fluid and waste material pass into the ____________________ from tiny blood vessels in the peritoneal membrane.
8. The most common type of peritoneal dialysis is continuous ambulatory peritoneal dialysis. The dialysate stays in the abdomen for about ____________________ to ____________________ hours and is then drained from the abdomen.
9. The best donor organ in kidney transplant is usually someone from the same____________.
10. The major complication in kidney transplant is ____________________.

O. Use the stem to make a new word that fits the definition.

1. ____________________ uria — painful urination
2. ____________________ uria — scanty urine
3. ____________________ uria — little or no urine
4. ____________________ uria — too much urine
5. ____________________ uria — blood in the urine
6. ____________________ uria — protein in the urine
7. ____________________ uria — pus in the urine
8. ____________________ uria — sugar in the urine

P. Describe how the urinary system interacts with other body systems.

____

____

____

APPLYING THEORY TO PRACTICE

1. If a patient had a urinalysis done and plasma proteins and red blood cells were shown in the urine, it would indicate a problem with what part of the nephron?

___

2. What is the advantage of doing a urinalysis over other diagnostic tests?

___

___

3. In glomerular filtration, how much filtrate passes through in 6, 10, and 15 hours?

___

___

4. Leslie has kidney disease and may need dialysis. She wants to know exactly what the kidney does regarding blood purification. Explain by using the path of the formation of urine as your guide.

___

___

___

___

5. Margaret is pregnant and she seems to be having a kidney problem. What kidney disorder is common in pregnant women? What is the reason for a common urinary infection in females? Explain the condition and how to prevent it.

___

___

6. As the nurse clinician, when you visit the residents in an assisted living facility, you are frequently asked various questions. One of the most common questions is "Why do I have to get up so often at night to urinate" Residents also want to know what else they should be concerned about regarding their kidneys and other bladder problems. What information would you provide?

___

___

___

___

SURF THE NET

For additional information and interactive exercises, use the following key words:

- urinary system—organs and function
- kidneys—structure and function
- nephron—parts
- urine formation—filtration, reabsorption, and secretion
- path of urine formation
- urinary output
- control of urinary secretions—chemical control and nervous control
- aging's effect on the urinary system
- disorders of the system—acute and chronic kidney failure, uremia, glomerulonephritis, hydronephrosis, pyelitis, kidney stones, cystitis, neurogenic bladder, urethritis
- dialysis
- kidney transplants

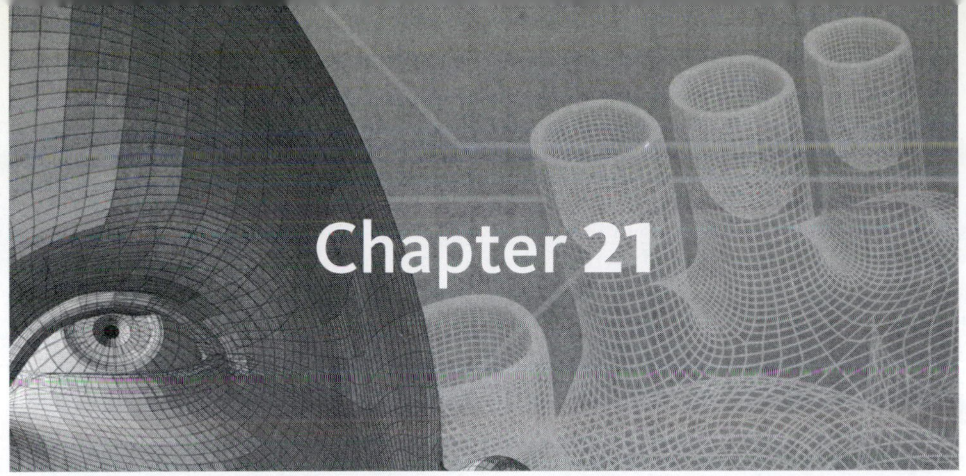

Reproductive System

OVERVIEW

Reproduction is the act of reproducing a new member of the species; in humans this is done by sexual intercourse.

Functions of the Reproductive System

Functions of the reproductive system include (1) housing the necessary organs capable of reproduction, and (2) the production of hormones necessary for the development of the reproductive organs and the secondary sex characteristics. The hormones are estrogen and progesterone in the female and testosterone in the male.

Reproduction Process. In the reproduction process, the *germ cells,* or *gametes,* are ova in the female and sperm in the male. Normal cell division is mitosis, a duplication of the 46 chromosomes. In human reproduction, meiosis occurs. *Meiosis* reduces the number of chromosomes in the germ cells to 23; when the ova and sperm unite, the fertilized egg contains 46 chromosomes, the same number as the other cells of the body.

Fertilization

In fertilization, the sperm is deposited in the vagina and travels up through the uterus to the fallopian tube. One milliliter of semen contains 100 million sperm. For fertilization to occur, the epithelial cells around the ova must be broken down. Hundreds of swarming sperm produce the enzyme necessary to penetrate the cells. One sperm then unites with the egg. Fertilization, the union of the sperm nucleus with the ovum nucleus to form a fertilized egg or *zygote,* occurs in the outer one-third of the fallopian tube. The ovum has two X sex chromosomes; the sperm has an X and a Y sex chromosome. In reproduction, a female comes from the union of two X chromosomes, the male from an X and Y chromosome. The chromosome of the male parent determines the sex of the child.

Fetal Development

The zygote travels through the fallopian tube and implants itself into the endometrial lining of the uterus and fetal development continues. See Table 21-1 for the phases of fetal development and Table 21-2 for the embryonic germ layers.

The female and male sex organs develop from the same embryonic tissue. For the first 2 months there is no gender difference; then the ovaries develop from the cortex and the testes develop from the medulla of the gonad embryonic tissue. Look at Figure 21-7 in the textbook to see how the undifferentiated external genitalia develop into fully differential structures.

Organs of Reproduction

The female reproductive system includes two ovaries, two fallopian tubes, one uterus, and one vagina. The male reproductive system includes two testes, seminal ducts, glands, and the penis.

Female Reproductive System

Ovaries. The ovaries are the primary sex organs of the female; they produce germ cells and the hormones estrogen and progesterone.

Graafian follicle: each ovary contains thousands of follicles, which when influenced by the follicle-stimulating hormone (FSH) of the pituitary are responsible for the process of the development of the ova into mature ova. The follicles also produce estrogen.

Ovulation: the follicle enlarges, migrates to the outside of the ovary, and breaks open, releasing the ovum from the ovary.

Corpus luteum: the name given to the ruptured graafian follicle after ovulation; these cells produce progesterone.

Fallopian Tubes. Fallopian tubes, or oviducts, are attached at one end to the uterus; the other end curves over the ovary. The fimbriated ends of the fallopian tube catch the ovum when ovulation occurs. The tubes propel the ova down the tube to the uterus.

Uterus. The uterus is a muscular organ that can greatly expand to accommodate a fetus. It is divided into three parts:

Fundus: bulging, rounded, upper part.

Body: middle part.

Cervix: lower, narrow portion that extends into the vagina.

The **uterine wall** is comprised of three layers, the outer serous layer, or *visceral;* the middle muscular layer, the *myometrium;* and the inner mucous layer, the *endometrium,* which changes in consistency each month.

Vagina. The vagina is the short canal that extends from the cervix of the uterus to the vulva. The *hymen* is a semipermeable membrane found at the entrance to the vagina.

External Female Genitalia. The external female genitalia, or *vulva,* contains the external organs of the reproductive system:

Mons pubis: a mound of fatty tissue over the pubic bone, covered with coarse hair.

Vestibule: area surrounding the openings of the urethra and the vagina; within the vestibule is a thin fold of tissue, the hymen.

Clitoris: small structure above the urethral opening; contains many nerve endings.

Labia majora and *labia minora:* folds of skin surrounding the vagina.

Bartholin's glands: mucous glands at the entrance to the vagina.

Perineum: area between the vagina and the rectum.

Breasts. Breasts are accessory organs of the reproductive system. They produce milk after childbirth. The *areola* is the dark area that surrounds the nipple.

The Menstrual Cycle

In the menstrual cycle, a mature egg develops and is ovulated every 28 days, beginning at puberty. The menstrual cycle is divided into four stages: follicle, ovulation, corpus luteum, and menstruation.

In the **follicle stage,** FSH secreted from the pituitary gland stimulates a graafian follicle in the ovary. The follicle grows, producing *estrogen,* and the egg cell matures. Estrogen stimulates the endometrium lining and is necessary for secondary sex characteristics. The follicle stage lasts 10 days.

In the **ovulation stage,** the estrogen blood level rises and the pituitary stops producing FSH and starts producing luteinizing hormone (LH). The combination of hormone activity causes the follicle to rupture, and a mature ovum is released (*ovulation*). The ovulation stage occurs around the 14th day of the cycle.

In the **corpus luteum stage,** after ovulation, LH stimulates the graafian cells to change to cells called the *corpus luteum,* which produce *progesterone.* This hormone maintains the growth of the endometrium and inhibits FSH; this stage lasts 14 days.

In the **menstruation stage,** if fertilization does not occur, the progesterone level rises, inhibiting the LH hormone. As LH drops, the corpus luteum disintegrates and the lining of the endometrium breaks down and is discharged through the vagina. *Menstruation* has occurred. Menstruation occurs and the estrogen level drops, causing FSH from the pituitary to start the cycle again. See Figure 21-12 in the textbook for an overview of the menstrual cycle.

Menopause

Menopause is the time in a female's life when the menstrual cycle ceases; it occurs between 45 and 55 years of age. Physiological changes occur in the reproductive organs. "Hot flashes" and some psychological changes may also occur.

Male Reproductive System

Testes. Testes are the primary male reproductive organs. They lie outside the body in the *scrotum* (an external sac). They produce sperm and testosterone and are divided into partitions or lobules.

Seminiferous tubules are found in each lobule; FSH stimulates the production of *sperm* in cells that line the tubules.

Interstitial tissue supports the seminiferous tubules. The cells produce *testosterone,* necessary for the growth and development of reproductive organs and secondary sex characteristics.

In the descent of the **testicles,** the testes, which develop in the abdominal cavity, move downward into the scrotum in the last 3 months of embryonic life. If the testes do not descend, the condition is known as *cryptorchidism.* This condition must be corrected, or spermatogenesis will not occur.

Epididymides. The epididymides are overlying structures to which the testes are attached. They are formed by networks of seminiferous tubules.

Ductus Deferens, Seminal Vesicles, and Ejaculatory Ducts. The *ductus deferens* or *vas deferens* are a continuation of the epididymis; they serve as storage sites for sperm cells and excretory ducts of the testes. The vas deferens enter the abdominal cavity in the inguinal area, wrap around the bladder, and meet the seminal vesicles. The *seminal vesicles* are two highly convoluted membranous tubes that produce seminal fluid, which is added to the sperm cells. *Ejaculatory ducts* are formed by the vas deferens and the seminal vesicles. They descend into the prostate gland to join with the urethra.

Penis. The penis is the external organ of the male reproductive system. It contains erectile tissue. The *foreskin* is the loose-fitting skin that covers the end of the penis. *Circumcision* is a procedure in which the foreskin is removed.

Prostate Gland. The prostate gland is located under the urinary bladder. It surrounds the opening of the bladder leading to the urethra and secretes a fluid that enhances sperm mobility.

Bulbourethral or Cowper's Glands. The bulbourethral or Cowper's glands are located on either side of the urethra below the prostate gland; they add an alkaline fluid to semen.

Semen. Also known as seminal fluid, semen is a mixture of sperm cells and secretions of the seminal vesicle, prostate, and bulbourethral glands. Semen provides energy and is a transport medium for sperm.

Erection and Ejaculation. When the male is sexually aroused, nerve impulses cause the erectile tissue to engorge with blood, which makes the tissue increase in size and become firm. Stimulating the glans penis results in stimulation of the seminal vesicles, impulses are sent to the ejaculatory center, and orgasm occurs. Secretions stored in the vas deferens, ejaculatory ducts, and prostate gland are forcibly expelled through the urethra and the engorgement ceases.

Impotence. Impotence is the inability to have or sustain an erection. *Primary* impotence is when the male has never had an erection. *Secondary* impotence is current impotence. Transient periods of impotence are not a dysfunction. The cause of impotence is mostly organic; treatment includes penile implants, injections, and oral medications.

Contraception

Contraception is the conscious decision not to reproduce. Abstinence, a healthy choice, is voluntarily refraining from intercourse. See Table 21-5 in your textbook for other methods of contraception.

Infertility

Infertility is the inability to reproduce. Causes may be damage to the fallopian tubes, low sperm count, hormonal imbalance, and other disorders. Treatments include the following:

Fertility drugs promote ovulation by stimulating hormones.

Artificial insemination involves placing semen into the vaginal canal by a cannula and syringe around the time of ovulation.

Surgery to open blocked tube is called laparoscopy.

Assisted reproductive techniques include the following:

In vitro fertilization involves the use of ovulation-inducing drugs to stimulate the development of multiple ovarian follicles. A laparoscopy is done to remove the follicles and extract the ova. The ova are cultured in vitro with sperm; if fertilization is successful, the zygote at the four- to eight-cell stage is transferred to the uterus.

Gamete intrafallopian tube transfer is when the zygote is transferred into the end of the fallopian tube.

Disorders of the Reproductive System

Disorders of the Female Reproductive System.

Amenorrhea: absence of menstruation; normal in pregnancy.

Dysmenorrhea: painful menstruation.

Menorrhagia: excessive or heavy menstrual bleeding that may lead to anemia.

Premenstrual syndrome (PMS): symptoms exhibited just before the menstrual cycle.

Leukorrhea: whitish discharge from the vagina.

Fibroid tumors: benign growths that occur in the uterine wall.

Endometriosis: endometrial tissue outside the uterine cavity. The tissue responds to hormonal changes. Tissue outside the uterus allows no way for the blood to leave the body, resulting in internal bleeding, inflammation, and pain.

Breast cancer: the most common cancer in women. Early detection is critical. Women should do breast self-exams, as well as have annual *mammograms* after the age of 40.

Endometrial cancer: usually occurs after menopause.

Ovarian cancer: leading cause of cancer death in women between the ages of 40 and 65.

Cervical cancer: can be detected by a *Pap smear,* which is a sample of cell scrapings of the cervix and cervical canal.

Infections of the Female Reproductive Organs.

Pelvic inflammatory disease (PID): infection that occurs in the reproductive organs and spreads to the fallopian tubes and peritoneal cavity. It is treated with antibiotics.

Salpingitis: inflammation of the fallopian tubes.

Toxic shock syndrome: bacterial infection, by the organism *Staphylococcus.*

Vaginal yeast infection: caused by fungus; symptoms are itching, burning, redness, and leukorrhea.

Male Reproductive Disorders.

Epididymitis: painful swelling in the groin and scrotum caused by infection.

Orchitis: infection of the testes; complication of mumps.

Prostatitis: infection of the prostate gland.

Benign prostatic hypertrophy (BPH): indicates an enlarged prostate, which occurs in most men after the age of 70; urinary problems develop.

Prostate cancer: most common cancer in men after the age of 50. Males over age 40 should have annual rectal exams as well as a prostate-specific antigen blood screening test, which detects an abnormal substance released by the cancer cells.

Sexually Transmitted Diseases. Sexually transmitted diseases (STDs) are also known as *venereal diseases.* They are transmitted through the exchange of body fluids, such as semen, vaginal fluid, and blood. The most common are chlamydia, genital herpes, and genital warts. Protection from STDs includes abstinence and practicing safe sexual behavior. All STDs must be treated, because they may lead to sterility in females.

Chlamydia is the major cause of urethritis, bacterial vaginitis, and PID. Up to 80% of affected women and 25% of men have no symptoms.

Genital warts can appear on the shaft of the penis or inside the vagina. The disease may be asymptomatic; diagnosis is made by examination.

Genital herpes is a viral infection; blister-like areas may appear on the genitalia and cause a burning sensation. Symptoms may disappear after 2 weeks, but may reappear throughout the lifetime.

Gonorrhea is a bacterial infection. Males have painful urination and a discharge of pus from the penis; females may be asymptomatic. It is treated with antibiotics.

Syphilis is a bacterial STD, treated with antibiotics.

Trichomoniasis vaginalis infection is caused by a protozoan, and is treated with antibiotics.

The Effects of Aging on the Reproductive System

Hormone production declines with aging, and there may be atrophic changes. In the female, menopause occurs; in the male, changes are more gradual.

ACTIVITIES

A. Describe the functions of the reproductive system.

____

____

____

____

____

B. Select the letter of the choice that best completes the statement.

1. The specialized sex cells or germ cells are also known as
   a. gonads.
   b. testicles.
   c. ovaries.
   d. gametes.
2. In the formation of the germ cells, the specialized cell division process is known as
   a. mitosis.
   b. spermatogenesis.
   c. meiosis.
   d. oogenesis.
3. In the male, there is one pair of single sex chromosomes, an X and a Y, and
   a. 22 autosomal pairs.
   b. 22 autosomal single chromosomes.
   c. 23 autosomal pairs.
   d. 23 autosomal single chromosomes.

4. Spermatozoa entering the female reproductive tract live for
   a. 1–2 days.
   b. 2–3 days.
   c. 3–4 days.
   d. 1 week.

5. In one ejaculation, 100 million sperm may be deposited in 1 ml of seminal fluid. A person is considered sterile if the sperm count is less than ___ million per milliliter.
   a. 10
   b. 20
   c. 30
   d. 40

6. Sperm may die before they can approach the ovum for all of the following reasons, *except*
   a. high temperature of the female abdomen.
   b. high acidity of the secretions in the vagina.
   c. specialized lining of the uterus.
   d. lack of the propulsion ability.

7. For fertilization to occur, the layer of epithelial cells must fall away from the ovum. This layer is called
   a. the corona radiata.
   b. the zona pellucida.
   c. hyaluronidase.
   d. hyaluronic acid.

8. True fertilization occurs when the sperm nucleus and the egg nucleus unite to form a fertilized egg cell, or
   a. gamete.
   b. gonad.
   c. zygote.
   d. embryo.

9. The process that gives rise to all three germ layers is known as:
   a. trophoblast.
   b. blastocele.
   c. gastrulation.
   d. chorionic villi.

10. The gender of the child is determined by
    a. the chromosome of the male parent.
    b. the chromosome of the female parent.
    c. either the male or female parent.
    d. the timing of pregnancy.

C. Label the structure of the sperm and ovum.

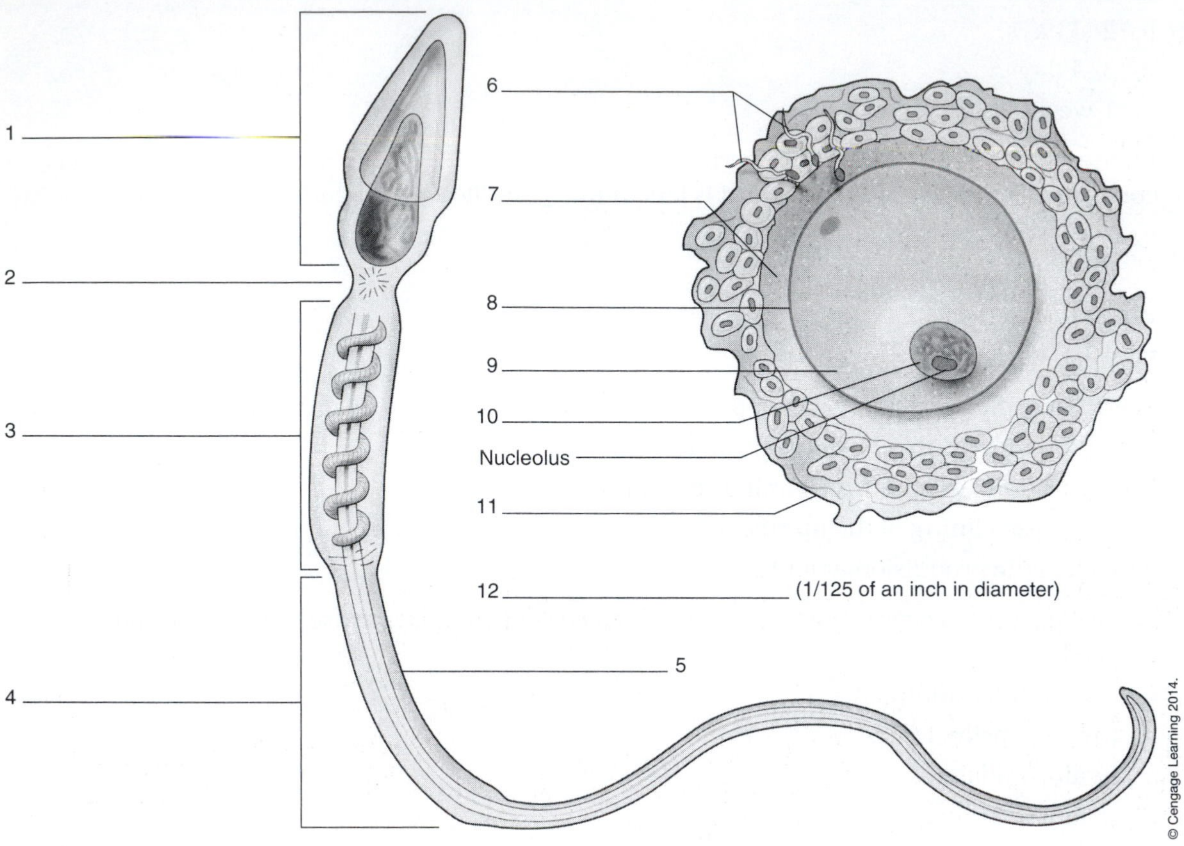

D. Complete the following statements regarding fetal development.

1. For the first 2 months, the embryo develops without a(n) ____________________ identity.
2. The structure that anchors the placenta to the uterine wall is the _ ____________ _______.
3. Implantation of the zygote occurs__ to _ days after ovulation.
4. The embryonic germ layers that form from 13 to 28 days after ovulation are the ____________________, ____________________, and ____________________.
5. The skin, pituitary glands, and parts of the nervous system derive from the ____________________ layer.
6. The lining of the lungs, urethra, digestive tract, and bladder derive from the ____________________ layer.
7. The muscles, bones, blood, heart, and lungs derive from the ____________________ layer.
8. The thick layer of hair covering the fetus is called ____________________.
9. The protective covering on the skin of the fetus at the end of the 5th month is called ____________________ ____________________.
10. A baby born at the end of the ____________________ month can live outside the uterus.

E. The undifferentiated external genitalia develop into fully differentiated structures. Complete the following statements.

In the male:

1. The tubercle becomes the ____________ ____________.
2. The folds become the ____________ ____________.
3. The swelling becomes the ____________.

In the female:

1. The tubercle becomes the ____________.
2. The folds become the ____________ ____________.
3. The swelling becomes the ____________ ____________.

F. Label the female organs of reproduction.

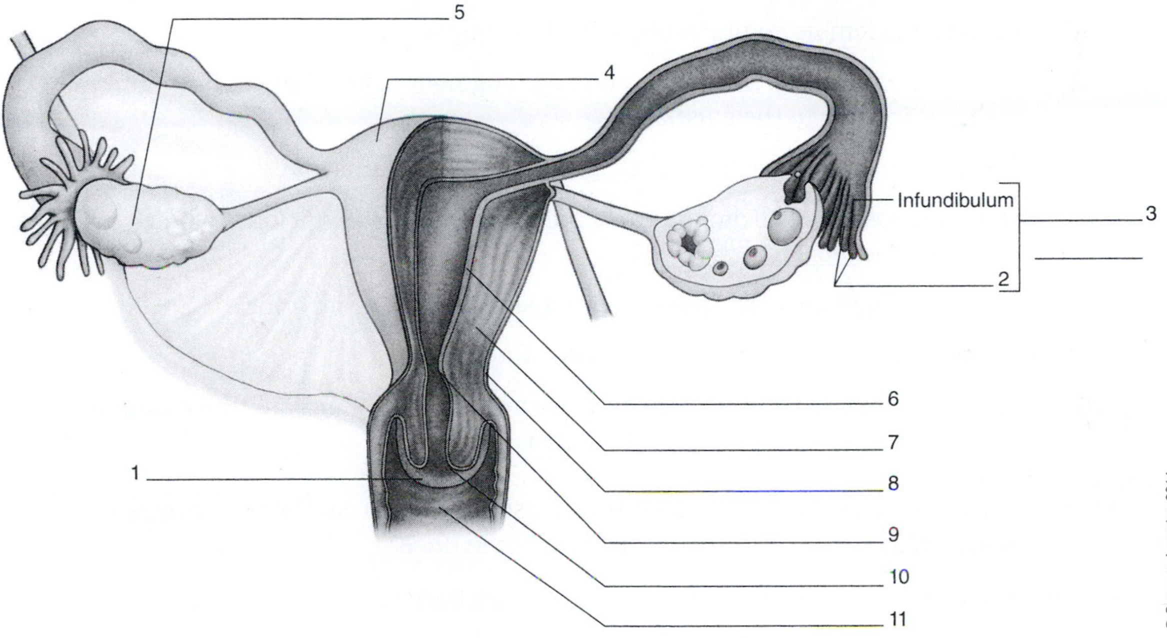

G. Match the numbers on the previous diagram with the following descriptions.

________ a. Produce ova and the hormones estrogen and progesterone

________ b. Oviducts; carry the ova to the uterus

________ c. Smooth, muscular layer of the uterus

________ d. Inner mucous layer of the uterus

________ e. Short canal that extends from the cervix to the vulva

________ f. Bulging, rounded part of the uterus

________ g. The narrow portion of the uterus that extends into the vagina.

________ h. Outer end of the oviduct that curves over the top edge of each ovary with fringe like folds

H. Name three functions of estrogen and three functions of progesterone.

____

____

____

____

____

____

I. Mark the underlined word or words in the following statements either true or false. Correct any false statements.

________ 1. The reproductive years begin at the time of puberty and menarche.

________ 2. Fertilization of the ovum takes place in the inner third of the oviduct.

________ 3. The hymen found at or near the entrance to the vaginal canal has some openings that allow for the menstrual flow.

________ 4. The external female genital is also called the vulva.

________ 5. The area surrounding the urethra and the vagina is called the vestibule, and the urethra is inferior to the vagina.

________ 6. Above the urethral opening is the clitoris, which contains many nerve endings.

________ 7. Extending posteriorly from the mons pubis are 2 longitudinal folds of hair-covered skin called the labia minora.

________ 8. The Bartholin glands are found on either side of the vaginal orifice.

________ 9. The area surrounding the nipple is called the areola.

________ 10. Prolactin from the posterior lobe of the pituitary gland stimulates the mammary glands to secrete milk following childbirth.

J. Select the appropriate word or words about the menstrual cycle from the following list to complete the statements. A word may be used more than once.

corpus luteum	decreasing	discharged	decrease
endometrium	estrogen	FSH	fallopian tube
follicle	follicles	implantation	LH
menstruation	one	ovaries	ovulation
pituitary	progesterone	puberty	rupture
uterine	uterus	5	4
10	12	14	15
17			

1. The menstrual cycle starts at ____________________. The average age for menstruation to begin is between ____________________ and ____________________.

2. Changes that occur during the menstrual cycle involve hormones from the ____________________ gland and the ____________________.

3. The four stages of the menstrual cycle are ____________________, ____________________, ____________________ ____________________, and ____________________.

4. ____________________ from the ____________________ gland is secreted on day 5 of the cycle.

5. It reaches the ovary through the bloodstream and stimulates several ____________________; however, usually only ____________________ matures.

6. As the follicle grows, an egg cell develops inside, and the follicle fills with a fluid containing ____________________.

7. The ____________________ stimulates the lining of the uterus to thicken with mucus and a rich supply of blood vessels to prepare the ____________________ for the ____________________ of a fertilized egg.

8. The follicle stage lasts ____________________ days.

9. When the ____________________ level increases in the blood, the pituitary stops secreting ____________________.

10. The ____________________ hormone is now secreted by the pituitary.

11. The three hormones circulating in the blood at this time are ____________________, ____________________, and ____________________ in different concentrations.

12. On day 14, this combination stimulates the mature follicle to ____________________, releasing the egg into the ____________________ ____________________.

13. This event is called ____________________.

14. After ____________________, LH stimulates the cells of the ruptured follicle to divide quickly; this mass of cells is now called the ____________________ ____________________.

15. The ____________________ ____________________ produces a hormone called ____________________, which maintains the growth of the endometrium.

16. Progesterone inhibits the release of ____________________.

17. The corpus luteum stage lasts about ____________________ days.

18. If fertilization does not occur, the progesterone reaches a level in the bloodstream that inhibits ____________________ secretion from the pituitary.

19. With the drop in LH, the corpus luteum breaks down ____________________ progesterone levels.

20. As the progesterone level decreases, the endometrial lining breaks away from the ____________________ wall and is ____________________ from the body with the unfertilized egg.

21. This is the menstrual stage and lasts about ____________________ days.

22. The estrogen level is also ____________________ at this time, which then stimulates the pituitary to secrete ____________________ and the cycle begins again.

K. Label the ovary, showing the development of the graafian follicle.

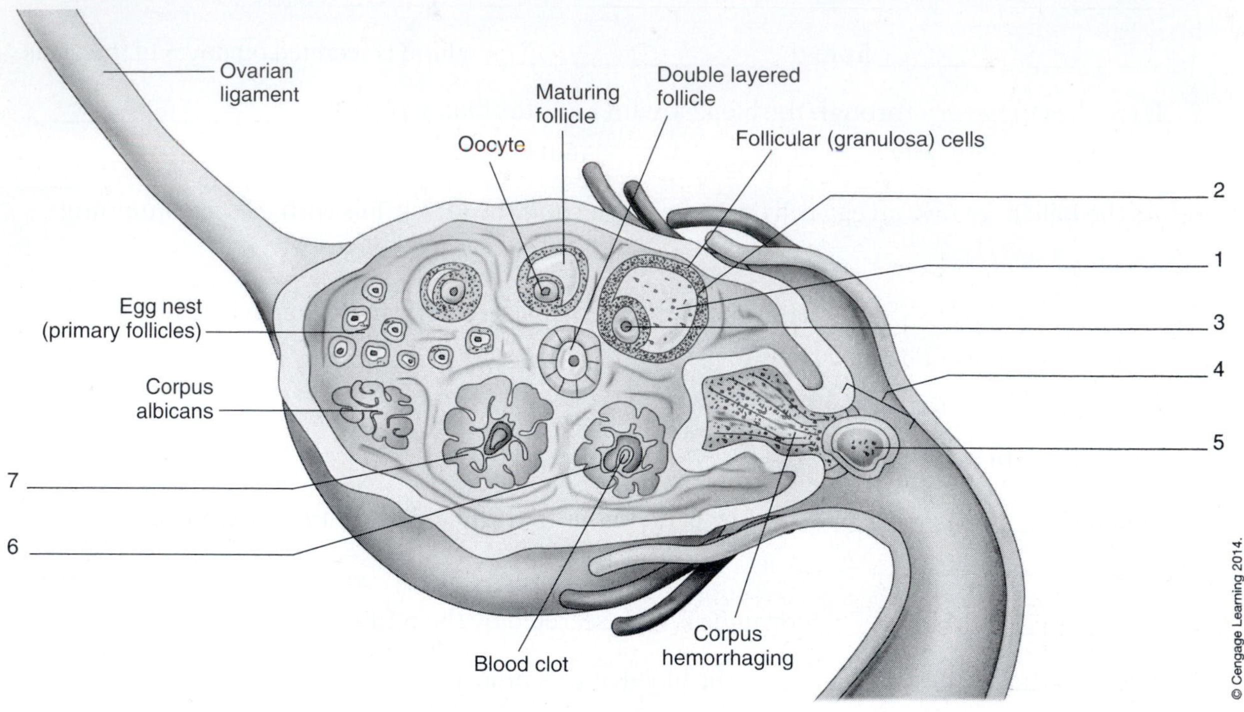

L. Answer the following questions about menopause.

1. Define menopause.

____

____

2. Describe the anatomical changes that occur during menopause.

____

____

____

3. Describe the physiological changes that occur during menopause.

____

____

____

4. Describe the psychological changes that occur during menopause.

____

____

____

____

M. Label the male reproductive system.

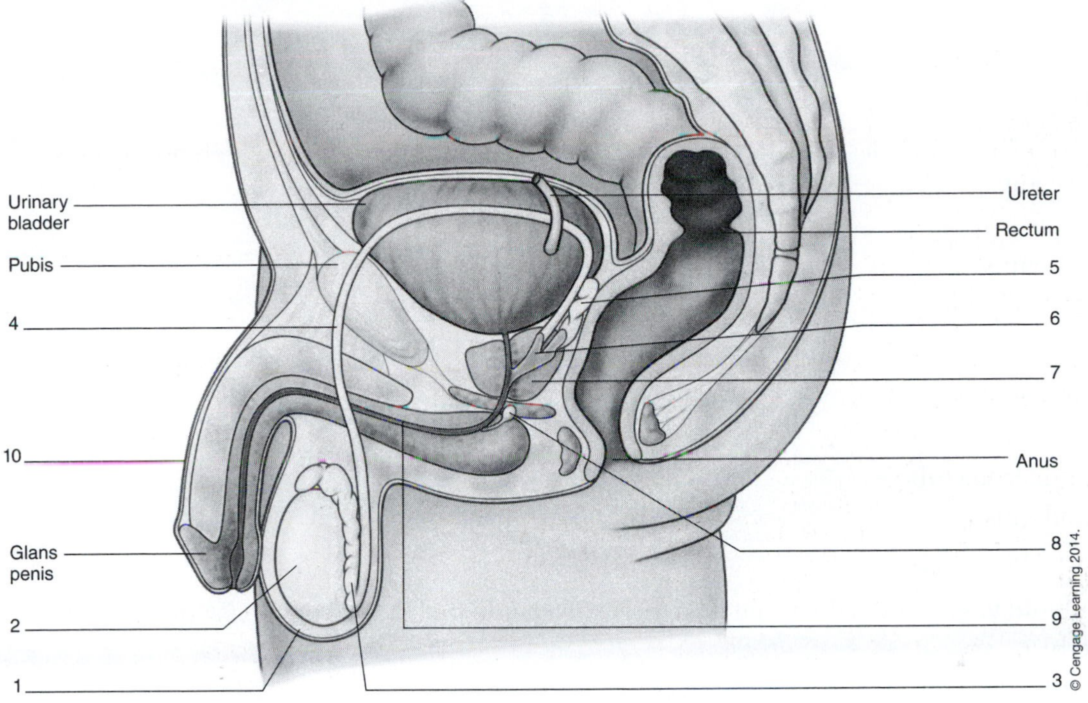

N. Select the letter of the choice that best completes the statement.

1. The testes produce the male gametes and the male hormone testosterone; they are encased in a pouch called the
   a. testicular.
   b. epididymis.
   c. scrotum.
   d. seminal ducts.
2. The pathway of sperm is through a series of ducts in which of the following orders?
   a. Epididymis, seminal ducts, ejaculatory ducts, and urethra
   b. Epididymis, ejaculatory ducts, seminal ducts, and urethra
   c. Seminal ducts, epididymis, ejaculatory ducts, and urethra
   d. Epididymis, urethra, seminal ducts, and ejaculatory ducts
3. The testes are attached to an overlying structure called the
   a. epididymis.
   b. tunica albuginea.
   c. lobule.
   d. seminiferous tubules.
4. Each testicular lobule contains seminiferous tubules that produce sperm under the influence of
   a. LH.
   b. FSH.
   c. ICSH.
   d. testosterone.

5. In males, mature sperm formation requires about _____ days.
   a. 50
   b. 28
   c. 74
   d. 24
6. The seminiferous tubules are supported by tissue called the __________, which produces testosterone.
   a. rete testis
   b. epididymis
   c. tunica albuginea
   d. interstitial
7. The vas deferens are continuations of the
   a. interstitial tissue.
   b. seminiferous tubules.
   c. epididymis.
   d. rete testis.
8. The seminal vesicle has a duct that leads away from it to join the vas deferens and form the
   a. urethra.
   b. ejaculatory duct.
   c. prostatic urethra.
   d. penis.
9. The ejaculatory ducts descend into the prostate gland to join with the
   a. penis.
   b. ureter.
   c. urethra.
   d. prepuce.
10. The prostate gland is located
    a. superior to the bladder.
    b. inferior to the bladder.
    c. posterior to the rectum.
    d. lateral to the rectum.

O. Compare and contrast the following.

1. Prostate gland/bulbourethral gland

____

____

2. Progesterone/testosterone

____

____

3. Menstruation/menarche

____

____

4. IVF/GIFT

____

____

5. Primary impotence/secondary impotence

____

____

P. Circle the correctly spelled word in each of the following statements.

1. Benign tumors of the uterus are known as (fibroids, fiboids).
2. Breast cancer can be detected in its early stage if women have routine mammograms and do breast exams by (palpating, palpatating) their breasts.
3. A mammogram is recommended on an (anuall, annual) basis for all women over the age of 40.
4. (Cervical, Cervixal) cancer is seen in women between the ages of 30 and 50.
5. To diagnose cancer of the cervix, a (Papinacolaou, Papanicolaou) smear is done.

Q. Match the word or words in Column A with the correct descriptions in Column B.

	Column A	Column B
1.	_________ PID	a. failure to sustain an erection
2.	_________ toxic shock syndrome	b. human papilloma virus
3.	_________ vaginal yeast infection	c. blister-like areas in the genitals
4.	_________ genital warts	d. pelvic inflammatory disease
5.	_________ prostatitis	e. most common STD
6.	_________ impotence	f. itching and burning of the vulva
7.	_________ endometrial ablation	g. test to determine cervical cancer
8.	_________ genital herpes	h. inflammation of the prostate
9.	_________ Pap smear	i. treatment for menorrhagia
10.	_________ chlamydia	j. staphylococcus bacterial infection

R. Find the word that matches each description and then use it in the crossword puzzle. Definition blanks indicate the number of letters in the answer.

1. Term used to describe the absence of the menstrual cycle
   Answer (10) _ _ _ _ _ _ _ _ _ _
2. Term used to describe painful menstruation
   Answer (12) _ _ _ _ _ _ _ _ _ _ _ _

3. Minor surgical procedure to allow for direct visualization of the abdominal cavity
   Answer (11) ___________

4. Procedure to remove only the tumor in breast cancer
   Answer (10) __________

5. Abnormal or excessive bleeding
   Answer (11) ___________

6. Inflammation of the testicle
   Answer (8) ________

7. Inflammation of the fallopian tubes.
   Answer (11) ___________

8. Treatment for prostate cancer that freezes and destroys cancer cells
   Answer (11) ___________

9. A genital sore that occurs in syphilis
   Answer (7) _______

10. Endometrial tissue found outside the uterus
    Answer (13) _____________

11. A sexually transmitted disease that may be asymptomatic in females
    Answer (9) _________

12. Failure to conceive despite effort for at least 1 year
    Answer (11) ___________

S. Answer the following questions about sexually transmitted diseases.

1. Define what is meant by the term *sexually transmitted disease (STD)*.

____

____

____

2. Describe some symptoms of STDs that may occur.

____

____

____

3. Explain how to prevent STDs.

____

____

____

T. Use the words from the following list to complete the story about reproduction.

abdominal	endometrium	seminal vesicles
alkaline	cervix	testicular
bladder	fertilization	urethra
Cowper's gland	fallopian tube	vagina
ductus deferens	egg	uterus
epididymis	sperm	

THE BEGINNING OF LIFE

I was waiting and waiting to start a new life;
it finally happened when my host married a wife.

I started out life in a testicular cell,
and became a mature ______________ in a place called the ______________.

I left this long and tubelike place,
and traveled up the ______________ ______________ into the
______________ space.

I traveled in my tube around the ______________ head, neck, and tail.
and got squirted with fluid that made me hearty and hale.

First came fluid from the ______________ ______________;
it was the first big drink since I left the testicle.

The tunnel I traveled went through a tight spot,
the prostatic ______________, where I received another ______________ pop.

I'm now ready to leave, but before I go—
__________________ __________________ gives me an alkaline bath to make me fast, not slow.

I couple with the host's new wife;
they are both eager to begin a new life.

I squeeze up through the __________________, a muscular tube,
and enter the __________________, pretty well lubed.

I swim up the __________________, which is shaped like a balloon,
taking a look at the place I hope to move into soon.

The __________________ lining is thick in preparation
to receive me and the ovum after __________________.

I move through the __________________ __________________ and see a(n)
__________________ shining bright, which I know I will be able to penetrate tonight.

This is wonderful: We two have become one.
And now another new life has begun.

U. Describe how the reproductive system interacts with other body systems.

____

____

____

APPLYING THEORY TO PRACTICE

1. Rebecca, age 13, questions Jodi, her mother, regarding menstruation. She is concerned that her body will look different. Jodi explains to Rebecca some of the physical and emotional changes that will occur when menstruation starts. List the changes that will occur.

   ____

   ____

   ____

2. Medical assistants have many roles in the health care profession. On career day, Lauren, a medical assistant, gives a presentation on the role of a medical assistant and the preparation for this type of health career. What information does Lauren include in her presentation?

   ____

   ____

   ____

3. Some men are afraid of having a physical examination for BPH or prostate cancer. They fear the treatment for these conditions will cause impotence. Dr. Joseph, a urologist, is concerned that men will not be checked for prostate cancer because of this fear. He is asked to address a group of local businessmen and discuss this topic. What information can Dr. Joseph give to the group?

____

____

____

____

____

4. Many women experience a problem with heavy bleeding called menorrhagia. This problem frequently leads to anemia and discomfort. What is the current treatment for this problem?

____

____

____

____

5. In the course of human growth and development, certain physical, mental, emotional, and social tasks must be accomplished. List each stage of development, the age of each stage, and at least one physical, mental, emotional, and social task that must be accomplished during each stage.

____

____

____

____

____

SURF THE NET

For additional information and interactive exercises, use the following key words:

- reproductive system—function
- reproductive process—fertilization and fetal development
- female organs of reproduction—structure and function
- menstrual cycle
- male organs of reproduction—structure and function
- infertility
- effects of aging on the reproductive system
- diseases of the female reproductive system
- diseases of the male reproductive system
- sexually transmitted diseases—types and prevention

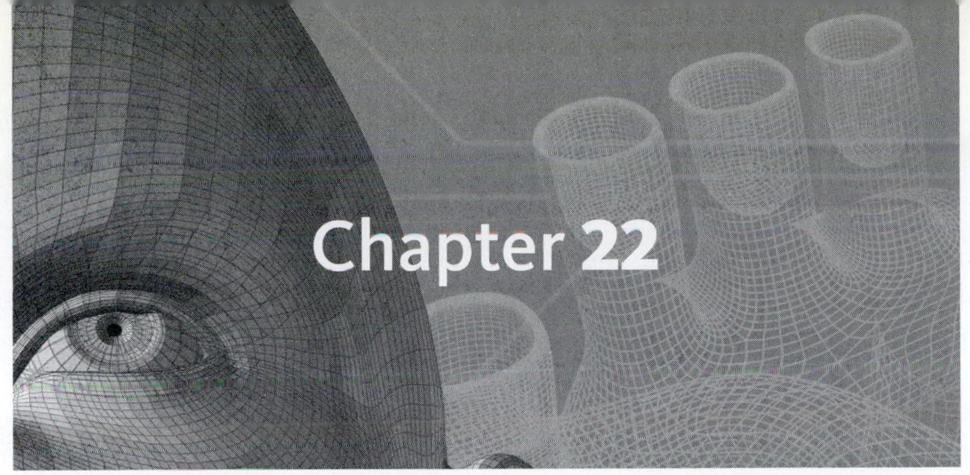

Genetics and Genetically Linked Diseases

OVERVIEW

Genetics is the branch of biology that studies how the genes are transmitted from parents to offspring.

Chromosomes are the structures found in the nucleus of each germ cell that contain DNA.

A **gene** is a small unit of DNA found along the length of the chromosome. It carries information for the cellular synthesis of a specific protein.

Types of Mutations

Mutations are the appearances of new and different traits caused by changes in the chromosome. Types of mutation include the following:

Gene mutation: a new or altered gene is produced to replace a normal or preexisting gene.

Chromosomal mutation: change in the number of chromosomes found in the nucleus or a change in the structure of a whole chromosome.

Types of gene mutation include the following:

Somatic cell: mutation that occurs in individual body (somatic) cells. It is not inherited (e.g., skin changes as we age).

Lethal gene: results in death in utero or later in life.

Human Genetic Disorders

A **genetic disorder** or **hereditary disorder** is caused by a variation in the genetic pattern, whereas a *congenital disorder* evolves during fetal development and is not related to a genetic malformation. Genetic disorders include the following:

Phenylketonuria (PKU): human metabolic disorder caused by an enzyme deficiency, where amino acids cannot break down, causing mental retardation.

Sickle cell anemia: abnormal hemoglobin molecule in red blood cell; common in individuals of African descent.

Tay-Sachs disease: deficiency of a lysosomal enzyme that breaks down fat; the fat molecules then accumulate in the brain cells and destroy them.

Huntington's disease: degeneration of the central nervous system.

Duchenne's muscular dystrophy: muscles suffer loss of protein and the contractile fibers are eventually replaced by fat and connective tissue, rendering the skeletal muscles useless.

Cystic fibrosis: the lining of the digestive tract, ducts of the pancreas, and respiratory tract produce thick mucus that blocks the passageways.

Thalassemia (Cooley's anemia): blood disorder found in people of Mediterranean descent.

Hemophilia: sex-linked disorder; person is unable to produce factor VIII, which is necessary for blood clotting; mothers can pass this disease to sons.

Chromosomal Aberrations. *Down's syndrome (mongolism)* involves an extra chromosome designated as chromosome 21. *Mutagenic agents* speed up the occurrence of mutations.

Genetic Counseling

Genetic counseling involves talking with parents or prospective parents about the possibility of genetic disorders.

Genetic Testing. Genetic testing includes the following diagnostic tests done during pregnancy to determine genetic problems:

Amniocentesis is the withdrawal of amniotic fluid during week 16 of pregnancy and can determine the presence of as many as 200 possible genetic disorders.

Chorionic villi sampling may be done as early as 8 to 10 weeks into the pregnancy; a sample of fetal cells is removed from the fetal side of the placenta.

Genetic Engineering

Genetic engineering is gene transfer from the cell of one species to another or isolating a specific gene and growing copies of it. Examples of the products of genetic engineering include interferon, human insulin, and human growth hormone.

Gene Therapy

Gene therapy is a technique used for correcting defective genes responsible for disease.

ACTIVITIES

A. Use the words from the following list to complete the statements. Words may be used more than once.

adulthood	dominant	lethal	RNA
childhood	embryology	mitosis	somatic cell
chromosomes	fertilization	mutation	synthesis
chromosomal	gene	recessive	teens
DNA	genetics	reproductive	

1. The process by which an egg and a sperm unite is called ____________________.
2. A gene is an area of ____________________ that carries information for the cellular ____________________ of a specific protein.

3. Due to the combined influence of all of the genes on all of the ____________________, a new individual is formed.

4. The branch of biology that studies how genes are transmitted from parents to child is ____________________.

5. The inheritance of a changed or mutated gene will cause the appearance of a new and different trait called a(n) ____________________.

6. When there is a change in the number of chromosomes, it is a(n) ____________________ mutation.

7. Mutations that occur such as how the skin changes as we age, are called ____________________ ____________________ mutations.

8. A gene that results in death is called a(n) ____________________ gene. It may occur during embryonic development or later in life.

9. Most persons carry two to three ____________________ genes; two similar ____________________ genes must be present in an individual for the gene to be expressed.

10. Lethal genes that exert their influence later in life are Tay-Sachs disease (death occurs during the ____________________ years), Duchenne's muscular dystrophy (death usually occurs during the ____________________ or ____________________ years), and Huntington's disease (death occurs during the ____________________ years).

B. Select the letter of the choice that best completes the statement.

1. A genetic disorder is caused by a condition
   a. that occurs in the first trimester.
   b. that occurs during delivery.
   c. that occurs in the last trimester.
   d. resulting from a variation in the genetic pattern.

2. PKU is caused by an enzyme deficiency in which
   a. the red blood cell forms a sickle shape.
   b. lipids accumulate in the brain.
   c. amino acids build up in the brain.
   d. the muscles atrophy.

3. At birth, infants are tested for the genetic disorder
   a. PKU.
   b. sickle cell anemia.
   c. Huntington's disease.
   d. Down's syndrome.

4. In __________________, a missing enzyme causes lipid molecules to accumulate in the brain.
   a. Tay-Sachs disease
   b. cystic fibrosis
   c. hemophilia
   d. PKU

5. Degeneration of the central nervous system occurs in
   a. Tay-Sachs disease.
   b. cystic fibrosis.
   c. thalassemia minor.
   d. Huntington's disease.

6. Duchenne's muscular dystrophy affects the
   a. contractile fibers of skeletal muscle.
   b. respiratory passages, which become thick with mucus.
   c. smooth muscle of the digestive tract.
   d. limbs, causing spastic paralysis.

7. In cystic fibrosis, the linings of exocrine glands become filled with mucous plugs. The system most affected is the __________________ system.
   a. muscular
   b. circulatory
   c. digestive
   d. central nervous

8. Cupping and clapping is the treatment of choice for
   a. Huntington's disease.
   b. Tay-Sachs disease.
   c. cystic fibrosis.
   d. Down's syndrome.

9. In Down's syndrome, the chromosomal aberration that occurs is
   a. a pair of chromosomes adhering to each other.
   b. a missing chromosome.
   c. nondisjunction of sex chromosomes.
   d. an extra chromosome.

10. When a cell or group of cells is exposed to radiation or chemicals, the speed of mutation
    a. is not affected.
    b. increases.
    c. decreases.
    d. depends on the age of the individual.

C. Answer the following questions concerning genetic disorders.

1. In sickle cell anemia, what does the rapid destruction of sickle cells cause?

____

2. Clumping of red blood cells causes damage to what systems of the body? What is the resulting disorder?

____

____

3. Name two genetic disorders that involve the red blood cells.

____

____

4. Name three genetic disorders that involve the central nervous system.

____

____

____

5. Describe three tests done during genetic counseling.

____

____

____

APPLYING THEORY TO PRACTICE

1. Describe gene therapy. List the people who may be especially interested in this topic.

____

____

____

SURF THE NET

For additional information and interactive exercises, use the following key words:

- genetics
- gene mutations
- genetic disorders—phenylketonuria, sickle cell anemia, Tay-Sachs disease, Huntington's disease, Duchenne's muscular dystrophy, cystic fibrosis, thalassemia, hemophilia
- chromosomal aberration—Down's syndrome
- genetic counseling
- genetic testing
- gene therapy